Starting Research in Clinical Education

Starting Research in Clinical Education

EDITED BY

Eliot L. Rees

Lecturer in Medical Education
School of Medicine
Keele University;
National Institute for Health and Care Research (NIHR) Academic Clinical Fellow in General Practice
Research Department of Primary Care and Population Health
University College London
London, UK; and
Education Research Committee, Association for the Study of Medical Education (ASME)

Alison Ledger

Associate Professor and Academic Lead for Staff Development
Academy for Medical Education
The University of Queensland
Brisbane, Australia; and
Chair, Education Research Committee, Association for the Study of Medical Education (ASME)

Kim A. Walker

Senior Lecturer and Lead for Faculty Development
Centre for Healthcare Education Research and Innovation (CHERI)
University of Aberdeen
Aberdeen, UK; and
Director of Publications, Association for the Study of Medical Education (ASME)

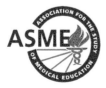

WILEY Blackwell

This edition first published 2024

© 2024 The Association for the Study of Medical Education (ASME).

The right of Eliot L. Rees, Alison Ledger, and Kim A. Walker to be identified as the authors of the editorial material in this work has been asserted in accordance with law.

Registered Offices

John Wiley & Sons, Inc., 111 River Street, Hoboken, NJ 07030, USA

John Wiley & Sons Ltd, The Atrium, Southern Gate, Chichester, West Sussex, PO19 8SQ, UK

For details of our global editorial offices, customer services, and more information about Wiley products visit us at www.wiley.com.

Wiley also publishes its books in a variety of electronic formats and by print-on-demand. Some content that appears in standard print versions of this book may not be available in other formats.

Library of Congress Cataloging-in-Publication Data applied for

[PB ISBN: 9781119861980]

Cover Design: Wiley
Cover Image: © fotodelux/Getty Images

Set in 9.5/11.5pts PalatinoLTStd by Straive, Pondicherry, India

SKY10054666_090623

Contents

List of contributors, vii
Foreword, xi
Preface, xiii
Acknowledgements, xv
Companion website, xvii

PART I: Research design

1 Getting started in clinical education research, 3
Jennifer Routh and Robert K. McKinley

2 Constructing a research question, 13
*Megan Anakin, Joanne Robertson-Smith,
and Tim J. Wilkinson*

3 Clarifying research paradigms and design, 21
J. Cristian Rangel, Meredith Young, and Lara Varpio

4 Using educational theory in research
and scholarship, 31
Clare Morris and Nick Schindler

5 Involving stakeholders, 39
*Katherine A. Moreau, Catherine M. Giroux,
and Kaylee Eady*

6 Sampling and recruiting participants, 47
*Jennifer Cleland, Kirsty Alexander,
and Amudha Poobalan*

7 Conducting ethical research, 57
Anne-Marie Reid and Susan Jamieson

**PART II: Evidence synthesis and
mixed methods**

8 Evidence syntheses: choosing an approach, 69
*Catherine M. Giroux, Susanne Mak, Rebecca
Ataman, and Aliki Thomas*

9 Evidence synthesis: key steps and design
considerations, 79
Claire Duddy and Sophie Park

10 Realist research: unpicking the influence
of context, 89
Claire Duddy and Geoff Wong

11 Mixed methods research: the sum is greater
than the parts, 99
*Catherine Scarff, Christy Noble, Koshila Kumar,
and Wendy Hu*

12 Action research: improving clinical education
programmes, 107
Janet Lefroy and Emma Collins

13 Online data collection: emerging
possibilities, 115
Dominique Harz and Kristina Dzara

PART III: Qualitative research

14 Interviews and focus groups: guided
conversations, 127
Lucy Wallis, Becky Petley, and Rachel Locke

15 Visual elicitation: techniques for digging
deeper in qualitative interviews, 137
*Gerard J. Gormley, Sayra Cristancho,
and Katherine Crook*

16 Ethnography: sense and sensibilities
in conducting fieldwork, 145
Lisa Dikomitis and Brianne Wenning

17 Narrative research: from the general to the
particular, 155
*Kathleen E. Leedham-Green, Alexandra Wright,
and Giskin Day*

18 Approaches to thematic analysis: becoming
a knowing researcher, 165
Virginia Braun and Victoria Clarke

19 Behind the scenes of qualitative analysis:
learning from new researchers' struggles, 175
*Anne de la Croix, Malou Stoffels,
and Jan Willem Grijpma*

PART IV: Quantitative research

20 Survey research: uses and misuses, 183
*Patrick G. Corr, Radwa Aly,
and Anthony R. Artino, Jr.*

21 Experimental methods: more than simply
testing hypotheses, 191
Peter Yeates and Rebecca Edwards

22 Statistical analysis: unpacking
uncertainty, 201
*Christy K. Boscardin, H. Carrie Chen,
and Justin L. Sewell*

23 Big data: where to start and what to expect, 213
*Milou Silkens, Asta Medisauskaite,
and Chris McManus*

**PART V: Succeeding in clinical education
research**

24 Maximising opportunities and overcoming
challenges, 227
Susil Pallikadavath and Simon Gay

25 Managing your project, 235
Michelle D. Lazarus and Georgina C. Stephens

26 Writing your dissertation, 245
Frederick Speyer, Benjamin Davies, and Sarah Yardley

27 Writing for publication, 253
Amaya Ellawala and Aileen Barrett

28 Disseminating your findings, 261
Jonathan Guckian and Teresa Chan

29 Developing your career, 271
*Gillian Vance, Sarah Simpson, Sue Jackson,
and Richard Conn*

Conclusion, 283

Index, 285

List of contributors

Kirsty Alexander
ScotGEM Lecturer in Medical Education
School of Medicine
University of Dundee
Dundee, UK

Radwa Aly
Executive Director of Clinical Research
School of Medicine & Health Sciences
The George Washington University
Washington DC, USA

Megan Anakin
Senior Lecturer and Education Adviser
Dunedin School of Medicine
University of Otago
Dunedin, New Zealand

Anthony R. Artino, Jr.
Professor and Associate Dean for Evaluation and Educational
Research
School of Medicine & Health Sciences
The George Washington University
Washington DC, USA

Rebecca Ataman
PhD Candidate
School of Physical and Occupational Therapy
McGill University
Montreal, Quebec, Canada

Aileen Barrett
Editor in Chief
The Clinical Teacher
Assistant Scheme Director, GP Training (South-East)
Academic Lead, Research, Policy and Information
Irish College of General Practitioners
Dublin

Christy K. Boscardin
Professor and Director of Student Assessment
School of Medicine
University of California, San Francisco
San Francisco, CA, USA

Virginia Braun
Professor of Psychology
School of Psychology
Waipapa Taumata Rau The University of Auckland
Auckland, New Zealand

Teresa Chan
Associate Professor
Department of Medicine; and
Associate Dean of Continuing Professional Development
Faculty of Health Sciences
McMaster University
Hamilton, Ontario, Canada

H. Carrie Chen
Professor of Paediatrics and Senior Associate Dean of Assessment
and Educational Scholarship
School of Medicine
Georgetown University
Washington DC, USA

Victoria Clarke
Associate Professor in Qualitative and Critical Psychology
School of Social Sciences
University of the West of England
Bristol, UK

Jennifer Cleland
President's Chair in Medical Education and Vice Dean (Education)
Lee Kong Chian School of Medicine
Nanyang Technological University
Jurong West, Singapore

Emma Collins
Lecturer in Nursing and Professional Doctorate Candidate
School of Nursing & Midwifery
Keele University
Newcastle under Lyme, UK

Richard Conn
Clinical Senior Lecturer in Paediatrics
School of Medicine
Ulster University
Derry, Northern Ireland

Patrick G. Corr
Assistant Professor of Clinical Research and Leadership
School of Medicine & Health Sciences
The George Washington University
Washington DC, USA

Sayra Cristancho
Associate Professor
Schulich School of Medicine & Dentistry
Western University
London, Ontario, Canada

Katherine Crook
PhD Graduate
School of Medicine
University of Leeds
Leeds, UK

Benjamin Davies
General Practitioner Partner
Fremington Medical Centre
Barnstaple, UK

Giskin Day
Principal Teaching Fellow
Imperial College London
London, UK

Anne de la Croix
Assistant Professor
Research in Education
Amsterdam UMC location Vrije Universiteit
Amsterdam, The Netherlands

Lisa Dikomitis
Professor of Medical Anthropology and Social Sciences and Director
of Research
Kent and Medway Medical School
University of Kent and Canterbury Christ Church University
Canterbury, UK

Claire Duddy
Realist Reviewer and NIHR Pre-Doctoral Fellow
Nuffield Department of Primary Care Health Sciences
University of Oxford
Oxford, UK

Kristina Dzara
School of Medicine
Saint Louis University

Kaylee Eady
Assistant Professor of Health Professions Education
Faculty of Education
University of Ottawa
Ottawa, Ontario, Canada

Rebecca Edwards
PhD Candidate
School of Medicine
Keele University
Newcastle under Lyme, UK

Amaya Ellawala
Lecturer in Medical Education
Health Professions Education Unit
Hull York Medical School
York, UK

Simon Gay
Professor of Medical Education (Primary Care)
Leicester Medical School
University of Leicester
Leicester, UK

Catherine M. Giroux
Postdoctoral Fellow
Institute of Health Sciences Education
McGill University
Montreal, Quebec, Canada

Gerry J. Gormley
Professor of Simulation and Clinical Skills
School of Medicine, Dentistry and Biomedical Sciences
Queen's University Belfast
Belfast, Northern Ireland

Jan Willem Grijpma
PhD Candidate and Teacher Trainer
LEARN! Academy
Vrije Universiteit
Amsterdam, The Netherlands

Jonathan Guckian
Advanced Medical Education Fellow
Leeds Institute of Medical Education
University of Leeds
Leeds, UK

Dominique Harz
Adjunct Instructor of Graduate Program in Orthodontics
Department of Orthodontics
Pontificia Universidad Católica de Chile
Santiago, Chile

Wendy Hu
Professor of Medical Education and Associate Dean
School of Medicine
Western Sydney University
Sydney, New South Wales, Australia

Sue Jackson
Associate Professor of Adult Nursing
Department of Nursing Midwifery & Health
Northumbria University
Newcastle upon Tyne, UK

Susan Jamieson
Professor of Health Professions Education
School of Medicine, Dentistry & Nursing
University of Glasgow
Glasgow, UK

Koshila Kumar
Sub-Dean (Academic) Development and Associate Professor
Division of Learning and Teaching
Charles Sturt University
New South Wales, Australia

Michelle D. Lazarus
Associate Professor & Director of the Monash Centre for Human
Anatomy Education
Department for Anatomy and Developmental Biology
Monash University
Clayton, Victoria, Australia

Kathleen E. Leedham-Green
Senior Teaching Fellow
Medical Education Research Unit
Imperial College London
London, UK

Janet Lefroy
Professor of Medical Education
School of Medicine
Keele University
Newcastle under Lyme, UK

Rachel Locke
Deputy Head of School
School of Sport, Health and Community
University of Winchester
Winchester, UK

Susanne Mak
Assistant Professor and Associate Director of Occupational Therapy
Programme
School of Physical and Occupational Therapy
McGill University
Montreal, Quebec, Canada

Robert K. McKinley
Emeritus Professor of Education in General Practice
School of Medicine
Keele University
Newcastle under Lyme, UK

Chris McManus
Professor of Psychology and Medical Education
Research Department of Medical Education
University College London
London, UK

Asta Medisauskaite
Senior Research Fellow
Research Department of Medical Education
University College London
London, UK

Katherine A. Moreau
Associate Professor of Health Professions Education
Faculty of Education
University of Ottawa
Ottawa, Ontario, Canada

Clare Morris
Course Director for MSt Medical Education
Institute of Continuing Education
University of Cambridge
Cambridge, UK

Christy Noble
Clinical Learning & Assessment Lead
Academy for Medical Education
The University of Queensland
Brisbane, Australia

Susil Pallikadavath
National Institute for Health Research (NIHR) Academic Clinical
Fellow in Cardiology
NIHR Biomedical Research Centre for Cardiovascular Disease
University of Leicester
Leicester, UK

Sophie Park
Professor of Primary Care and Medical Education
Research Department of Primary Care and Population Health
University College London
London, UK

Becky Petley
Lecturer in Psychology
Faculty of Sport, Health and Social Sciences
Solent University
Southampton, UK

Amudha Poobalan
Senior Lecturer in Public Health
Centre for Healthcare Education Research and Innovation
University of Aberdeen
Aberdeen, UK

J. Cristian Rangel
Assistant Professor
Department of Innovation in Medical Education
University of Ottawa
Ottawa, Ontario, Canada

Anne-Marie Reid
Professor of Medical Education
Leeds Institute of Medical Education
University of Leeds
Leeds, UK

Joanne Robertson-Smith
Professional Practice Fellow, Simulation Educator and Clinical Nurse
Educator
Otago Clinical Skills Laboratories
University of Otago and Te Whatu Ora – Southern
Dunedin, New Zealand

Jennifer Routh
PhD Candidate in Veterinary Education
School of Veterinary Medicine
University of Surrey
Surrey, UK

Catherine Scarff
Senior Lecturer in Medical Education
Melbourne Medical School
University of Melbourne
Melbourne, Victoria, Australia

Nick Schindler
Postgraduate Tutor in Medical Education
Institute of Continuing Education
University of Cambridge
Cambridge, UK

Justin L. Sewell
Professor of Medicine
School of Medicine
University of California, San Francisco
San Francisco, CA, USA

Milou Silkens
Research Fellow
Department of Health Services Research and Management
City, University of London
London, UK

Sarah Simpson
Associate Clinical Lecturer in Paediatric Dentistry
School of Dental Sciences
Newcastle University
Newcastle upon Tyne, UK

Frederick Speyer
PhD Candidate
School of Medicine, Dentistry and Biomedical Sciences
Queen's University Belfast
Belfast, Northern Ireland

Georgina C. Stephens
Senior Lecturer
Monash Centre for Human Anatomy Education
Monash University
Clayton, Australia

Malou Stoffels
PhD Candidate and Education Consultant
Research in Education
Amsterdam UMC location Vrije Universiteit
Amsterdam, The Netherlands

Aliki Thomas
Associate Professor
School of Physical and Occupational Therapy and Institute of Health
Sciences Education
McGill University
Montreal, Quebec, Canada

Gillian Vance
Professor of Medical Education
School of Medicine
Newcastle University
Newcastle upon Tyne, UK

Lara Varpio
Professor
Department of Pediatrics
University of Pennsylvania and
Co-Director of Research in Medical Education
The Children's Hospital of Philadelphia
Philadelphia, PA, USA

Lucy Wallis
Research Associate in Qualitative Health Services Research
Bristol Medical School
University of Bristol
Bristol, UK

Brianne Wenning
Lecturer in Global Health
Kent and Medway Medical School
University of Kent and Canterbury Christ Church University
Canterbury, UK

Tim J. Wilkinson
Professor of Medicine and Medical Education and Deputy Dean
Education Unit
University of Otago
Christchurch, New Zealand

Geoff Wong
Associate Professor of Primary Care
Nuffield Department of Primary Care Health Sciences
University of Oxford
Oxford, UK

Alexandra Wright
Fifth Year Medical Student
Faculty of Medicine
Imperial College London
London, UK

Sarah Yardley
Associate Professor of Palliative Medicine
Marie Curie Palliative Care Research Department
University College London
London, UK

Peter Yeates
Senior Lecturer in Medical Education Research
School of Medicine
Keele University
Newcastle under Lyme, UK

Meredith Young
Associate Professor
Institute of Health Sciences Education
McGill University
Montreal, Quebec, Canada

Foreword

The Association for the Study of Medical Education (ASME)'s mission is to 'advance scholarship in medical education' through a wide range of activities – events, awards, resources, and the work of special interest groups and committees. It was during an away day of one of these groups, the Educational Research Committee, when the idea for this publication truly evolved. As a committee, we were reflecting on the popularity of the 'getting started in clinical education research' workshop regularly offered at ASME's Annual Scholarship Meeting and Researching Medical Education conferences. We were struck by the levels of interest, energy, and ambition of colleagues taking their first steps into educational research and wondered how we might extend the reach of the workshop to others embarking on similar journeys. We talked about our own pathways into clinical education research, crossing disciplinary boundaries, and research traditions encountering new theoretical and conceptual tools. We reflected on the hurdles we had faced, the things we wished we had known, and the guidance we wished we had been able to access.

Gradually, the idea for this book took shape. We wanted to offer something that could provide a foundation for new researchers, which would appeal to those undertaking research degrees in clinical education as well as those 'going it alone'. We wanted it to be accessible and practical, to include specific examples and suggestions that would help our imagined readership design, implement and write up their studies. . .and gradually the book took shape.

It is a privilege to be writing the foreword to the imagined book, now very tangible and I congratulate the editors on the work they have done to bring together what I believe will become another of the 'go-to' publications for our community of scholars.

I believe *Starting Research in Clinical Education* to be a scholarly text, one that embraces the full extent of Boyer's (1990) typology of scholarship as discovery (fostering research that can shape and inform our educational practices), integration (drawing on inter-disciplinary and inter-professional dialogue), and application (fostering engagement, dialogue, and knowledge-exchange). One way I might support my claim is to look to the authorship of the chapters contained within; for me, there are a number of noteworthy characteristics. The first is that the chapters bring together experienced and early career researchers; researchers close to the experience of the anticipated readership to help ensure chapters were accessible, invitational, and useful. Furthermore, the authorship goes some way to redressing a growing commentary on the characteristics of authors in our community, be it around gender, geography, or disciplinary field. Albert et al. (2020) noted that medical education researchers tend to draw upon a narrower knowledge field than their peers in higher education, suggesting this impedes inter-disciplinary knowledge exchange. In contrast, the authors of these chapters span an impressive mix of disciplines. It creates a heady mix of expertise, reflecting a depth of understanding of context, practice and, I would suggest, praxis. Praxis, for me at least, is about the ways we embody and enact theory, and how we thoughtfully and creatively direct our activity at purposeful change. I believe this book contains a wide range of tools that will equip new members of the clinical educational research community to achieve just that.

Professor Clare Morris
Past Chair of
ASME Education
Research Committee

References

Albert, M., Rowland, P., Friesen, F. et al. (2020). Interdisciplinarity in medical education research: myth and reality. *Advances in Health Sciences Education* 25: 1243–1253.

Boyer, E.L. (1990). *Scholarship Reconsidered*. Carnegie Foundation for the Advancement of Teaching.

Preface

The idea for this book was conceived from a discussion at an Italian restaurant the night before the Association for the Study of Medical Education (ASME)'s Researching Medical Education conference in 2019. We were discussing resources for clinical education students. ASME has already produced two excellent books: *Understanding Medical Education,* which serves as the authoritative guide to teaching and learning approaches in medical education; and *Researching Medical Education,* which offers a range of theories and how they can be best deployed to conduct rigorous research.

However, we perceived there was an unmet need for a single coherent research methods resource for the students we supervise in clinical education programmes. The response was 'let's do it'. Now, after a couple of more visits to that Italian restaurant and some concentrated work in between, we are delighted to see this book come to fruition.

Starting Research in Clinical Education is the definitive practical guide to designing, conducting, and reporting clinical education research projects that address important topics and employ rigorous methods. We chose the term *clinical education research* to encompass research related to the learning or development of students or professionals within any healthcare profession worldwide. Sometimes the terms research, scholarship, and evaluation are used interchangeably. We think there is an important difference in that research aims to answer a specific question and generate new knowledge that can inform wider practice. While the book is focused on research, many of the methods and principles discussed can be used for rigorous educational evaluation and scholarship.

Our ethos, from conception through to publication, has been to ensure this book meets the needs of new researchers in clinical education. We recognise, however, that these new researchers come from many different backgrounds. Some may be undertaking education fellowships or intercalated or postgraduate degrees in clinical education, medical education, dental education, or health professions education. Others may be coming to education research later in their clinical or academic careers. This book is the ideal resource for those embarking on their first clinical education research projects or using methods with which they are unfamiliar. The authors draw on examples of previous projects to illustrate the important factors to consider when designing studies and the strengths and challenges of different methodological approaches. On the companion website, we provide information, activities, and exercises for you to work through in order to help support your thinking in research design.

When inviting authors, we were keen to ensure we were drawing on both the wisdom of experienced researchers and the recent insight of early career academics. You will find, therefore, that most chapters have been authored by a combination of senior and junior contributors. We hope this helps in making sure the content balances credibility and accessibility.

Similarly, we wanted to ensure we had diversity in our authorship team in terms of geography and disciplinary background. We were delighted to include a global team of chapter authors from 44 different institutions in 9 different countries. Likewise, we have authors from the whole spectrum of disciplinary backgrounds including anatomy, anthropology, dentistry, education, global health, medicine, nursing, occupational therapy, physiotherapy, psychology, public health, and veterinary medicine.

Each chapter has been peer reviewed by at least two other chapter authors (one early career and more experienced researcher) as well as the three editors. We are extremely grateful for the energy and enthusiasm that authors put into both reviewing and responding to the reviews they received. We believe this has significantly strengthened the individual chapters and the book as a whole.

Moving on to the structure and how to use the book. *Starting Research in Clinical Education* is divided into five parts. The first, research design, takes you through all the stages of designing a clinical education project. Chapter 1 explains how to get started and identify a topic to research. Chapter 2 then explores how to move from a research topic to a clearly articulated research question. Chapter 3 aims to clarify research paradigms and design to ensure these are coherent with your research question and methods. Chapter 4 considers approaches to using educational theory within research. Chapter 5 discusses the importance of involving stakeholders in your research, how to identify who these might be, and how to involve them meaningfully. Chapter 6 describes different approaches to sampling and recruiting participants for your study. Chapter 7 explores the origins and principles of ethics in research and how these should be applied in the design, conduct, and reporting of your research. We consider that no matter what research methods you decide to use, these seven chapters in Part I are all essential reading.

The next three parts explore common research methods within clinical education research which we have grouped into three approaches: Part II evidence syntheses and mixed methods, Part III qualitative research, and Part IV quantitative research. These parts do not intend to be comprehensive. Rather, they intend to discuss the prevailing methods within clinical education research to give you ideas of the opportunities available and how these might best be used. We consider these three parts as akin to a tasting menu. They should give you enough information about different methods to whet your appetite and to have an idea of which might be most appropriate for your research question. They should provide sufficient information to get started with the method and point you in the direction of more detailed resources to refer to as your research progresses.

Part V then offers guidance for how to succeed in your clinical education research project. Chapter 24 explains how to maximise opportunities along the way including how to choose and work with your supervisor. Chapter 25 introduces you to principles of project management to help you keep on track throughout your research. The next three chapters cover different approaches to dissemination. Chapter 26 is suited to anyone doing a project as part of a degree course that needs to write a dissertation or thesis. Chapter 27 discusses different types of journal publication, the journal submission, and peer review process and enhances your chances of publishing. Chapter 28 considers a range of approaches to dissemination including different types of conference presentations, social media, and multimedia. Finally, Chapter 29 discusses how to build on the success of your first project and develop a career in clinical education research. Again, regardless of which method you eventually select, the chapters in Part 5 should all be of use. While some of these chapters may appear to fit at the end of the research

process, we encourage you to read these at the start to plan for later success.

Within each chapter you will find a number of common features. *Learning objectives* are clearly articulated and outline what you should expect to achieve from reading the chapter. Each chapter also has *Top tips*, *Common pitfalls*, and *Ethical issues*. These are nuggets of practical wisdom specific to the method or aspect of research in the chapter and are tailored to the clinical education context. Many chapters also have additional reading or resources available on our companion website. These are signposted within the chapters, but we also encourage you to peruse the site to see what may be of use to you. You will also find that some chapters signpost to specific resources for further reading. These are recommended for anyone who chooses to use that method for their research or wants a more comprehensive understanding.

When reading through the chapters, and in particular the *Top tips* and *Common pitfalls*, you will find there are some recurring messages. First, good research results from teamwork and collaboration. This can mean working as part of a larger team or could simply be working with a supervisor. To quote John Donne, 'no man is an island' – don't try and go it alone. Having colleagues to work with makes the research more enjoyable and allows you to share your challenges and successes. Second, the clinical education community is extremely welcoming and supportive. Do reach out to people and start to develop a network. This will help your research, make the process more enjoyable, and support you in growing your career.

We hope you enjoy reading this book as much as we have enjoyed creating it. Furthermore, we wish you every success with your first clinical education research projects. We look forward to hearing and reading all about them. Good luck!

Eliot L. Rees
Alison Ledger
Kim A. Walker

Acknowledgements

The idea for this book was sparked by discussions at ASME Education Research Committee meetings, Researching Medical Education conferences, and conversations with our own research students over the years. We, therefore, acknowledge our colleagues and students, past and present, whose experiences informed many of the decisions we made along our editing journey.

Thank you to all our chapter contributors for agreeing to our invitations and for collaborating with us over the past two years. We were delighted to recruit such a diverse authorship team who not only prepared their own chapters but also provided thoughtful feedback on others, strengthening the book as a whole. We are extremely grateful for the work everyone undertook to get the book to print stage. Thanks also to some additional reviewers, who offered valuable opinions when called upon: Kevin Eva, Hannah Gillespie, Victoria Leigh, and Jessica Penney.

Companion website

Starting Research in Clinical Education provides the starting point for you in your research journey. Naturally, any book is constrained by its length, therefore we have additionally developed a companion website to complement the information in the book. The companion website provides you with access to additional reading and resources which aim to deepen your understanding of the topics covered within the book. Not all chapters have companion website material, but those which do offer you further information, videos, exemplars, and case studies to reinforce and enhance your understanding of the concepts in the book. These are clearly signposted within the text and organised by chapter on the companion website. We hope the companion website encourages you to pursue further learning and development.

URL: www.wiley.com/go/clinicaleducation

PART I

Research design

1 Getting started in clinical education research

Jennifer Routh and Robert K. McKinley

Learning objectives

By the end of this chapter, you should be able to:
- Describe the basic features and aims of education research.
- Evaluate possible research topics of interest.
- Conduct a preliminary critical literature review to inform the early stages of research planning.
- Recognise the importance of collaboration, supervision, and mentorship in clinical education research.

Why do you want to do clinical education research?

Even before you start getting started, it is important to consider why you want to do clinical education research. There are many possible answers to this question. While some may appear more noble than others, they are all valid. You may have a burning desire to answer a question or solve a problem. You may seek personal development by expanding your knowledge or skills, developing relationships, or advancing your career. You may want to gain academic credentials such as publications and may perceive that education research might be an easier way to do it than in other disciplines (hint: it is probably not!). What is most likely is that you are motivated by a combination of these factors. Are these enough to sustain your enthusiasm for a process that may take more time, effort, and perseverance than you expected?

So, you have got the enthusiasm and are being honest with yourself about your motivation and stamina. Hopefully, this chapter will set you on your way to getting started.

Defining clinical education research

What is research?

Research is the search for trustworthy answers to problems. Good research is not haphazard, it is particular and rigorous. The Oxford English Dictionary defines research as the 'systematic investigation or inquiry aimed at contributing to knowledge of a theory, topic, etc., by careful consideration, observation, or study of a subject' [1].

Research is exciting. It can also be intimidating. From being someone who searches for, critiques, synthesises, and uses knowledge, you become a knowledge maker. This demands diligence and respect for the scientific method. It is a process that starts with constructing a research question that matters. You then address the question by systematically collecting and analysing appropriate data. Finally, you disseminate your findings, thus adding to the sum total of human knowledge. Your findings may influence practice, policy, or future research. With this comes great responsibility.

What is education research?

Education research is research into, on, or about any aspect of education with the aim of understanding, informing, or improving its practice [2]. It is a relatively young field that emerged from philosophy, sociology, psychology, anthropology, and history during the twentieth century [3], and these disciplines continue to inform our research today. This is a reflection of education's complexity and the resulting need to research it from multiple perspectives.

Education research may seem quite alien if you are used to biomedical research. The latter is built on the assumption that there is a single 'truth' that can be understood through objective observation.

Starting Research in Clinical Education, First Edition. Edited by Eliot L. Rees, Alison Ledger, and Kim A. Walker.
© 2024 The Association for the Study of Medical Education (ASME). Published 2024 by John Wiley & Sons Ltd.
Companion website: www.wiley.com/go/clinicaleducation

Educational settings are complex social systems and cannot be completely understood from a single perspective or 'lens'. What you observe is affected by the 'lens' you use: psychological, sociological, or anthropological lenses will reveal different insights on the same problem. Further, as the observer, you cannot be entirely separate from the system being examined: you may be outside the system being observed but your unique experiences affect not only what you see but the meaning you make of it. This apparent subjectivity does not align with what many biomedical scientists see as 'good science' consisting of objective, quantitative, repeatable measurement. However, understanding people and their complex thoughts, actions, interactions, and relationships which lie at the heart of education requires multiple perspectives, each of which contributes to our broader understanding of the whole.

What sort of questions can education research answer?

Broadly, education research can:
- Describe (what was done or is happening?)
- Justify (did it work?)
- Clarify (why or how did it work?) [4]

Through answering these questions, your intention may be to change the practice of an aspect of education, e.g. making classroom teaching more effective. Your intention may also be to inform political, social, or cultural change, e.g. to increase the diversity of students who enter higher education. Education research can be transformative, aiming to enable education stakeholders to play an active role in researching matters that affect them (see Chapter 5).

What is clinical education research?

Clinical education encompasses everything to do with learning to deliver healthcare, including undergraduate education, postgraduate training, and continuing professional development. Clinical education research aims to advance understanding about clinical education and develop trustworthy knowledge, replacing tradition, intuition, and dogma as the basis of what and how we teach [5]. The scope of clinical education research extends further than workplace-based learning, to include selection and recruitment, curriculum design, teaching and learning approaches, assessment, professionalism, fitness to practice, career choices, transitions, well-being, and beyond [6]. The output of this research can be far-reaching, with direct benefits to patients, learners, individual clinicians, or entire health and education systems.

What makes good clinical education research?

Coe defined six characteristics of education research, which also apply to clinical education research [2].

Systematic

Good education research is systematic rather than slapdash. Your decisions ought to be deliberate and in service of the research question but also comprehensive and careful so that others can have confidence in your answers. This requires you to be careful and to use methods which are accepted as rigorous by other researchers in our field [3].

Critical

A critique of what has gone before, including previous claims, assumptions, or methods, will enhance the quality of your research. You should not simply accept conclusions offered by other authors, rather you ask whether there is an alternative explanation. For example, you may consider that their findings are the result of their particular perspective or methodology and other approaches may provide alternative insights.

Evidential

Evidential means that recommendations are substantiated. Research findings provide a solid basis for moving practices away from those based on tradition, opinion, or anecdote to evidence-based education. Original research creates this evidence, but originality does not necessarily mean researching a completely new topic; it can build on the work of other researchers. Your contribution to education research is therefore part of an ongoing scholarly conversation [7], and it can have a greater impact when it builds on what has been done before.

Theoretical

Your research should have a theoretical basis. A theory is 'an abstract description of the relationships between concepts that help us to understand the world' [8]. Theory helps you make sense of teaching and learning and can be built and tested through research (see Chapter 4). It also enables you to connect your research with existing knowledge and aids the transferability of your findings to other settings.

Transparent

There are three key considerations in relation to transparency. First, describing your research in sufficient detail to enable others to repeat it. Second, maintaining integrity: e.g. reporting inconsistencies in your data or changes in your project which could have affected the outcome. Finally, it means that you reflect on how your life experiences or personal philosophy might have impacted any aspect of your research, from the research question to dissemination (see Chapter 3).

Identifying a topic of interest

There are several 'prestudy tasks' [9] to complete before you commence your research journey. This starts with choosing your general topic of interest. From here, you will develop your specific research questions (see Chapter 2).

Your topic should be both interesting and worthwhile. The results of your research should matter to both you and your intended audience. The topic may emerge from everyday problems and your reflections on personal experiences: what interests you? What irritates you? What concerns you? As a note of caution, you must be able to distinguish between your emotional and intellectual motivations. Proving or validating your own experiences or preconceptions is unlikely to lead to a fruitful research endeavour, unless the topic is also important to others [9]. You must be open to having your views disproven!

While important, reflection on experience is not the only source of research ideas [10]. Sources include discussions with stakeholders, such as educators who research, learners, patients, or policymakers: what are they thinking about? What are their suggestions for good research projects? (see Chapter 5). You should also review academic journals, social media, and medical journalism: are there current topical debates that need answers?

Theory, models, and conceptual frameworks can provide new insights or lines of inquiry into problems in clinical education (see Chapter 4). Just as in physics, where you might test Newton's laws by collecting real-life data, you can test theories in your own educational settings. These might be from within clinical education (e.g. experience-based learning [11]) or drawn from other fields (e.g. situated learning theory [12]). The particular benefit of basing your research on theory is that you are helping to build a coherent body of work [13], and your research should be applicable outside the specific context of your study.

Undertaking a preliminary literature search

Once you have identified a topic of interest, you need to find out what is already known about it. Time, talent, and commitment are precious commodities that should not be wasted on reinventing the wheel.

It is imperative to discover what is already known about the topic and, perhaps more crucially, what is not known. You need to ensure that there is a 'gap' [7]. In a well-studied field, finding the gap is challenging. In an understudied field, the challenge is to ensure the gap matters.

There is an entire research discipline devoted to the systematic search for, appraisal, and synthesis of academic literature, the outcomes of which are research projects in themselves (see Part II of this book). This is not always necessary at the start of a project. However, conducting a preliminary literature search is essential. It does not need to be comprehensive, but it should at least aim to answer these questions:

- What research has been published on this topic, and where are the gaps?
- Are there conflicting findings in previous studies that could be further investigated?
- What sorts of research aims, objectives, questions, and methods have been used?

How do I search the literature?

Although your first instinct may be to turn to a familiar search engine (e.g. Google), this is likely to result in thousands of results, which will range from papers in high-quality scientific journals to material from sources with less rigorous quality control. Instead, we recommend using tools for searching the formal academic literature. These fall into two groups: indexing services and scholarly literature search engines.

Indexing services (e.g. PubMed) enable you to search a database of journals systematically using subject-specific search terms. This enables you to streamline your search and ensure you are only retrieving reports published in the academic literature. However, there are two cautions when searching for them. First, no database indexes all journals. Therefore, it is good practice to search multiple databases to maximise your chances of finding relevant material. Second, your choice of search terms is critical and may not align with keywords in individual papers or the terms within the indexing service. To overcome this, we recommend considering synonyms and combining terms with Boolean operators (e.g. AND/OR/NOT) [14].

If you have access to a university or health library, you will be able to search academic databases which require subscriptions (e.g. SCOPUS, EMBASE) and draw on librarians for support. Your library might have its own search engine, which allows you to access results from all of its subscribed databases at once, and they can provide links to full texts seamlessly without multiple login steps. Your library may also offer training on how to use the databases and help with constructing search terms.

Scholarly literature search engines, such as Google Scholar, Microsoft Academic, and Semantic Scholar, are freely accessible. These are easy to use if you are familiar with using generic search engines, can be used with both natural language and keyword searching, and provide links to freely available full texts. However, these will return many more results than the indexing services, meaning you will retrieve more irrelevant material. Furthermore, you cannot limit the search by subject area or material type, nor can you only search titles and abstracts.

I have got my search results, what do I do now?

If you have no results, we counsel caution. If there appears to be very little or nothing published, we urge you to stop and think 'why?' Is it because your idea is truly novel? Is that likely? Or is it an important topic that is very difficult to research? Or is it irrelevant and not worth researching? Or has your search strategy failed to find the appropriate studies?

Alternatively, you may have thousands of results. This does not mean that there is no need for further research on the topic, but the challenge then is to identify the important gaps. In this case, we would encourage you to identify and focus on review articles first to get a feel for the field. While they summarise what is known, review articles can identify gaps in knowledge that may help you to focus on a particular area. It is also worthwhile looking at the methodologies that have been used. Are there key techniques that you will need for your own project? Or are there novel methodologies with which you could generate meaningful insights?

The optimum situation is when you find a manageable number of publications. Your search terms should have found any relevant review articles, but you should have assimilated individual papers too, particularly those published more recently than the reviews. Consider the research questions which have been asked, the methods applied, the results, and the author's ideas about the next steps in research. As you start to identify key authors or papers, look at the literature they cite and the literature which has cited them. That will help you understand how research in your chosen area has developed and continues to evolve. Tools such as Google Scholar or http://connectedpapers.com can help with this.

No matter how many results you have, you will need a process for reviewing them. We suggest you

do this in two distinct stages. The first is to identify papers which are *likely* to be useful (screening), and the second is to decide whether they are useful or not (critical appraisal).

When screening your results, we suggest you initially scan titles and save those which seem relevant (see 'How do I keep track of the papers I have found?' section). Having identified a smaller subset as potentially interesting, the next task is to review the abstracts; this will enable you to further refine your selection. Subsequently, you should obtain and read the full papers. Many will be available either online or as printed journals through your library. If your library does not have a subscription which allows access, it is worthwhile searching for online versions using Google Scholar. Your library may be able to request a copy of the paper through an interlibrary loan service, although there is often a charge. If these routes fail, you can email the paper's corresponding author and request a copy.

Critical appraisal is the process of making a judgement of the quality of a paper and its relevance to your work. There are tools available for critically appraising academic literature (e.g. Critical Appraisal Skills Programme [15]). However, for the purposes of conducting your preliminary search, these may not be necessary. We suggest reading this literature with the following questions in mind:

- Is this paper relevant to my emerging research topic?
- Are the methods robust and trustworthy?
- What are the main findings and implications?
- Are the conclusions supported by the methods and results?
- How can this study inform my research topic or project design?

How do I keep track of the papers I have found?

We strongly encourage you to use citation management software from the start of your research journey. A good citation management package will allow you to import the citation details, the abstract, and often a PDF of the item. You can read the abstract and PDF, track what you have read, and add your own notes or keywords to help organise your library. However, the most useful feature of this type of software is the way it works with your word processor. They enable you to insert citations into your writing and to compile reference lists. These are formatted automatically and can be easily reformatted if needed. See the resource on the companion website for a comparison of different citation management applications.

Taking stock

At the end of your preliminary search, you should be able to identify the existing research around your topic of interest and where the gaps are. You should have an understanding of the range of methodologies employed and formed opinions on the strengths and weaknesses of previous work.

Do not be too modest about the validity of your perspective as a novice clinical education researcher. Regardless of your experience, your perspective is new and therefore valuable. We encourage you to engage in debates, defend your ideas, and be ready to listen and learn.

Research aims and objectives

Once you have a topic, you can start to construct the aims and objectives of your research, which will inform the specific research questions (see Chapter 2).

Research aims, objectives, and questions are intimately connected and will direct how your research will be conducted. Definitions and examples for each are provided in Table 1.1. Your research aim represents the overarching purpose of your research stated in general terms [16]. Possible aims include adding to the knowledge base, achieving a personal, social, institutional, and/or organisational impact, measuring change, understanding a complex phenomenon, testing new ideas, generating new ideas, or examining the past [17]. The focus required for good research means that there is usually only one aim per study.

Your research objectives will be determined by your aim. Each study will usually have two to three research objectives to keep the project manageable. They will use action verbs to describe the tasks that must be completed to achieve your aim and answer your research question(s). They should be specific, measurable, appropriate, realistic, and time specific (SMART) [16, 18]. It is a good idea to number them for reference in research proposals, study protocols, and ethics applications.

Constructing a good research question is usually much more challenging than stating aims and objectives and is the focus of Chapter 2. They are critical, the 'linchpin of the research process' [19]. They will orientate your study, directly determine your methodology and methods, and the wording of your research questions can make or break your project. It is worth investing considerable time and effort to get it right.

We acknowledge that there is debate about whether aims, objectives, and questions are always required: it may not be necessary to have both objectives and questions [16, 20], but we suggest having both is good practice (Table 1.1).

Table 1.1 Definitions and examples of the key terms in the planning of a research project

Term	Brief definition	Example
Topic of interest	A broad topic of clinical education that is interesting and worthwhile exploring.	Medical specialty stereotypes.
Research aim	The overarching purpose. What is the big picture? What do you aim to achieve in performing this research?	To explore stakeholders' perceptions of medical specialty stereotypes.
Research objective(s)	The intermediary steps required to achieve your overarching aim. What do I need to do to achieve my aim and answer my questions? Usually numbered and written in terms of action verbs.	1 To characterise, from the perspectives of key stakeholders, what collective medical specialty stereotypes exist. 2 To explore the differences in the perspectives of medical specialty stereotypes between stakeholders.
Research question(s)	A recasting of each research objective as one or more questions, which if answered, will address at least part of each objective. They should be relevant, feasible, and focused (see Chapter 2).	1 What stereotypes do patients, medical students, clinical trainees, and consultants hold of internal medics, radiologists, pathologists, and surgeons? 2 How do medical specialty stereotypes compare across patients, medical students, clinical trainees, and consultants?

Reflecting on your resources

You now need to critically examine your topic and see if it is fit for purpose for a research project. The following questions may help you decide. We encourage you to discuss these questions with an experienced supervisor or mentor (see the next section).

- *Can you manage the scope of the project?* Initially, many projects are just too big, and you may need to focus on only one aspect of your research topic. Think about the breadth and depth and whether you need to reduce these to make the project manageable from the outset [21].
- *Do you have the relevant skills and expertise to perform the research to a good standard?* If not, you either

need to develop these or recruit a co-researcher with the required skills to help.

- *Do you have the time to do the research?* If your research is part of a formal programme of study, you will usually have a deadline. This may not be true of extracurricular research, but in this case, you may not have enough capacity to do the research well. You also need to consider your research participants' availability, which may be constrained by curriculum timetables, rotas, holidays, or exam periods. You need to accommodate these in your plans for data collection.
- *What resources do you have available?* You may find that there are resources that are required in order to complete your study. Resources could include financial, technological, or human. Financial resources can pay for participant incentives, travel, transcription, and patient involvement. Technological resources include hardware (e.g. recording devices, and computers) and software (e.g. statistical and qualitative data analysis packages). Human resources provide expertise (e.g. supervisors, collaborators, statisticians, librarians, and research design experts).
- *Will you be able to collect/access the data you need?* You may need to work with gatekeepers (people who can grant or deny you access to potential participants or data sets). Remember, it is not just programme leads who are gatekeepers, you may have to build a relationship with the professional and support staff responsible for providing information essential to your study. It is worthwhile contacting all gatekeepers as early as possible, ideally meeting face to face to promote trust. This also allows the gatekeeper to ask questions and provides an opportunity for you to learn about the site, participants, or data that you want access to. This can be invaluable when making recruitment and sampling decisions later on (see Chapter 6) [22].
- *What are the ethical considerations and can you manage them?* A good rule of thumb is that all research which involves gathering data from human participants requires research ethics approval no matter how innocuous the research question may seem (see Chapter 7). The routes to ethics approval vary depending on where you will conduct your research and may be a local, regional, or national procedure depending on the topic of your research, your participants, and how you will recruit them. It is essential that you familiarise yourself with the process which will apply to your project. Ethics review also takes time, often much more time than you expect, so make sure you start the

process early to prevent delays or missing later deadlines. It can pay dividends to get the application as 'right' as possible the first time it is submitted, to prevent delays in multiple rounds of edits. This is where an experienced supervisor or utilising your institution's advisory service can be really helpful.
- *Will your findings be useful to others?* This helps to answer the 'so what?' question. It is important that you use your time, talent, and energy wisely, on projects that have the potential for impact. The impact need not be big but it should exist.

Getting help

The prospect of your first research project can be intimidating: there are many choices to be made and many pitfalls to avoid, and the simplest approach is not always the best. We would encourage you to seek help and support early in your research journey. If your project is part of a course of study (e.g. a bachelor's or master's degree project), you will have a supervisor: use them. If your project is extracurricular, it is still important to find someone to help.

How do I find someone to help?
If you do not have an allocated supervisor, we suggest two approaches. If you are studying or working for an academic or healthcare organisation, there are likely to be staff who have a research interest in education or training. Talk to your colleagues to find out who they are and ask for an introduction or search your institution's website to get their contact details. If this is not fruitful, make an appointment with your local director or head of education/training, who could signpost you in the right direction.

If your search in-house is unsuccessful, you can move on to other sources of support. Look at the websites of organisations such as universities with faculties of health professions education, national medical education organisations (e.g. the Association for the Study of Medical Education, or its equivalent in other countries), or professional bodies and colleges. What are their research interests? Do they have an education research group? Do they hold research meetings, seminars, or webinars? Make contact, tell them you are interested in getting started in education research, and ask whether you can either attend their events or meet someone to discuss research. Additionally, social media platforms (e.g. Twitter) can be incredibly fruitful sources of professional connections.

How should I prepare for my meeting?

If someone is willing to give you their time, you should make the most of it. Consider what you need from them. This could range from you wanting to help them with one of their research ideas, to you wanting their help with your research idea. Preparation before meeting them will pay dividends.

If your desire is to work with them on one of their research ideas, review their website, peruse their publications, and read some recent papers. This will enable you to check if your interests align and have an informed conversation when you meet.

If you have a firm research idea, prepare a short, written pitch. Aim to demonstrate that you have reviewed the literature and have an idea of how you would approach the problem. Send it in advance of your meeting and be prepared for challenge. Challenge should not be perceived as hostility, rather as an expression of interest in your idea. Common challenges include:

- 'It has been done before'. If you have been reasonably thorough in your literature search, this should be unlikely, but it is not impossible. Ask by whom and if you recognise the reference, clarify the gap you have identified. If you do not recognise the source, acknowledge that and follow it up. However, if the person you are meeting knows the literature well, it is likely they have ideas for next steps in researching this topic. This is a golden opportunity to discuss how you could work together to research other, related, questions.
- 'It is too big or not focused enough'. This is probably the most common challenge. The essence of good research is to find 'simple' questions which start to address complex problems. Do not be afraid to ask, 'how can or where should I focus?'
- 'It is not possible'. This is probably the most difficult challenge to meet. You may have ideas for methodologies or perspectives which have not been applied to this problem. It is important that you can explain these clearly.
- 'Have you thought about. . .'. This can be frustrating initially. You may feel that you are being pushed away from what you really want to pursue. However, you are getting feedback which can be valuable, particularly if their idea is a good one. This signifies interest and a desire to support you in developing your idea.
- Conflicting advice. There are different ways of approaching the same research idea, and researchers might present you with alternatives to consider which are mutually exclusive! Ultimately, it is your research project. We encourage you to seek advice but be prepared to choose the best path for you, considering factors such as resources and feasibility.

What can I expect from the meeting?

It is reasonable to expect they will engage with you and your ideas in a positive and productive manner. This may vary from a suggestion to meet someone else with an interest in your topic, to a suggestion of other literature to look at, to advice on how to refine your research's scope, and perhaps an invitation to come back and see them again. All of these are positive outcomes, even if they mean more work for you. You may feel that you have been supported, your ideas validated, and your confidence boosted. However, if your ideas have been challenged, you could feel the opposite and that you or your ideas have been rejected. It is important to look past this. Their aim will be to make your work the best it can be, both in terms of rigour and impact.

Finalising your idea

After considering the scope, individuality, feasibility, and impact of your research topic and performing a preliminary literature review, consulting relevant stakeholders and, if necessary, recruiting others to your team, you should be ready to commit to your research idea . . . or not! Now is the time to make changes if things are not quite right. Consider how you could tweak the project to improve its suitability, this most commonly involves narrowing down the scope. You can also decide to let things go completely, but it is important to then move on to a new idea. Choosing your research topic is an important decision to get right.

Summary

This chapter has introduced you to the first steps in clinical education research (Figure 1.1). Your next and very critical step is to formulate and finalise your research question(s) (see Chapter 2). The research question(s) and objectives will inform your design choices (see Chapter 3) and theoretical underpinnings (see Chapter 4). We encourage you to engage with stakeholders throughout the research process (see Chapter 5) and carefully consider how best to sample and recruit participants (see Chapter 6). Underpinning all of this must be an ethical approach to your research (see Chapter 7). We encourage you to start this journey with a balance of realism and optimism. It will demand your talent, time, and enthusiasm, but we believe that the rewards are commensurate with the effort you will expend.

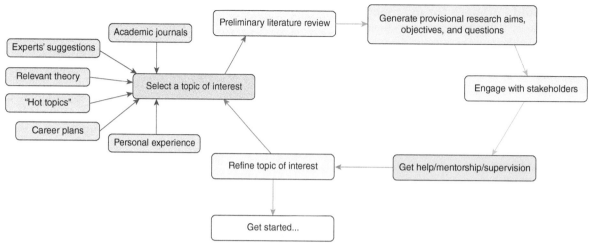

Figure 1.1 The first steps in clinical education research.

Top tips

- Be realistic! Start with a small but high-quality research project – do a little, well.
- Review dissertations of previous students on your programme, or other similar subjects. This may help you better understand what the finished product will look like.
- Start a research diary as soon as possible and use it to generate and keep track of thoughts and ideas.
- Reflect on your motivations for conducting research and consider how much time you have to dedicate to this.

Common pitfalls

- It can be tempting to rush into projects without discussing them with experienced researchers or reading the literature. This early work will pay dividends later.
- Research rarely takes a smooth path. Try not to be disheartened if your initial ideas are challenged.
- For a first project in clinical education, it is unlikely that you will be able to reach all the gold standards. It is reasonable to consider what is practical within the scope of your time and resources.

References

1 OED Online (2021). Research, n.1. http://www.oed.com/view/Entry/163432 (accessed 29 October 2021).

2 Coe, R. (2021). The nature of educational research. In: *Research Methods & Methodologies in Education* (ed. R. Coe, M. Waring, L.V. Hedges, and L. Day Ashley), 5–14. London: SAGE Publications Ltd.

3 Bridges, D. (2006). The disciplines and discipline of educational research. *Journal of Philosophy of Education* 40 (2): 259–272.

4 Cook, D.A., Bordage, G., and Schmidt, H.G. (2008). Description, justification and clarification: a framework for classifying the purposes of research in medical education. *Medical Education* 42 (2): 128–133.

5 Suter, W.N. (2012). *Introduction to Educational Research: A Critical Thinking Approach*. Thousand Oaks, CA: SAGE Publications Ltd https://doi.org/10.4135/9781483384443.

6 Incubator for Clinical Education (2020). Is my work ClinEdR?. https://research.ncl.ac.uk/clinical-education-research-incubator/abouttheincubator/what-is-clinedr (accessed 18 July 2021).

7 Lingard, L. (2015). Joining a conversation: the problem/gap/hook heuristic. *Perspectives on Medical Education* 4 (5): 252–253.

8 Varpio, L., Paradis, E., Uijtdehaage, S. et al. (2020). The distinctions between theory, theoretical framework, and conceptual framework. *Academic Medicine* 95 (7): 989–994.

9 Glesne, C. (2011). Prestudy tasks: doing what is good for you. In: *Becoming Qualitative Researchers: An Introduction*, 4e (International ed.), 27–62. Boston, MA: Pearson.

10 Machi, L.A. and McEvoy, B.T. (2016). Step one: select a topic. In: *The Literature Review: Six Steps to Success*, 17–36. Thousand Oaks, CA: SAGE Publications Ltd.

11 Dornan, T., Conn, R., Monaghan, H. et al. (2019). Experience based learning (ExBL): clinical teaching for the twenty-first century. *Medical Teacher* 41 (10): 1098–1105.

12 Lave, J. and Wenger, E. (1991). *Situated Learning: Legitimate Peripheral Participation*. Cambridge: Cambridge University Press.

13 Bolander Laksov, K., Dornan, T., and Teunissen, P.W. (2017). Making theory explicit – an analysis of how medical education research(ers) describe how they connect to theory. *BMC Medical Education* 17 (1): 18.

14 Haig, A. and Dozier, M. (2003). BEME guide no. 3: systematic searching for evidence in medical education – part 2: constructing searches. *Medical Teacher* 25 (5): 463–484.

15 Critical Appraisal Skills Programme (2022). CASP checklists. https://casp-uk.net/casp-tools-checklists (accessed 14 July 2022).

16 Doody, O. and Bailey, M.E. (2016). Setting a research question, aim and objective. *Nursing Research* 23 (4): 19–23.

17 Newman, I., Ridenour, C.S., Newman, C. et al. (2003). A typology of research purposes and its relationship to mixed methods. In: *Handbook of Mixed Methods in Social and Behavioral Research* (ed. A. Tashakkori and C. Teddlie), 167–188. Thousand Oaks, CA: SAGE Publications Ltd.

18 Doran, G.T. (1981). There's a S.M.A.R.T. way to write management's goals and objectives. *Management Review* 70 (11): 35.

19 Bryman, A. (2007). The research question in social research: what is its role? *International Journal of Social Research Methodology* 10 (1): 5–20.

20 Thomas, D.R. and Hodges, I.D. (2010). Developing research aims and objectives. In: *Designing and Managing Your Research Project: Core Skills for Social and Health Research*, 38–47. London: SAGE Publications Ltd.

21 White, P. (2008). What makes a research question? In: *Developing Research Questions: A Guide for Social Scientists*, 33–58. Basingstoke: Palgrave Macmillan.

22 Day Ashley, L. (2021). Planning your research. In: *Research Methods & Methodologies in Education* (ed. R. Coe, M. Waring, L.V. Hedges, and L. Day Ashley), 33–42. London: SAGE Publications Ltd.

2 Constructing a research question

Megan Anakin, Joanne Robertson-Smith, and Tim J. Wilkinson

Learning objectives

By the end of this chapter, you should be able to:
- Identify and develop a problem worth researching.
- Describe the features of a good research question.

- Articulate a feasible, interesting, novel, ethical, and relevant research question.
- Evaluate a research question.

Introduction

The research question is the cornerstone of any research project. The importance of taking time to construct a good research question cannot be overstated. A question that is too broad will make it challenging for you to choose appropriate methods to study your topic and may be impossible to answer meaningfully. A question that is too narrow risks being meaningless to others. Spending time constructing a research question will also help you communicate clearly when you seek supervisors or collaborators, recruit participants, and write up your study. This effort early in the research process will pay dividends later. It will keep you focused.

In Chapter 1, you were introduced to how to identify a topic to research. This chapter will illustrate the steps required to go from an idea for a topic to a clearly articulated research question.

What is a research question?

A research question identifies a problem about a topic so it can be addressed using systematic methods of investigation. Such a problem or topic could be a challenge you have experienced in your educational practice, an issue that concerns teachers or learners, or an educational idea or phenomenon that could be better understood. How you articulate your question directs you to appropriate methods to answer it. It guides how you interact with study participants to generate information with them and helps keep you focused on how and why you are studying your chosen issue or problem.

Examine the five pairs of research questions shown in Table 2.1. Can you identify the topic and the problem that the author wants to investigate? Consider the differences between each pair of research questions. In column A, the problems the researcher wants to address may be clear, however, there is important information missing. In column B, details are included that enable the reader to make inferences about possible study designs, participants, and central concepts that will be investigated. In question 1A, it appears that two instructional methods will be compared; however, question 1B provides the context and subject area. It also identifies that assessment data will be gathered. You might be able to predict a possible hypothesis and infer that the data will be analysed using statistical methods. In question 2A, only a glimpse of a possible problem is provided: that students might not like their placements. However, there is no indication of which group of students the researcher might be interested in studying. The reader may not understand what is meant by the term 'placement'. Question 2B provides a description of the term 'placement' because it specifies the features of hospital wards as the clinical learning environment that is the setting for the proposed study. Notice the difference between pairs of questions 3–5 and see if you can identify the key words that add clarity and specificity to produce focused research questions.

Starting Research in Clinical Education, First Edition. Edited by Eliot L. Rees, Alison Ledger, and Kim A. Walker.
© 2024 The Association for the Study of Medical Education (ASME). Published 2024 by John Wiley & Sons Ltd.
Companion website: www.wiley.com/go/clinicaleducation

Table 2.1 Examples of general and focused research questions

	A: General	B: Focused
1	Is an online module better than lectures?	Does an online module about oral pathology result in higher assessment scores for dental students than when the same knowledge is presented as a series of lectures?
2	What do students like about placements?	What features of hospital wards do dietetic students find helpful for learning?
3	How do students perceive feedback from teachers?	How do physiotherapy students interpret feedback from their supervisors in community placement settings?
4	How do students and teachers talk about a management plan for a patient?	How do medical students and consultants resolve identity tensions when discussing a management plan for an elderly patient in a busy hospital ward environment?
5	How do students learn professional behaviour?	How do nursing students learn to collaborate with colleagues to care for a person in an end-of-life hospice setting?

Defining the problem

To help you identify keywords to construct a focused research question, it is helpful to invest time thinking about how you might express the problem you would like to investigate. As the famous quote goes, 'If I had eight hours to chop down a tree, I would spend the first six sharpening my axe' [1]. This same approach can apply to research planning. It can be tempting to launch into a project and think about the purpose later. Equally, you might be tempted to choose a research method and think about the goal of your study later. You should be aware that there are important drawbacks if you use these two approaches to constructing a research question. You may end up with a purpose-less project or a study where the goals and methods

are not aligned. To avoid these drawbacks, consider investing your time to define the problem that you would like to investigate. This investment will be time well spent because it can help you identify an appropriate theoretical perspective, consider possible study designs, and assist you to make decisions about how you carry out your project. We encourage you to consider this phase of research as time to define the problem.

One way to define the problem is to discuss your ideas with a colleague. Consider this hypothetical scenario: Sam is running a six-week-long course and wants to research it. Sam wonders if the starting point is to administer a questionnaire to students to collect information about whether they liked the course or not. Sam explains this idea to their colleague. Their conversation is presented in Box 2.1.

BOX 2.1   Illustrated case study of a clinical educator defining their research problem.

Charlie: *What do you want to do with the answer? For example, if you found that three-quarters of students like the course, what might you do with that information?*

Sam: *I could compare the three-quarters of students who like the course with the one-quarter who do not.*

Charlie: *But what do you want to do with that information? What is the problem you want to solve?*

Sam: *Why do I need to solve a problem? I want the students to tell me what is going well and what I can do to improve my course.*

Charlie: *That is an important part of your teaching practice to know more about. Some people might consider that evaluation rather than research. It might be easier to explore how your students are experiencing your course if you narrow your focus. What information do you have already? What do others know about this topic more generally?*

Sam: *Great idea, I need to think about it.*

Time passes.

Sam: *I have thought about narrowing the focus of my research. Now I am curious to know why some students seem very engaged in the course, whereas others are not.*

Charlie: *Sounds like you have identified a problem. Your research area is becoming more focused. What do you mean by engagement?*

Sam: *Hmm. Do we not all share the same definition of engagement?*

Charlie: *Why do you not read about engagement and let me know what you find out?*

Sam explores the clinical education research literature. Sam notices that student engagement has been studied in a variety of ways and researchers have offered different definitions. At first, Sam feels confused but persists with reading and thinking about the literature about engagement. Finally, an article catches their interest because it describes how student engagement is enhanced when active learning strategies are used by teachers [2]. Active learning strategies require students to complete tasks that are challenging and relevant to them. Sam explains these ideas to Charlie.

Charlie: *That is great! Reading and drawing on the literature really helps focus and develop a question. How might you use these ideas to study engagement?*

Sam: *But I still want to improve my course.*

Charlie: *When conducting an educational research project, you can be practical and theoretical at the same time. This means you can use the project to improve your course AND contribute to our theoretical understanding about engagement.*

Sam: *Theoretical?*

Charlie: *The findings that result from your project might be of interest to others. Other educators might want to apply your ideas to their courses. Other researchers might be able to build on how you define and study engagement. Theory helps you to explain to others how and why students are engaged in your course. It helps others determine how applicable your findings might be in their contexts.*

Sam thinks about how to balance theory and practice. Sam remembers being intrigued about challenging tasks when reading the literature.

Sam: *Now I am wondering if I should explore how I can provide the optimal amount of challenge to students in my course. How would I know if tasks have the optimal amount of challenge to keep students engaged?*

Charlie: *What is one way you might gather information to answer this question?*

Sam: *I am wondering if maybe I should ask my students. I could add questions to the course evaluation questionnaire that ask students to rate statements about how challenging assignments and activities were for them.*

Charlie: *Do you want to know if students agree or disagree with statements that you write about the assignments and activities in the course? Or, do you want to know why students may experience particular aspects of the assignments and activities in the course to be more challenging that others?*

Sam: *I want to know about why students are challenged by certain parts of my course.*

Charlie: *Then maybe you need to re-think using a questionnaire to gather information to answer your research questions. A questionnaire might not allow you to gather the type of information you need to better understand how or why students find certain parts of your course challenging (or not).*

Sam: *I might have to read more about how others have studied and think about student engagement and challenging tasks, so I know what needs to be explored next. I am not so sure that a course evaluation questionnaire will give me the answers I am looking for.*

In this scenario, Charlie supports Sam to define a problem worth studying. The conversations helped Sam to develop and focus ideas, consider and reconsider methods, and generate possible research questions. Discussing your ideas with others will help clarify your thinking and define your problem which you can then fine tune into a research question. When you present a draft research question to a colleague, examine their reaction. If your conversation about the problem is lukewarm or generates 'ho hum' responses, then the following questions might help to further develop the research question, 'Who cares about this question and why?', 'What might people do with the answer?', 'How might the answer change how people think about the problem?' These questions will help you construct a research question that is important and relevant to others.

From problem to question

Having identified a topic for research and defined the problem, the next step is to articulate it in the form of a research question. A good research question is fundamental to any research. It can help you describe the relevance and merit of your project to others in the form of a succinct explanation or 'elevator pitch' that includes the impact of your research [3].

Cummings et al. describe five characteristics of a good research question using the mnemonic FINER [4] (Table 2.2).

The first thing to consider is the feasibility of the question. Would you have sufficient time, expertise, and resources to answer the question. As alluded to earlier, often research questions need focusing to make them manageable. It is better to have a focused

Table 2.2 FINER research questions

Characteristic	Feature
Feasible	Likely to be able to recruit sufficient participants to answer the question Research team has the right expertise Will have sufficient time and resources Manageable in terms of scope Fundable (if required)
Interesting	The answer will be of interest to the research team
Novel	Will add new insights
Ethical	A study that a research ethics committee will approve
Relevant	Likely to have impact on policy, practice, or future research

Source: Adapted from Cummings et al. [4].

question that you are able to answer than to have a more nebulous question that remains unresolved.

Next, it should be of interest to you and your supervisor or research team. It will be easier to persevere when faced with difficulties if you are working on a project you are interested in. One way to check for interest is the 'Oooh' test. Ask yourself, 'Does this research question deeply interest me? Am I excited by this research question?' If the answer is, 'Yes!' then you will probably be able to find the personal motivation to persist with a study that addresses that research question. If the answer is, 'No' or even, 'Hmmm', then reconsider your research question or put it aside until you can answer affirmatively. The 'Oooh' test also helps you to detect if the research question is aligned with your own view of knowledge and the world around us. A negative answer might be an indication of a mismatch between the phrasing or focus of the question and your perspective about how you can study it that should be resolved.

Your research question should enable you to provide new knowledge to the field. Occasionally, this will be through researching a previously unresearched area. More likely, however, this will be taking a new perspective on a problem using different methodological or theoretical approaches.

For any research question, it must be able to be answered using a study that would be approved by a research ethics committee. See Chapter 7 for detailed guidance about conducting ethical research.

A good research question will address a problem that is relevant and important to your educational community [5–7]. This community might be local and composed of colleagues in your workplace.

Your community might be regional or global and represented by policies and strategic priorities of national or international organisations. A good research question should be able to pass the 'So what?' test. If you can confidently answer this test with supporting evidence and logic, then your research question will likely be viewed as relevant and important to your research community. A good research question and its feasibility will then guide the choice of study design [8].

Getting help

Supervisors and collaborators can help you understand how the wording of your research question conveys your implicit perspective (see Chapter 3) and suggests the methods most appropriate for your study. A question such as, 'What assignments and activities do students find challenging in the course?' suggests a 'fact finding' perspective that could be addressed by using a questionnaire that will be analysed quantitatively to yield numerical results. Whereas a question like, 'Why do students find certain parts of my course challenging?' might suggest a perspective that seeks to interpret the experiences of students that might be best understood by talking with them or observing their behaviour when doing assignments and activities in the course.

Colleagues can help you keep an open mind when constructing a research question. When working alone, it can be difficult to sustain curiosity and motivation to keep exploring options. It can also be challenging to think about your topic or problem from different perspectives. You may find that you finalise your research question too quickly. To remain open to alternatives, ask yourself, 'What possibilities am I closing off by answering this question?' or 'What might I be missing?'. Better yet, find a supervisor or colleague with whom to discuss these questions.

Colleagues can help you better understand whether answering the question will contribute new knowledge and whether it is likely to have the potential to influence policy, practice, or future research. They may be able to point you in the direction of literature that you would not have instinctively considered, but that may be helpful when you are finalising your question.

Beyond the question

During a project, your research question can be used to check that decisions made while gathering and interpreting data are aligned [5, 9]. Markers or reviewers will ask: Does your introduction lead to, and justify the research question? Will the methods answer the question? Are the results explained by the methods? Are there methods with no results? Is the discussion based on the results and does it link back to your question? Although you may consider these alignment issues to be self-evident, it has been our experience that some 'drifting' of alignment can occur if the question is not well defined. One way to keep alert to possible drift is by keeping your research question visible when you write about your project. This visibility can be achieved by sticking a small note to the computer screen with the research question written on it.

The types of decisions available to you will depend on the study design of your research project. The term 'study design' refers to the set of methods and procedures that you use to generate and analyse data. With hypothesis-driven study designs, the research question is used to generate one or more hypotheses that determine the sequence of procedures to ensure the results are valid and reliable [10]. Hypothesis-driven study designs typically involve research questions that are usually fixed from the start of the study. With exploratory study designs, the research question is also used to guide the methods selected. However, the research question may need to be refined or revised during data analysis if the findings are unanticipated. It is quite common and permissible for the research question to evolve as your study develops. However, if the research question changes, then you will need to check that your study remains internally consistent. Ask yourself, 'Are the methods, results, and conclusions still aligned to this new research question?' The appropriateness of altering a research question during a project depends on the researchers' perspective. This perspective includes what a person considers to be knowable and what it means to know something (see Chapter 3).

When your project is completed, the research question will help you make decisions about how you communicate your results to others [7, 11]. It will help you to construct a coherent report of your research, write an achievable statement about the aim of your study, and decide which procedures need to be described in detail so a reader can understand and potentially replicate the methods used to conduct your study. By revisiting your research question, it will remind you to select, define, and use a limited set of terms to describe the main elements of your study. The research question can also be used to inform how you might structure the presentation and discussion of the results of your study.

Questions to avoid

So far, we have discussed the features of high-quality research questions. It is also worth highlighting some of the common limitations in research questions that can lead to flawed research designs. We encourage you to avoid these when you refine and focus your research questions.

Focusing on learner reactions

Student reactions are important when planning learning activities, but they can be over-interpreted when they are used as research data. A focus on educational factors or outcomes will be of greater interest to people beyond your classroom or workplace. Kirkpatrick presents a hierarchy of outcome measures to help you consider the type of evaluation information you suggest by your research question [12]. The least impactful evidence involves student reactions that can be generated by questions such as 'Did students like the activity?' and 'Did students find the activity difficult?'. More interesting evidence involves gathering information about outcomes with questions such as 'Did the activity change students' behaviour?' and 'Did the activity alter organisational performance?'.

Using self-reported outcome data

Constructing research questions that focus on student self-perceptions of learning can be similarly problematic as to questions that focus on student reactions. The answer to 'Did you learn anything?' can be inaccurate. Evidence to support this claim comes from a study involving *The Dr Fox Lecture* [13]. In this study, a person provided a lecture that was deliberately designed to be entertaining and persuasive, but the content was intended to be meaningless, contradictory, and confusing. Students highly rated the quality of the lecture and its impact on their learning. Likewise, students rated a session more highly if cookies were provided compared with one where they were not [14]. One way to avoid this pitfall is to construct your research question using 'Why?' and 'How?' rather than 'What'. For example, 'Why did this strategy work?' or 'How did this strategy work?' can be more illuminating than 'What happens when I use this teaching strategy?'. Another suggestion for producing impactful evidence is to ask, 'What happens if I use this teaching strategy rather than that one?'

Another common flaw is to equate confidence with competence [15]. Students' greater confidence with a topic after an intervention can sometimes be misinterpreted as indicating they learned something. Students who know little can often be naively confident, while those who know more may have developed insight and will have a decline in confidence. Later, a competent person may end up being confident again. This relationship between confidence and competence is known as the Dunning–Kruger effect [15]. The message here is not to presume that an increase in confidence is necessarily related to an increase in competence. Educational phenomena can be difficult to define and distinguish from one another. Once again, our advice is to take the time to discuss the key terms and concepts in your research question with others and investigate how they have been used and studied in the clinical education research literature.

Comparing something with nothing

In order to overcome the weakness of using self-reported outcome data, some researchers will use assessment data to try to demonstrate the merit of their educational interventions. A flaw that often arises here is when the comparison is between some educational intervention and none. Consider the example of a case-based workshop on blood transfusion. It could be tempting to develop an assessment and compare the outcomes between those that had the workshop and those that did not. Similarly, it might be tempting to test the learners before and after the workshop and compare the outcomes. Both of these designs will be comparing some teaching interventions with no teaching intervention. The workshop would have to be pretty bad for learners to perform worse after it. If you are planning on undertaking a 'justification' study [6], it is better to consider comparing different educational approaches (e.g. case-based workshop versus online learning module).

Assuming shared understandings

Another flaw can arise if you assume that everyone agrees upon the meanings of words. As an example, the word 'learning' can be used as a verb to refer to a process of constructing new capabilities, and it can be used as a noun to refer to new capabilities a person possesses. The participants in your study might hold different views of learning. One student may view learning as the score on a test. Another student might see learning as knowing something new. Yet another student might define learning as seeing the world in a different way. Likewise, different definitions of learning have been proposed and studied by educational researchers. About a century ago, John Watson defined and studied learning as a change in behaviour [16]. In contrast, a contemporary definition informed by cognitive psychology states that learning is 'to add knowledge and skills to long-term memory. If nothing has been added to long-term memory, nothing has been learned' [17].

Learning has been defined for a Western schooling context as 'a student must have sufficient surface knowledge before moving to deep learning and then to the transfer of these understandings' [18]. Given this diversity of definitions for learning, do not be surprised if a colleague misunderstands the intended focus of your research question. For example, consider the different possible ways that the research question could be interpreted: 'How do students learn to behave professionally?' Consider this flaw as an opportunity to understand how your research question can be interpreted by the context of possible theories, goals, and outcomes for your study. Explaining your research to others can often unmask implicit assumptions and areas where there is not a shared understanding of terminology. It is common for people to present their research after it has been completed. However, you can also gain great value from presenting the research before it is done. The questions generated by audience members at such presentations can reveal areas of ambiguity. Another way is to ask yourself, 'What would this phenomenon look like if I were to observe it happening?' In the case of learning, ask, 'What does learning in this situation look and sound like?' More importantly, do other people think learning looks and sounds the same way you have suggested?

Evaluating your research question

Once you have constructed a good research question, it is now time to test it. First, revisit the 'So what?' test. Ask yourself, 'Other than me, who else might care about this research question?' Consider the answer to 'Would someone working in a different part of the world find this question interesting?'. The answer to these questions will help you consider the relevance of your research question in terms of the teaching you are doing, the impact on your clinical team and workplace, the recognition of your study by the clinical education community, and, at an even greater scale, the change in the world that will make it a better place for everyone.

Next, you can use a checklist to help you evaluate your research question, examples of which can be found in the general research design [19] and clinical education literature [20, 21]. Alternatively, Box 2.2 presents a set of reflective prompts to help you evaluate your research question.

Summary

After reading this chapter, we hope you appreciate that the time invested to generate and think about ideas, define the problem, and discuss possible

---

BOX 2.2   Reflective prompts to help you evaluate your research question.

Is my research question. . .
- Relevant? Will others think it is interesting and important?
- Focused? Is it specific or narrow enough that I can imagine possible methods to study the topic or problem?
- Feasible? Is it possible to conduct this research? Do I have access to resources and participants? Do I have enough time to devote to answering this question? Is this question worth the time and resources that are required to be invested in it?
- Rigorous? Can I choose or develop appropriate methods to answer this question? Will the methods generate data and results that are aligned to the question?
- Original or novel? What will the answer to my question add to what is already known?
- Ethical? Will I be able to conduct a study in a way that is safe for my participants?
- Linking theory and practice? What view of education is framing my research question and how does it relate to education practices around me?
- Clarity? Is my research question well-articulated? How do other people interpret my research question and was that as I intended?

---

research questions with colleagues will be time well spent. We have outlined common pitfalls to avoid and suggested ways to evaluate your research question. It is typical to become stuck at in the beginning of a research endeavour, but the techniques covered in this chapter can assist you in breaking free of this impasse. We hope you find these suggestions useful to help you construct a research question that will be relevant, focused, and feasible.

Top tips

- Use an appropriate framework to help you in constructing your research question.
- Present your developing question to supervisors or peers, and use feedback to enhance clarity and specificity.
- Make sure you understand the nature of the problem you want to research.

Common pitfalls

- Focusing on student reactions or self-perception at the expense of educational factors or outcomes.
- Asking a question that is only of interest to your local institution or programme. Consider the potential relevance of your research to others.
- Asking a question that is too broad and infeasible to answer. Reflect on what is possible within your available resources.

Ethical issues

- Make sure you can answer your research question ethically. For example, it can be inequitable to randomly assign learners to different interventions.
- If evaluating your own teaching practice, consider the degree to which participants will offer honest information that addresses your research question. It may be that you need to refine your research question or ask someone else to help to collect the data you need.
- Acknowledge those who have supported you to develop your research question, and if appropriate, invite them to collaborate.

References

1 Allen, R.G. (1983). Wealth is thoughts not things. In: *Creating Wealth*. New York, NY: Simon and Schuster.
2 Graffam, B. (2007). Active learning in medical education: strategies for beginning implementation. *Medical Teacher* 29 (1): 38–42.
3 Morgan, W.R. and Wright, E.S. (2021). Ten simple rules for hitting a home run with your elevator pitch. *PLoS Computational Biology* 17 (3): e1008756.
4 Cummings, S.R., Browner, W.S., and Hulley, S.B. (2013). Conceiving the research question and developing the study plan. In: *Designing Clinical Research*, 4e (ed. S.B. Hulley, S.R. Cummings, W.S. Browner, et al.), 14–22. Philadelphia, PA: Lippincott Williams & Wilkins.
5 Cleland, J.A., Jamieson, S., Kusurkar, R.A. et al. (2021). Redefining scholarship for health professions education: AMEE guide no. 142. *Medical Teacher* 43 (7): 824–838.

6 Cook, D.A., Bordage, G., and Schmidt, H.G. (2008). Description, justification and clarification: a framework for classifying the purposes of research in medical education. *Medical Education* 42 (2): 128–133.

7 Norman, G. (2014). Data dredging, salami-slicing, and other successful strategies to ensure rejection: twelve tips on how to not get your paper published. *Advances in Health Sciences Education* 19 (1): 1–5.

8 Zaniletti, I., Devick, K., Larson, D. et al. (2022). Study types in orthopaedics research: is my study design appropriate for the research question? *The Journal of Arthroplasty* 37: 1939–1944.

9 Varpio, L., Paradis, E., Uijtdehaage, S., and Young, M. (2020). The distinctions between theory, theoretical framework, and conceptual framework. *Academic Medicine* 95 (7): 989–994.

10 Creswell, J.W. and Creswell, J.D. (2018). *Research Design: Qualitative, Quantitative, and Mixed Methods Approaches*, 5e. Thousand Oaks, CA: SAGE Publications.

11 Lea, S.J., Stephenson, D., and Troy, J. (2003). Higher education students' attitudes to student-centred learning: beyond 'educational bulimia'? *Studies in Higher Education* 28 (3): 321–334.

12 Kirkpatrick, D.L. and Kirkpatrick, J.D. (1998). *Evaluating Training Programs: The Four Levels*, 2e. San Francisco, CA: Berrett-Koehler.

13 Naftulin, D.H., Ware, J.E., and Donnelly, F.A. (1973). The Doctor Fox lecture: a paradigm of educational seduction. *Journal of Medical Education* 48: 630–635.

14 Hessler, M., Pöpping, D.M., Hollstein, H. et al. (2018). Availability of cookies during an academic course session affects evaluation of teaching. *Medical Education* 52 (10): 1064–1072.

15 Kruger, J. and Dunning, D. (1999). Unskilled and unaware of it: how difficulties in recognizing one's own incompetence lead to inflated self-assessments. *Journal of Personality and Social Psychology* 77 (6): 1121–1134.

16 Moore, J. and John, B. (2017). Watson's classical S–R behaviorism. *The Journal of Mind and Behavior* 1: 1–34.

17 Clark, R., Kirschner, P.A., and Sweller, J. (2012). Putting students on the path to learning: the case for fully guided instruction. *American Educator* 36 (1): 5–11.

18 Hattie, J.A. and Donoghue, G.M. (2016). Learning strategies: a synthesis and conceptual model. *npj Science of Learning* 1 (1): 1–3.

19 O'Leary, Z. (2017). *The Essential Guide to Doing Research*, 3e. SAGE Publications.

20 Dine, C.J., Shea, J.A., and Kogan, J.R. (2016). Generating good research questions in health professions education. *Academic Medicine* 91 (12): e8.

21 Mattick, K., Johnston, J., and de la Croix, A. (2018). How to. . . write a good research question. *The Clinical Teacher* 15 (2): 104–108.

3 Clarifying research paradigms and design

J. Cristian Rangel, Meredith Young, and Lara Varpio

Learning objectives

By the end of this chapter, you should be able to:
- Define key concepts in research design.
- Describe two research paradigms commonly used in clinical education (post-positivism and constructivism).
- Recognise the importance of aligning research questions and designs with a specific paradigm.
- Identify the most common research tools associated with each paradigm.
- Differentiate the markers for rigour in post-positivism and constructivism.

Introduction

Research design is often equated with the scientific method, where the researcher constructs a hypothesis, designs an experiment, and tracks observations to either prove or disprove the hypothesis. This approach is foundational to many discoveries in the natural and physical sciences because it is well suited to identifying patterns in the material world (e.g. taking medication x can treat disease y). However, the problems clinical education researchers wrestle with rarely follow clear-cut, predictable causal patterns that can be objectively observed and measured. Sometimes, clinical education research involves the quantification of human practices, for example, assessing behaviours or skills [1], or examining causal connections between one event (e.g. duty hours) and an outcome (e.g. medical error [2]). Some clinical education researchers explore aspects of human interactions, relationships, and experiences (e.g. the power dynamics in interprofessional healthcare teams [3]), or develop understandings of deeply personal impacts of educational practices (e.g. the lived experiences of shame in residency [4]). Given this heterogeneity, the clinical education research enterprise must include research designs that involve objective quantification of patterns in behaviour or relationships, and those that explore and identify the ways that people produce consequential meaning out of their everyday experiences.

In this chapter, we introduce some of the considerations that shape research design, highlighting the differences that make a difference between studies that use objective quantification and those that explore the subjective experiences of people. We focus on two schools of thought (post-positivism and constructivism) and explore how these paradigms shape the ways in which clinical educators ask questions, how scholars in each of those paradigms think differently about the nature of their objects of study, and how such ways of thinking shape research design choices – from research protocols to tools used to gather and interpret data. We will highlight the differences between these two paradigms in the kind of data researchers gather, how they interpret such data, the role of theory, and the scope of conclusion they propose to the field. All these elements are the building blocks of research design.

To ground our foray into the intricacies of research design, we begin by defining the term *research design*. Then we present a case-study vignette from which we will illustrate how we think through research designs – one from an objective quantification orientation (post-positivism) and one from a subjective exploration orientation (constructivism). Research design comes with a set of terms, some of which may be unfamiliar. These terms are defined in Table 3.1, including references for those who wish to read further.

Starting Research in Clinical Education, First Edition. Edited by Eliot L. Rees, Alison Ledger, and Kim A. Walker.
© 2024 The Association for the Study of Medical Education (ASME). Published 2024 by John Wiley & Sons Ltd.
Companion website: www.wiley.com/go/clinicaleducation

Table 3.1 Table of definitions for research design

Paradigm	A specific way of formulating and justifying the things we know, the things we can know, and the ways in which we can get to know the world around us [5]
Ontology	The conceptualisation of the nature of reality. It asks: What is/exists? Is reality singular and stable or multiple and ever-changing? [5]
Post-positivist ontology	A post-positivist ontology assumes that reality is external to the individual, singular, identifiable, and often quantifiable, even if imperfectly [6]
Constructivist ontology	A constructivist ontology assumes that individuals experience the world differently and thus construct subjective meanings out of their personal experiences [7]
Epistemology	The conceptualisation of the nature of knowledge: how do we know what is/exists? How do we generate new knowledge? [5]
Post-positivist epistemology	Guided by the assumption that reality is singular, identifiable, and quantifiable, this epistemological stance aims to develop knowledge about 'reality' that is as accurate as possible. It recognises the imperfections in our current theories, tools, techniques, and of scientists themselves [6]
Constructivist epistemology	Guided by the assumption that reality is experienced differently by differently located individuals (based on class, race, gender, sexuality, social status, etc.), a constructivist epistemology sees reality as multiple and as negotiated by different people. Thus, reality is always in flux and context based [7]
Methodology	The systematic, coherent, justified, and explicitly stated theoretical, conceptual, and research procedures of the research design. These building blocks of research design must be aligned within their own paradigm and be internally consistent – from the research question posed, to data type selection, to gathering tools utilised, to data analysis procedures and reported limitations [5]
Methods	The specific techniques, procedures, protocols, and tools utilised for data collection and analysis

What is research design?

Research design is the underlying structure of a study that integrates all elements of a specific research project in a logical manner so that the study findings are considered to be credible [8]. The design creates a coherent structure linking a research problem or a phenomenon of interest, a specific question or set of questions, a justifiable methodological approach (methodology), and a plan for collecting and analysing data to build new knowledge (method) [9, 10]. The integration of these four elements is essential for the internal coherence of the study. When a research design makes these logical connections explicit, it serves two important functions: '(1) to provide answers to the research questions and (2) to provide a road map for conducting a study' [11]. A clearly reported research design helps others to evaluate the quality of findings in terms of originality of insights, and generalisability or transferability in the field. This is no small feat. Achieving coherence requires you to reflect on and answer several questions, including the following:

- What dimensions of a problem or phenomenon do you want to better understand?
- What kind of knowledge do you hope to produce with your research?
- What kind of methodology will enable you to generate this knowledge?
- What will inform your data collection and analysis?
- What markers of rigour will establish that you conducted high-quality research?

Researchers working to generate objective quantifications from a post-positivist paradigm will answer these questions very differently than those seeking to explore the experiences of individuals via a constructivist paradigm. In this chapter, we use the following case vignette (see Box 3.1) to illustrate key differences between these research paradigms, with reference to the five questions above. Through this case, we will demonstrate how researchers in different paradigms can investigate in the same research topic with different goals – objective quantification (post-positivist) or exploration and identification of subjective experiences (constructivist).

BOX 3.1   Case-study vignette

After years of planning, a large academic teaching hospital began the first stages of implementing a new electronic health record (EHR) in the wards. The transition to the new EHR has not been as smooth as expected by the leadership. The complaints are many and varied, suggesting that many hospital staff felt ill-prepared for the transition. For example, staff have written to complain about feeling undertrained, overwhelmed by the many steps that it takes to go through the functions of the platform, disconnected from their care team collaborators, and concerned about the impact of the new system on patient safety.

In addition, some have suggested that they have transformed from clinicians to data-entry personnel. The hospital's director of education calls you to her office to discuss these complaints. You learn that the hospital provided more than the recommended number of user training sessions suggested by the EHR developer of the platform (a highly ranked provider who has outfitted several larger hospitals with this EHR). In these sessions, the developer taught attendees how to use the platform and how to safeguard patients' safety. You also learn that, for 12 months prior to implementation, the hospital offered many opportunities for hospital staff to engage in the mandatory EHR training. Training was available via many modalities including: 4 hours of in-classroom training; 40 × 1 hour self-paced videos; unspecified numbers of tip-sheets; and at least one simulated patient case for each specialty. The director shares that she has had informal accounts of staff who engaged in extra non-compulsory training and have had fewer complaints about the transition. She asks you to design a research programme to understand:

1 The relationship between the amount of training completed and users' satisfaction with the EHR.

2 The relationship between modalities of training (i.e. classroom, video tutorials, simulation, case studies, etc.) and users' skills with the EHR.

3 How the EHR may be influencing care team collaborations.

4 How the EHR may be impacting patient safety.

The findings from this research will inform revisions to the training protocols to improve effective use of the EHR and to improve user satisfaction during the next phase of implementation of the EHR in the wards.

Post-positivist research design

What dimensions of the problem/phenomenon do you want to investigate?

In the case, the director has a clear set of objectives in mind: to revise training protocols to improve the effective use of the EHR and to improve user satisfaction during the next phase of implementation of the EHR in the wards. You can also see that the director has some hypotheses in mind. She suggests that there is a likely relationship between:

- The amount of time completed in training and users' satisfaction with the EHR.
- The modalities of training and the users' skills using the EHR.

These aspects of the problem can be clearly defined, measured, analysed, and interpreted to provide answers to specific hypotheses. These targets can be transformed into measurable dimensions reflecting the users' skills and experiences. These measures could include data within the EHRs themselves, surveys, training logs, and other quantitative data collection instruments. Given these considerations, you could answer the director's questions 1 and 2 using a post-positivist research design that engages quantification and hypothesis testing approaches to research. For example, you could focus on answering: Does the time spent by clinicians in EHR training relate to users' satisfaction with the EHR?

To begin to answer this research question, a quick review of the fundamentals of the post-positivist stance is important. Researchers working in this tradition engage in research from the understanding (i.e. belief, assumption) that there is a single reality that is experienced by all. In the post-positivist tradition, there is a 'truth' that we can identify and understand; often understood through measurement. However, post-positivists understand that they will never fully or perfectly understand the truth or our reality because our theories, tools for data collection, techniques for data analysis, and the scientists themselves are imperfect. But this acknowledgement of imperfection leaves an opportunity for improvement – as our theories, research tools, and techniques improve, so will our understanding of our external reality. Therefore, while any study you do can generate insights, these insights will be your best approximations of reality and are always open to falsification (i.e. being proven wrong) or refinement (i.e. improved through new findings). This is the *ontology* that a post-positivist researcher brings to the research design, and therefore, these beliefs, values, and assumptions are woven through that design.

A post-positivist ontology means you are looking to understand a component of the objective external reality: e.g. how the amount of time spent in EHR training relates to clinicians' overall satisfaction with the EHR. This means that you need to transform the concepts you are interested in to operationalised, and often quantified, targets. For example, if your hypothesis (drawn from previous research or observation) focuses on the amount of time in training, then you need to determine how time will be measured in the same way for all participants to allow for comparison (e.g. hours? number of modules completed?). You would also need to determine how satisfaction will be conceptualised (e.g. general satisfaction? self-perceived ease of searching/entering into the EHR? satisfaction in comparison to previous record keeping?), and how data will be collected, analysed, and interpreted to understand participant satisfaction. The director has hypothesised that user satisfaction increases proportionally with increasing time spent in training. You can also hypothesise that user satisfaction will vary with the time spent in different kinds of training (e.g. self-paced videos might generate more satisfaction than the in-classroom trainings) and by the specific characteristics of individual trainees (e.g. age, gender, qualifications/degrees, and years of experience in their current clinical setting). To address our vignette, you will not collect data on users' EHR-based *skills*; instead, the variables you will use are focused on user's characteristics, their perceived satisfaction, and how that relates to time in training. As these examples illustrate, you should strive to ensure that the variables you choose to include in your design are directly aligned with the hypothesis that your data will test.

What kind of knowledge do you hope to produce with your research?

Researchers working within a post-positivist *epistemology* recognise that research findings are likely to be imperfect, but they can contribute to the progression of knowledge. This means researchers rely on the work that has preceded their own investigations. For this reason, they are in a state of continually revising their assumptions and improving the collective understanding of reality. This slow, continued refinement of our understanding is achieved by refining or disconfirming current theories, hypotheses, or understandings of reality.

Guided by this set of assumptions about the knowledge we can produce, you may develop a research design that identifies the relationship between individuals' time spent in EHR training and their satisfaction with the EHR. You would acknowledge and accept that your findings are what you know for now – that is, they will hold until they are inevitably refined or overturned by new understandings. This means that the study findings do not 'prove' anything about reality (that is far too definitive). Instead, your findings will 'suggest', 'indicate', or 'likely support' a particular interpretation and acknowledge the possibility of other interpretations in light of new data.

What kind of methodology will enable you generate this knowledge?

The post-positivist methodology (see Table 3.1) is not a singular entity; post-positivism can lead you to choose from a range of approaches. What these methodologies have in common is a design that builds on existing knowledge, and that aims to

better describe our external reality. The focus is on using, testing, or refining *theory* (see Chapter 4) to explain observations, draw causal inferences, and better understand phenomena [12]. Furthermore, these methodologies can use different kinds of data: quantitative data, qualitative data, or combinations of these data. Post-positivism is not indicated by the kind of data that is used, but by the way that data is interpreted and understood. From a post-positivist stance, data can be used to describe a phenomenon, explain a relationship, predict future behaviour, or refute an assumption or theory. In clinical education research using post-positivist approaches, data can be collected in a variety of ways, including through assessments, surveys, experiments, or naturalistic observations, or from archives (e.g. databases or health record data). Qualitative data can be collected and interpreted from a post-positivist frame such as linguistic or content analysis [13].

Returning to the case, you could use a cross-sectional study design to assess the relationship between participants' time spent in EHR training and their satisfaction with the EHR. Your hypothesis could be derived from the theory of planned behaviour [14]. In this theory, the adoption of a new behaviour (in this case, the use of the EHR) is predicted by a person's intention to engage in that behaviour. This intention depends on several determinants, including an individual's *attitudes* (i.e. the level to which an individual favours a behaviour) and *perceived behaviour control* (i.e. an individual's perception of the difficulty or ease of performing a behaviour). This theory has been used to study clinicians' adoption of EHRs in other healthcare systems [15].

You could conceptualise user satisfaction as existing along a gradient and then use a Likert scale survey (see Chapter 20) to ask about participants' levels of satisfaction with several specific EHR-based clinical tasks (i.e. on a scale from 1 to 5, where 1 = not satisfied at all and 5 = extremely satisfied). For your data collection tools, you could choose to use a survey asking users how much time they spent in each kind of EHR training (i.e. classroom, video tutorials, simulation, case studies, etc.), presenting time as a series of discrete variables (e.g. 0–5; 6–10; 11–15 hours, etc.).

What will inform your data collection and analysis?

One of the core values of post-positivism is that knowledge is built slowly and incrementally; therefore, previous work must inform data collection and analysis. The strength of the literature review and the argument for how this study fits in the lineage of work that came before are important steps in the research process. The conceptual framework (i.e. the justification for why a study should be conducted) is vitally important in post-positivist research as there is an expectation you will build on, and contribute to, the existing body of knowledge [12, 16]. The literature review can help to refine a research question (see Chapter 2), identify the variables of interest and whether they have been quantified in the past, so that current work can explore relationships that have been underexplored, or underspecified, and even challenge existing theories in the field.

As explained above, the focus of post-positivist research is on theory testing, refinement, and clarification. That means that your work should have a clearly articulated theoretical framework, which outlines your chosen theory, how it will be used to better understand your phenomenon of interest, and how it will be operationalised within your study. Analysis and interpretation of findings are always grounded in the chosen theory. In this case, you could identify literature in the area of health informatics and technology adoption, and in the fields of education, business, and psychology through your chosen lens of the theory of planned behaviour.

The research questions you ask and the study design you develop to answer those questions will be shaped by your prior knowledge, your values, and your beliefs. If you hold post-positivist values (*axiology*), you will be keen to protect your research design from any potential biases and systematically control for them. You will endeavour to mitigate the influence of those biases but will openly report the limits of these efforts when disseminating your research. You will try to distance yourself from the research participants to minimise bias that could arise from pre-existing relationships (e.g. using survey tools for data collection rather than interviews), rely on standardised approaches to analysis, and use data collection tools that are as neutral as possible. You will also try to avoid influencing your participants. For instance, you may ask in your survey, 'How much time did you *spend* in classroom-based EHR training?' rather than, 'How much time did you *waste* in classroom-based EHR training?'. You will carefully consider language choices in your data collection tools, since value-laden questions might skew your findings. You will rely whenever possible on data that can be verified as accurate and collect evidence to support the interpretability of your findings.

What markers of rigour will establish that you conducted 'good' research?

Markers of rigour are the signs and signals that you look for to determine if the study has been done sufficiently well to be credible. There are several markers, which flow from the ontological, epistemological, and axiological roots of post-positivism. Post-positivism rests on the idea of an external reality that we can measure and understand, within the limits of our tools and abilities. This translates to markers of rigour such as documenting evidence of the accuracy of measurement (i.e. reliability, validity, and manipulation checks in experimental work). Also critical in post-positivism is the idea that any one project resides in a long lineage of work that has come before it, through relying on a well-established theory, deductively testing hypotheses, or situating a current project within the programme of work that preceded it. This translates into grounding the research design in previously published literature, establishing clear hypothesis development, description, and operationalisation and a detailed protocol that is open to critique and replication. These markers of rigour have been described as reproducibility (the ability to replicate a study if one wished) and generalisability (the assumption that similar findings could generalise from one context to another, so long as key variables are held constant). Examples of ways you could include these markers of rigour in the EHR case are offered in Table 3.2.

Constructivist research design

What dimensions of the problem/phenomenon do you want to investigate?

There are aspects of the case vignette that are either not readily amenable to quantitative measurement or where measurement gets us no closer to understanding the phenomena. The directors' last two areas of interest are not about measuring a cause-and-effect relationship. Instead, she is interested in the ways in which the new EHR shapes, in perhaps unexpected ways, the experiences and practices of care providers, including:

- How the EHR may be influencing care team collaborations.
- How the EHR may be impacting patient safety.

Certainly, it would be possible to quantify – via observations – the number of times members of a care team interact with each other before and after EHR implementations. However, such quantification may not get you closer to understanding the how or the unexpected ways the EHR has (or has not) impacted the content and quality of communication flows and their effects on collaboration, for example [17]. A research design that explores the subjective and unexpected experiences of users and that gathers rich detail about the work context may

Table 3.2 The markers of rigour in post-positivism in relation to specific values and illustrated with examples

Value	Markers of rigour	Examples
Objectivity	Accuracy of measurement, researcher at 'arm's length'	Evidence of reliability, validity, test–retest, multiple study cases, little reliance on self-report measures, efforts to reduce bias
Contextualisation	Situating the place of this study in a lineage or programme of work	Clear literature review, rationale for theory or methodological choices
Transparency	Others can examine, critique, and replicate work	Clear procedures and protocols, availability of materials and archived data
Reproducibility and generalisability	Findings will have meaning (sometimes predictive value) in other contexts	Multi-site studies, replication, and replicability, multiple measures
Humility	Researcher recognises limitations of current methods, tools, and interpretations	Justifications for methodological and analytic decisions, transparent limitations section

be more fruitful in understanding how different members of the care team have responded to the implementation of the EHR. To achieve these aims and objectives, you may pose the research question: 'What are clinicians' experiences of interprofessional team collaboration after the EHR implementation?'

To begin, a quick review of the fundamentals of the constructivist stance is required. Researchers working in the constructivist tradition hold very different assumptions than those working in post-positivist traditions [18, 19]. Within the constructivist paradigm, there is no single 'truth' to be discovered. Instead, researchers understand reality to be a product of individuals' engagement with other people, social groups, the physical world, and the common values, ideas, and discourses of their context [18]. The constructivist view of reality (i.e. *ontology*) posits that reality is an experience-driven phenomenon produced and negotiated by specific individuals, specific groups of individuals, and institutions within specific contexts (e.g. hospitals). Even though an external observer could identify patterns of human behaviour in response to an event or stimuli, every person's interpretation of such an event is potentially unique in its meaning and consequences. Individuals' unique histories and experiences shape their conceptualisation of what that experience 'is', and why specific parts of that experience matter. To be clear, researchers working within the constructivist paradigm focus on the social experiences of people as informed by the context in which they live. This is valuable in clinical education research because clinical education and practice are socially situated experiences.

Using a constructivist approach, you will be interested in understanding how specific individuals and groups of people in the hospital (e.g. doctors, nurses, physiotherapists, and pharmacists) perceive, experience, and engage with each other in their workplace via EHR technology. You will not begin your research with a hypothesis. Instead, you will build a study to enable participants to share their experiences of how the EHR impacts team collaboration, if at all. You will acknowledge that healthcare providers in different professions may face different types and degrees of challenges as users of the new EHR (i.e. it may require only one click for nurses to read doctors' notes, but it may require considerable navigational clicks for doctors to find the nurses' notes). Therefore, you will recruit participants from different professions who collaborate in interprofessional healthcare teams and sample broadly across other individual demographics (e.g. gender, level of digital fluency, race, and socio-economic status), level of seniority, and organisational considerations (e.g. hierarchies in the hospital, psychological safety of the workplace). Your objective is to design a study that enables a multi-faceted and meaningful understanding of the unique realities (including values, expectations, thoughts, emotions, and actions) of a diversity of study participants (both as individuals and as member of a particular professional group).

What kind of knowledge do you hope to produce with your research?

Researchers working within a constructivist epistemology begin with the premise that multiple realities are possible. This is the case because there are many individual-driven interpretations of experience. In the study you are developing, you will aim to capture a snapshot of the diversity of experiences of EHR users working in interprofessional healthcare teams. You will focus on communication disruptions and continuities and whether responsibilities unexpectedly shifted, changed, or intensified after the EHR implementation for different members of the interprofessional team. This is important because you need to consider that one EHR feature may streamline the data gathering for some healthcare workers but make the work of others more fragmented. In short, one person's perception of a 'solution' may be a 'problem' for someone else.

In constructivist research, you interact with participants to explore their realities. Therefore, your subjectivity is part of the knowledge created because you are in essence the data generation tool. The questions you ask, the prompts you use, the physical cues you give in the conversation: all of these features of data collection (and more) will involve you as co-generator of the data with the participant. What you know is always partial and evolving because an individual's experiences and interpretations of events change over time. The findings of the study will be bound to a specific time and place, though these findings may resonate with people's experiences in other contexts.

This does not mean that constructivist research is an 'anything goes' paradigm. It is, in fact, quite the opposite. Constructivist research requires you to be reflexive throughout the research process. Reflexivity is 'a set of continuous, collaborative, and multifaceted practices through which researchers self-consciously critique, appraise, and evaluate how their subjectivity and context influence the research processes' [20]. This reflexive stance and the acknowledgement and open disclosure of the subjective nature of experience of both researcher and the participants are important aspects of the axiology (i.e. values) of constructivist research. In relation to the case, you would ask questions such as

- How does my expertise and/or experience in clinical practice shape my questions and analysis?
- How does it shape my relationships with the study participants?
- How does my understanding of power differentials in interprofessional teams (e.g. doctors in relation to nurses) contribute to my understanding of responsibilities over tasks?
- How does my positive/negative view of new technologies shape my attitudes during data analysis?

What kind of methodology will enable you to generate this knowledge?
Constructivist research might set out to critique the limitations of phenomena studied in current scholarship, refine concepts, and/or develop new theories to explain different aspects of the human experience. Like in post-positivism, there are many possibilities when choosing a *methodology,* each connected to different disciplinary fields and histories (e.g. psychology, education, sociology, anthropology,

rhetoric, etc.). This methodological variety has important practical implications for research design. You must carefully consider the alignment of your research questions with your methodological choice, including the conceptual and methodological limitations of previous scholarship, how insights developed in different contexts (e.g. other disciplines or professions) will inform the study, and the need for new data collection methods to question common assumptions. For instance, if you have found theoretical or conceptual gaps in a particular field (e.g. training for new technologies in clinical education), you might set out to build a new theory in a specific context and so select a methodology that is designed to achieve that goal (e.g. constructivist grounded theory [21]). If you want to refine understanding of a concept that is a personally experienced phenomenon (e.g. shame, burnout), you might choose a methodology that was designed for that purpose (e.g. phenomenology [22]). Each of these choices must be informed by the existing body of research and your own research interests.

What will inform your data collection and analysis?
Constructivist research designs often include qualitative data collection and analysis methods. Common qualitative data collection methods in clinical education research include interviews and focus groups because these methods enable the researcher to gather rich context-based data of people's experiences and perceptions (see Chapter 14). Alternatively, the researcher could collect data via in situ observations, to identify and understand how people act, speak, and interact with one another under specific conditions and in a particular context. Another data collection method often used in constructivist research is the collection of readily available textual data, for example, emails, letters, meeting minutes, news reports, and patient records.

In the EHR study, you might draw from three different sources of data. First, you could gain ethical approval to access the emails and letters of complaints authored by clinical staff and sent to the hospital leadership and EHR implementation team. These texts could offer rich insights into how the clinical staff see potential risks to team collaboration arising from the new information flows post-EHR implementation. However, if the inclusion of emails is limited to complaints, we will be blind to the positive feedback that might be offered in other emails. It may be that positive experiences are common but those complimentary narratives are not being submitted to leadership. Therefore, for a more global view of how the EHR impacts team collaboration, you could interview a wide variety of EHR users. This second source of data could be collected from various interprofessional healthcare teams to understand their first-hand experiences of potential unintended consequences of the new technology. Finally, you could also use focus groups with clinical teams to allow them to collectively reflect on the impact of the EHR on their collaboration practices. Direct observations may not be feasible in this case because you may not be able to readily identify and observe moments when team collaborations occur in digital spaces.

Your original research question asked about clinicians' experiences of interprofessional team collaboration after the implementation of the EHR. The main aspects of this collaboration may be truly novel and context-specific; others may have been identified in other hospitals and professional fields [23]. When it comes to data analysis, you may keep theories and findings from existing other pre-existing literature in mind. You may choose to employ one of the family of thematic analysis approaches (see Chapter 18), teasing out matters of concern to the participants, while also considering existing theories and research in the field. In a constructivist study, using theory does not involve testing theory like in post-positivist research. Rather, you may be using a particular theory as a lens to help conceptualise or interpret different elements in the study data.

To reiterate messages from the earlier section on constructivist epistemology, the goal of analysis is to actively interpret meaning from the data collected. You are not aiming to find the correct interpretation, but to develop your own interpretation, shaped by your background, relationships and experiences, and the specific research context.

What markers of rigour will establish that you conducted 'good' research?

Since constructivism rests on the premise that reality is multiple and is understood through individuals' experiences of reality, constructivist research design must demonstrate that you attempted to capture a diversity of experiences from within the population of interest in the study (e.g. in our vignette-based study, we are interested in clinicians' experiences so we will seek participation from a diversity of clinical professions; however, we will not seek data from EHR implementors or vendors because they are outside of our population of interest). Therefore, in the study's dissemination manuscripts, you will aim to provide detailed information about the research process to ensure the transparency, authenticity, and sufficiency of the methodology selected; provide details on the application of data collection methods; and present an analysis that is coherent in relation to pertinent theories. Guidelines for reporting on research using quali-

Table 3.3 The markers of rigour in constructivism

Value	Markers of rigour
Reflexivity	The researcher carefully and consciously reflects and describes how their own subjectivity shaped the research design and resulting analysis
Authenticity	The researcher is genuine in explaining their position and including the voices of participants
Transferability	The research context and participant populations are described in sufficient detail, to allow others to determine whether the study is relevant to their contexts and populations
Credibility	The data collection and analysis process are explained in detail and demonstrate that the data interpretations are reasonable and supported by previous literature/theory

tative methodologies are available [23, 24]. However, it is important that learners understand that constructivist research does not rely on formulas or checklists to confirm the soundness of a given research design. Instead, rigour in this tradition is linked back to the ontological, epistemological, and methodological aspects of the study design (see Table 3.3).

Summary

In this chapter, we introduced two common and fundamentally different ways of thinking through research design in clinical education research. We have described the central differences between post-positivist and constructivist paradigms in terms of their assumptions of the nature of reality (i.e. *ontology*), the types of knowledge that they produce (i.e. *epistemology*), how they shape the processes and mechanism to produce new and meaningful knowledge (i.e. *methodology*), and the values and the role of research and the researcher (i.e. *axiology*).

Research design can be a very creative act, but this creativity must be grounded in solid foundations. These foundations include knowing how and why you are approaching a research problem in a certain way. To do so, you must ensure explicit alignment between the study's ontology, epistemology, axiology and interpretive framework (i.e. theories and concepts). This alignment ensures that the results and conclusions of your study can, on the one hand, advance the common areas of interest in the field, and on the other, open new venues for interrogating taken-for-granted ideas and practices in clinical education. For your findings to be seen as trustworthy and credible by your peers, build your study on solid foundations and be sure to refer to the markers of rigour relevant to your stated research paradigm.

Top tips

- Consider the nature of the research problem and question. Are you looking to measure or test a theory or hypothesis (post-positivism)? Or are you interested in subjective or unexpected experiences or developing a rich understanding of an education context (constructivism)?
- Review the ways your topic has been studied before. What theoretical assumptions have been made and what types of data have been explored?
- Aim for alignment of the components of the research design: question, data type, data collection, and analysis methods.
- Explain your research paradigm and methods in detail, so that your study can be judged according to appropriate markers of rigour.

Common pitfalls

- Rushing to decide on methods without considering an appropriate research paradigm. Your study will have stronger foundations if you take the time to align your ontology, epistemology, methodology, and methods.
- Applying familiar markers of rigour, rather than those that are appropriate for your chosen research paradigm. Be sure to design your study with reference to appropriate markers of rigour.
- Using terminology that you do not fully understand. Recognise that it takes time to grasp these concepts and revisit as needed.

Ethical issues

- Reflect on the ways you may influence the choice of research questions and methods, the data you produce, and the interpretations you present.
- In post-positivist research, aim to mitigate your influence and report any potential biases.
- In constructivist research, aim to be genuine and transparent in explaining your subjectivity, your methods, and how you reached your interpretations.

References

1 Schuwirth, L.W. and van der Vleuten, C.P. (2020). A history of assessment in medical education. *Advances in Health Sciences Education* 25 (5): 1045–1056.

2 Bolster, L. and Rourke, L. (2015). The effect of restricting residents' duty hours on patient safety, resident well-being, and resident education: an updated systematic review. *Journal of Graduate Medical Education* 7 (3): 349–363.

3 Paradis, E. and Whitehead, C.R. (2015). Louder than words: power and conflict in interprofessional education articles, 1954–2013. *Medical Education* 49 (4): 399–407.

4 Bynum, W.E. 4th, Artino, A.R. Jr., Uijtdehaage, S. et al. (2019). Sentinel emotional events: the nature, triggers, and effects of shame experiences in medical residents. *Academic Medicine* 94 (1): 85–93.

5 Varpio, L. and MacLeod, A. (2020). Philosophy of science series: harnessing the multidisciplinary edge effect by exploring paradigms, ontologies, epistemologies, axiologies, and methodologies. *Academic Medicine* 95 (5): 686–689.

6 Young, M.E. and Ryan, A. (2020). Postpositivism in health professions education scholarship. *Academic Medicine* 95 (5): 695–699.

7 Mann, K. and MacLeod, A. (2015). Constructivism: learning theories and approaches to research. In: *Researching Medical Education* (ed. J. Cleland and S.J. Durning), 49–66. Wiley Blackwell.

8 Dannels, S.A. (2010). Research design. In: *The Reviewer's Guide to Quantitative Methods in the Social Sciences*, 1e (ed. G.R. Hancock and R.O. Mueller), 343–355. New York, NY: Routledge.

9 Creswell, J.W. and Poth, C.N. (2016). *Qualitative Inquiry and Research Design: Choosing Among Five Approaches.* SAGE Publications.

10 Ringsted, C., Hodges, B., and Scherpbier, A. (2011). 'The research compass': an introduction to research in medical education: AMEE guide no. 56. *Medical Teacher* 33 (9): 695–709.

11 McGaghie, W.C., Bordage, G., Crandall, S., and Pangaro, L.N. (2015). Chapter 9: Research design. In: *Review Criteria for Research Manuscripts*, 2e (ed. S.J. Durning and J.D. Carline), 74–83. Washington, DC: Association of American Medical Colleges.

12 Varpio, L., Paradis, E., Uijtdehaage, S., and Young, M. (2020). The distinctions between theory, theoretical framework, and conceptual framework. *Academic Medicine* 95 (7): 989–994.

13 Denecke, K. and Deng, Y. (2015). Sentiment analysis in medical settings: new opportunities and challenges. *Artificial Intelligence in Medicine* 64 (1): 17–27.

14 Ajzen, I. (1991). The theory of planned behavior. *Organisational Behavior and Human Decision Processes* 50 (2): 179–211.

15 Hossain, A., Quaresma, R., and Rahman, H. (2019). Investigating factors influencing the physicians' adoption of electronic health record (EHR) in healthcare system of Bangladesh: an empirical study. *International Journal of Information Management* 44: 76–87.

16 Bordage, G. (2009). Conceptual frameworks to illuminate and magnify. *Medical Education* 43 (4): 312–319.

17 Alpert, J.M., Markham, M.J., Bjarnadottir, R.I., and Bylund, C.L. (2021). Twenty-first century bedside manner: exploring patient-centered communication in secure messaging with cancer patients. *Journal of Cancer Education* 36 (1): 16–24.

18 Creswell, J.W. (2003). *Research Design: Qualitative, Quantitative, and Mixed Methods Approaches*, 2e. Thousand Oaks, CA: SAGE Publications.

19 Mertens, D.M. (2005). *Research Methods in Education and Psychology: Integrating Diversity with Quantitative and Qualitative Approaches*, 2e. Thousand Oaks, CA: SAGE Publications.

20 Olmos-Vega, F.M., Stalmeijer, R.E., Varpio, L., and Kahlke, R. (2022). A practical guide to reflexivity in qualitative research: AMEE guide no. 149. *Medical Teacher* 45: 241–251.

21 Watling, C.J. and Lingard, L. (2012). Grounded theory in medical education research: AMEE guide no. 70. *Medical Teacher* 34 (10): 850–861.

22 Neubauer, B.E., Witkop, C.T., and Varpio, L. (2019). How phenomenology can help us learn from the experiences of others. *Perspectives on Medical Education* 8 (2): 90–97.

23 Barr, N., Vania, D., Randall, G., and Mulvale, G. (2017). Impact of information and communication technology on interprofessional collaboration for chronic disease management: a systematic review. *Journal of Health Services Research & Policy* 22 (4): 250–257.

24 O'Brien, B.C., Harris, I.B., Beckman, T.J. et al. (2014). Standards for reporting qualitative research: a synthesis of recommendations. *Academic Medicine* 89 (9): 1245–1251.

4 Using educational theory in research and scholarship

Clare Morris and Nick Schindler

Learning objectives

By the end of this chapter, you should be able to:
- Consider the different levels at which theory can operate within your writing.
- Identify the different ways in which theory can be deployed in clinical education research and scholarship.

- Articulate the ways your views on learning shape and inform your practice as an educator and researcher.
- Decide how to use theory in your research and scholarly activity.
- Choose appropriate theories to suit your views on learning.

Introduction

In this chapter, we explore the ways in which you can put theory to use in your clinical education research projects, with a particular emphasis on learning theory. The views you hold about learning will influence the ways you approach your work as an educator and clinical educational researcher [1]. Being able to articulate those views, making them explicit to yourself and to others, allows you to position your research within the contemporary literature and make informed choices about your research design.

We start with an outline of what we mean when we say theory and the levels at which it can operate in educational research. We have chosen to focus on learning theory, showing how you can relate your views of learning to those in the learning literatures. We do this by identifying the ideal-typical features of three educational schools of thought. We then move on to illustrate how you can use learning theories as theoretical, conceptual, and analytic tools to shape the design and implementation of your clinical education research project.

Putting theory to work in clinical education research

The thrill of discovering and using new research approaches can lead you to rush into the field, giving only passing consideration to what lies beneath the research design choices you have made. However, it is vital to get to the heart of our belief systems about the nature of truth and knowledge. These beliefs shape the ways we approach our research, knowingly or otherwise. Making your beliefs visible is part of the artistry of high-quality research. In Chapter 3, ontology, epistemology, methodology, and methods were introduced as the building blocks of research design. Crotty included a further element to research design, articulating your theoretical perspective (a well-developed theoretical position that helps make sense of the issues being researched) [2].

A well-designed research project achieves alignment between methodology, method, theoretical perspective, ontology, and epistemology. In much the same way as we seek constructive alignment in educational design (between teaching, learning outcomes, and assessment methods), we seek alignment in our research design. However, our field has been criticised for being under-theorised or for a tendency to evoke theory rather than use it in meaningful ways [3–5]. Taking time to stop, think, and articulate your theoretical perspective is part of the rigour of educational research. Indeed, no study is theory-free, as we all hold views of the world that will influence the ways we set out to make sense of it [6].

What is theory?

Theory is classically described as a logically related 'system of ideas' [4] or 'set of propositions' [7] that are brought together to explain a phenomenon.

Starting Research in Clinical Education, First Edition. Edited by Eliot L. Rees, Alison Ledger, and Kim A. Walker.
© 2024 The Association for the Study of Medical Education (ASME). Published 2024 by John Wiley & Sons Ltd.
Companion website: www.wiley.com/go/clinicaleducation

Theories have the potential to help explain how or why something functions in the way it does and can operate at different levels, with different degrees of explanatory power.

Grand theories have the highest level of abstraction and account for issues such as social structures and relations. These theories can offer ways into thinking and talking about complex issues such as power relations (e.g. Foucauldian theory), gender inequality (Feminist theory), or class and social relations (Marxist theory). Middle-range theories are more modest in scale and will typically draw on empirical research and focus on human interactions, e.g. Cultural Historical Activity Theory (CHAT), Actor Network Theory, or socio-cultural theory. Micro theories allow a focus at the individual level, e.g. symbolic interactionism or behaviourism [7].

Working with theory means making your assumptions explicit. One way to do this is by creating a theoretical framework for your study, where you identify and define the theories that underpin your work and explain how you are putting them to use in designing your study or developing your data collection tools [7]. In this way, theoretical perspectives are operationalised. We illustrate this later in the chapter, showing how learning theory can be put to use in research.

A review of the ways clinical education researchers work with theory suggests three key approaches [4]:

- Engaging in *close-up exploration,* drawing on theory explicitly in the design stages to explain a particular phenomenon.
- Offering *a specific perspective* on an aspect of medical education by explicitly building upon a deliberately chosen theoretical position.
- Adopting *a distanced perspective* where scholars draw upon what is already known in the field, through systematic or literature reviews and where theoretical perspectives function as a backdrop to what has gone before (see explanation of post-positivism in Chapter 3).

Decisions about the way (or ways) in which you will work with theory may therefore differ across studies or points in the research process and merit discussion with supervisors or co-researchers before commencing. Getting started in clinical education research is as much about engaging with new ways of looking at the world as it is about using new research approaches.

Working with learning theory

Your choice of theory (or theories) is important, as each has the potential to 'illuminate and magnify'

aspects of educational practice, whilst potentially leaving others in the dark [3]. Let us imagine you are designing a project focussed on how healthcare students learn in clinical environments. You are going to work purposefully with theory, in this case, middle to micro-range learning theory. You have not yet decided on your theoretical framework and want to try out options. There are, however, many ways in which you might seek to categorise or classify theories of learning and this is going to matter when it comes to laying out your theoretical framework.

One way might be to organise them according to their disciplinary origins. Hager [8], for example, looks at the influence of psychology and sociology on (work based) learning theory. He argues that psychological theories of learning, such as behaviourism and constructivism, have dominated the field, illuminating and magnifying the ways *individuals* act and think (with an emphasis on skill and knowledge acquisition). These theories would be helpful if, for example, the focus of your study was on how students draw upon schema and scripts when developing their clinical reasoning skills. Hager notes the limits of psychological theories of learning, particularly how they leave 'the significant role of social, cultural and organisational factors' in the dark [8]. Sociological and anthropological influences on learning are useful here, which underpin socio-cultural theories of learning such as Lave and Wenger's work on communities of practice [9]. So, if your interest was in how students develop their professional identity through placement experiences, you might turn to their work. The focus of your study will therefore give you clues to the theoretical perspective(s) you might draw upon, with the disciplinary origin of learning theories giving you clues to the kinds of issues they best support.

Another approach to categorisation is offered by Sfard, who invites us to 'bring to the open the tacit assumptions and beliefs that guide us' in our work as educators [1]. Sfard argues that these beliefs can be captured in two contrasting metaphors for learning, distinguished in part by the intended end point or goal of learning. If your guiding metaphor is *learning-as-acquisition*, you see the goal of learning as the attainment of something – knowledge, skills, appropriate professional attitudes (akin to psychological theories of learning, such as behaviourism, and cognitivism). If your guiding metaphor is *learning-as-participation*, you will see the goal of learning being full participation in a community (of practice), where learning is located in shared practice (drawing explicitly upon socio-cultural theory). Each metaphor sheds light on different elements or aspects of learning. In learning-as-acquisition, what is to be learned can be defined in advance, broken down into manageable units such as outcomes, or competencies. This would be helpful on a study exploring the best ways to teach healthcare students core clinical skills, for example. In learning-as-participation, learning is understood as the practices that allow 'newcomers' to become central to the work of the community over time (akin to apprenticeship). This would be helpful in a study of professional identity development.

A third approach to classification allows organisation across three educational schools of thought – cognitive-behavioural, socio-cultural, and cultural-historical. The cultural-historical category expands our views on learning, inviting consideration of the purposeful ways in which organisational culture and practice can be transformed, or expanded [10]. Such transformations are vital when circumstances change, and it is no longer possible to do things in the ways we have before. If your planned study was interested in what happened to clinical placements during the COVID-19 pandemic, for example, you might turn to CHAT.

Table 4.1 distils some of the distinctions between these schools of thought (and associated metaphors for learning) expressed as ideal-typical features. Each column might therefore be argued to offer up a theoretical framework, setting out the assumptions that underpin your approach.

In the next section, we illustrate, using case studies, the ways in which these different standpoints invite different approaches in the design and implementation of a research project.

Illustrative case studies

Context

Three new education researchers are interested in the teaching and assessment of communication skills in undergraduate clinical education. They are each in the process of designing their research projects for a master's in clinical education. They have identified the first three steps as being: the identification of their over-arching research question, defining the unit of analysis of their study, and from this, to make coherent methodological choices around approaches to data collection and analysis. Here, we aim to walk through each of our fictional researchers, and illustrate how, using their theoretical stance and assumptions about learning, they might approach this task.

Their supervisor has encouraged them to position themselves within the research, in other words, to make visible the factors that have shaped and informed their approach to the work. This typically includes an account of the theoretical perspective(s) you draw upon and may extend into your epistemological beliefs.

Positionality can be defined as 'an individual's world view and the position they adopt about a research task and its social and political context' [12]. Each of our researchers will approach their work drawing on a range of prior experiences, beliefs, and values. Borrowing from Bordage [3], positionality can be seen as the lens of your mind's eye. You can take on and off a variety of theoretical lenses as required, whilst your positionality or worldview remains a filter through which you experience everything. Researchers coming from

Table 4.1 Ideal-typical features of three educational schools of thought

School of thought (theoretical framework)	Cognitive-behavioural	Socio-cultural	Cultural-historical
Guiding metaphor	Learning-as-acquisition	Learning-as-participation	Learning-as-expansion
Goal of learning	Acquisition of knowledge, skills, etc.	Full participation in a shared practice	Transformation of practice (expansive learning)
Focus (who learns)	Individuals	Newcomers within a community of practice	Activity systems (organisations and collectives of people)
Emphasis	Accumulation (of knowledge, skills, attitudes)	Meaningful participation, *belonging* (to a community of practice), *becoming* (identity formation)	Analysis of existing practices and collective visioning of new practices
Relationship between learning and context	Transfer of learning to different contexts possible	Learning is context specific and situated	Expansive learning in response to the tensions and contradictions arising in practice/context

Source: Adapted from Morris [11].

different positions, for example, a medical student learning a skill compared to a researcher teaching that skill, may have different viewpoints based on their experiences. This is illustrated in more detail in the case study. There may be near infinite factors which inform your positionality, not least age, gender, ethnicity, and previous life experiences (including what you think of as, for example, 'good education' or 'good care'). As we introduce our three researchers, you might consider the factors that influence the ways they think about the issues at hand.

By making your own position explicit, you can recognise the strength of your lens, and where its blind spots might be. You can also signpost these considerations to others, who may interpret your work in a different light based on their own worldview and in doing so reveal contrasting and yet equally useful insights. Bradbury-Jones refers to early articulation of positionality as level five in their typology of theoretical visibility, 'where theory guides and directs the various phases of the research process' [13].

In the cases that follow, we focus on each of our fictional researchers' engagement with learning theory in the design stages. For the purposes of illustration, we have afforded each fictional researcher a worldview, aligned with the three educational schools of thought articulated in Table 4.1. In reality, your starting positions are likely to be less clear cut and will involve time spent thinking and discussing these issues with supervisors and fellow researchers. You may find it helpful to read clinical education research studies with a view to 'spotting' the theories they are working with, whether implied or clearly articulated.

Abdul
Positionality
Abdul is doing an intercalated degree course in clinical education. His medical school has a traditional pre-clinical/clinical divide, one that emphasises the application of theory to practice. Through studying clinical education, he recognises this approach is informed by cognitive-behavioural thinking, and this helps him make sense of how he is preparing to be a doctor. A central belief he holds is that individuals who study hard are able to acquire knowledge, which can then be applied to future examinations, clinical placements, and professional practice. Despite this, he has struggled to put the techniques taught in the medical school to effective use in clinical settings. Talking with his peers, he recognises that he is not alone in this struggle and does not feel that the Objective Structured Clinical Examinations (OSCEs) used to assess his skills reflect the realities of how they are used in practice.

Research question
At this point in the planning, Abdul has two possible studies in mind. One deals with the struggle of transferring taught skills into practice, the second is around their successful use in OSCEs. He, therefore, has two research questions in mind: The first is 'How well does communication skills teaching prepare medical students for clinical practice?' and the second is 'How does engagement in a communication skills course affect performance in OSCEs?' These questions arise because the assumption in behavioural and cognitive theory is that once the knowledge, skill, or attribute belongs to the learner, they can transfer it to other settings or contexts. This therefore means that what they learn during their course can be taken into practice and can be validly assessed in another context, such as an OSCE or in clinical practice, and the outcome can be related specifically to the course and how it is taught.

Identifying the unit of analysis
Once a research question has been established, or if you are having trouble refining a specific question, it is helpful to think about the object of the study (*unit of analysis*). This is the 'who' or 'what' in your research study and this too can be informed by the theories of learning you draw upon. Saljo explains:

> . . .every phenomenon lends itself to many conceptualizations. For instance, if one studies the traffic flow in urban areas, one attends to vehicles as parts of that system; how many they are, how much space they occupy, how fast they travel during peak traffic hours, and so on. There is no need for that particular inquiry to analyse the functionality of the electronic ignition system or the details of the tyres. The interesting unit is the vehicle as a functional element of a traffic system. [14]

For Abdul, the natural focal point for his research is that of the individual learner. This aligns well with the cognitive-behavioural theories he is drawn to and leads to his focus on how learners take the skills they have developed in theory (in a simulated environment) into the clinical workplace and how they perform on assessment of those skills.

Methodological choices
The next step is to design a study that flows from these starting points. There are many factors that shape your design choices, including their fitness for purpose and the available resources (pragmatism). However, as noted earlier, the aim is to seek a

degree of alignment, or coherence, between onto-logical and epistemological beliefs, theoretical per-spectives, methodology, and methods.

Abdul returns to his two possible research ques-tions and begins to test out ways he might seek answers to them. He has established his primary interest is in the individual, the skills they acquire and how they apply them, whether in practice or during an OSCE. This leads him to consider the fac-tors that might influence performance, not least the approaches used during the skills course. Each question leads him to different methodological approaches. His question 'How well does the teach-ing prepare medical students for clinical practice?' leads him to think about all the discussions he has had with his peers and the wide range of views expressed. This suggests a qualitative study, per-haps using interview methods and thematic analy-sis, where he can identify the factors that seem to influence a students' sense of preparedness.

The second question 'How does engaging with the course effect performance in OSCEs?' leads him to think about cause and effect, and a post-positivist framing for his work. The communication course is a relatively recent curriculum innovation, and he believes there will be data about student perfor-mance on OSCEs before and after its introduction. This possibility leans towards a quantitative study, involving statistical analysis of data.

These are two quite different methodological approaches that are possible to align to the same theoretical underpinning and focus. Establishing which route to choose early enables the researcher to focus their own skills and knowledge to best wield their chosen tools and explore their chosen line of enquiry.

Becky
Positionality
Becky trained as a speech and language therapist, before moving into clinical education and teaching on the communication skills course she now wishes to research. Working in a medical school, she feels like an outsider, not least as she received no formal training in communication skills herself. She recog-nises she developed and honed her own communi-cation skills initially on clinical placements, where she modelled her practice on that of her seniors, looking out for cues on how she was doing from patients, carers, and professionals around her. During her clinical education studies, she came across Lave and Wenger's [9] work on Communities of Practice and their ideas about learning as a social practice, the result of meaningful participation in those communities.

Research question
Becky has been strongly influenced by socio-cultural theories of learning and finds herself asking ques-tions about the ways in which medical students learn how to put their newfound communication skills to use in the clinical environment. Her socio-cultural stance leads her to question the assumption of transfer, recognising that learning is influenced by the contexts in which it is acquired and put to use. Her initial research questions seek to get to the heart of this issue, 'What factors influence the abil-ity of learners to put their learning to use in clinical environments?' or 'In what ways does participation in training shape the development of professional identity in medical students?'

Unit of analysis
Becky has come to see learning as something that arises from participation in communities of prac-tice, whether those involved in teaching (academic staff, simulated patients, and peers) or in practice settings (clinicians, patients, and families). Her interest in the experiences of learners is in relation to others around them (their participation). So, whilst the individual is still involved, they are no longer the primary unit of analysis. Like the engine in Säljö's car, individuals become an integral part of the phenomena, but not the specific focus for this particular study. Becky's focus is on how students can be supported to transfer their learning from one setting to another (see, for example, Brown [15]) or how they can make learning more authentic (see, for example, Kneebone et al. [16]).

Methodological choices
Becky's interest in socio-cultural theory comes from Lave and Wenger's work reimagining apprentice-ship, which they did by analysing ethnographic accounts of learning outside formal educational set-tings [9]. Becky wonders if she might be able to undertake an observational study to answer her question 'What factors influence the ability of learn-ers to put their communication skills to use in clini-cal environments?' She thinks about the possibility of nonparticipant observation, following students on their placements. She recognises that there are some practical barriers to this approach, and ethical ones too. She is, after all, in a power relationship with her learners and would not normally be in the clinical environment with them. This illustrates her reflexivity as a researcher (see Box 4.1).

Becky may alternatively decide she needs to cap-ture the views of the entire community of practice, seeking to interview students, communication skills faculty (including simulated patients), and clinical

BOX 4.1   Relationship between positionality and reflexivity

Positionality and reflexivity are interdependent and yet distinct [17]. If positionality is the world view of a researcher grounded in a specific socio-cultural context, then reflexivity is the ability of the researcher (or team) to reflect on their position within the research process, not least how their views on learning illuminate certain aspects whilst casting a shadow on others. Reflexivity involves a purposeful consideration of the impact of the researcher on the researched and vice versa. An understanding of theory can aid reflexivity, in providing the language to describe and interrogate your own, and others' views of learning.

teachers who support placements. This approach would work well as a response to the second possible research question 'In what ways does participation in the training influence the professional identity of learners in the workplace?' As Becky is explicitly drawing on socio-cultural theory, she might use some of the key ideas from this theory as sensitizing concepts [18] in her chosen approach to thematic analysis (see Chapter 18).

Christy
Positionality
Christy is a clinician educator, who leads the communication skills programme. They are curious to make sense of an apparent disjuncture between the ways students learn communication skills in the university and what they see happening in practice. They are questioning whether students are able to 'transfer' learning from their communication teaching sessions into the clinical workplace. They feel comfortable in challenging their assumptions of learning and are seeking to broaden their own horizons of theoretical understanding and are therefore interested in activity theory as it sees learning as happening within and across systems.

Research question
Christy has been reading about activity theory and the idea that learning happens within and between activity systems (such as the medical school and the clinical workplace). They have heard students talk about the ways they 'perform' communication skills in OSCEs and how this is different to how things are 'done' in practice. They might therefore ask 'How do students reconcile the differences between the ways they are taught communication skills and

what they see in practice?' or 'What do students learn about communication skills in practice and how might this shape the development of communication skills teaching in future?'

Unit of Analysis
In CHAT, the basic unit of analysis is defined as at least two interacting activity systems [10]. Christy can only make sense of the teaching and assessment of communication skills in the medical school with explicit reference to the practice of communication skills in clinical settings. Their research is likely to trace learners moving between settings and seek to make explicit the differences (tensions or contradictions) evident in and between these two settings (see, for example, Ajjawi et al. [19]).

Methodological choices and data analysis
CHAT is associated with an interventionist research methodology called The Change Laboratory [20]. The first steps in this approach involve an analysis of what is currently happening in practice, identifying contradictions or tensions existing within or between activity systems. Whilst Christy does not have the time, resources, or permissions to conduct a full Change Laboratory, they feel the analysis stages would help shed light on what is happening on the course, particularly how students are taking their learning from one setting to another. This fits both research questions, i.e. 'How do students reconcile the differences between the ways they are taught communication skills and what they see in practice?' and 'What do students learn about communication skills in practice and how might this shape the development of communication skills teaching in future?' Their analysis of the two interacting activity systems is informed by discussion with key people involved in the teaching, learning, and assessment of communication skills, including students, university-based educators, simulated patients, clinical placement supervisors, and others who interact with students in clinical environments (see, for example, Reid et al. [21]).

Summary

The views we hold of learning underpin every aspect of how we conceptualise, design, and implement clinical education research. Making these views explicit allows us to link them to learning theory, identify routes of enquiry, and select complementary methodological and analytic tools to inform our understanding and generation of new knowledge.

Understanding learning theory gives us better access to and appreciation of the toolbox of scholarly lenses, enabling us to see reality in different lights. We can select those which suit us best, those which are pragmatic and available to us, or those which deliberately subvert our assumptions and seek to make strange the everyday, in order to create new meaning.

Regardless of how we choose to use theory in our work, ensuring its inclusion from the outset enables us to justify our decisions to ourselves and others, viewing them in the light and enabling robust and thorough academic scrutiny.

Top tips

- Consider writing a position statement that makes visible the things you bring to your work as a researcher, including your views on learning.
- Seek alignment between the views you hold about the nature of knowledge (epistemology), your view on learning (theoretical perspectives), methodology (design choices), and methods (techniques used).
- Capture any changes in thinking throughout your study in your research diary. This will help you in articulating your reflexivity.
- Discuss your theoretical perspectives with your supervisor and peers and any collaborators.

Common pitfalls

- Rushing to start your research without first contemplating how you understand learning. Make time to think before you act.
- Choosing methodologies or methods that are at odds with your stated theoretical perspective. Strive to achieve alignment.

Ethical issues

- Always be mindful of the ethical issues arising from your theoretical, methodological, and methods choices.
- Reflect on any possible power relationships, for example, when observing your own learners as a researcher.

References

1 Sfard, A. (1998). On two metaphors for learning and the dangers of choosing just one. *Educational Research* 27 (2): 4–13.

2 Crotty, M. (1998). *The Foundations of Social Research. Meaning and Perspective in the Research Process*. London: SAGE Publications.

3 Bordage, G. (2009). Conceptual frameworks to illuminate and magnify. *Medical Education* 43 (4): 312–319.

4 Bolander Laksov, K., Dornan, T., and Teunissen, P.W. (2017). Making theory explicit – an analysis of how medical education research(ers) describe how they connect to theory. *BMC Medical Education* 17 (1): 18.

5 Teunissen, P.W. (2010). On the transfer of theory to the practice of research and education. *Medical Education* 44 (6): 534–535.

6 Rees, C.E. and Monrouxe, L.V. (2010). Theory in medical education research: how do we get there? Commentaries. *Medical Education* 44 (4): 334–339.

7 Varpio, L., Paradis, E., Uijtdehaage, S., and Young, M. (2020). The distinctions between theory, theoretical framework, and conceptual framework. *Academic Medicine* 95 (7): 989–994.

8 Hager, P. (2011). Theories of workplace learning. In: *The SAGE Handbook of Workplace Learning* (ed. M. Malloch, L. Cairns, K. Evans, and B.N. O'Connor), 17–31. London: SAGE Publications.

9 Lave, J. and Wenger, E. (1991). *Situated Learning: Legitimate Peripheral Participation*. Cambridge University Press.

10 Engeström, Y. (2011). Activity theory and learning at work. In: *The SAGE Handbook of Workplace Learning* (ed. M. Malloch, L. Cairns, K. Evans, and B.N. O'Connor), 86–104. London: SAGE Publications.

11 Morris, C. (2012). From time-served apprenticeship to time-measured training: new challenges for postgraduate medical education. Doctoral thesis. University of London. https://discovery.ucl.ac.uk/id/eprint/10020681.

12 Darwin Holmes, A.G. (2020). Researcher positionality – a consideration of its influence and place in qualitative research – a new researcher guide. *Shanlax International Journal of Education* 8 (4): 1–10.

13 Bradbury-Jones, C., Taylor, J., and Herber, O. (2014). How theory is used and articulated in qualitative research: development of a new typology. *Social Science & Medicine* 120: 135–141.

14 Säljö, R. (2009). Learning, theories of learning, and units of analysis in research. *Educational Psychologist* 44 (3): 202–208.

15 Brown, J. (2010). Transferring clinical communication skills from the classroom to the clinical environment: perceptions of a group of medical students in the United Kingdom. *Academic Medicine* 85 (6): 1052–1059.

16 Kneebone, R.L., Kidd, J., Nestel, D. et al. (2005). Blurring the boundaries: scenario-based simulation in a clinical setting. *Medical Education* 39 (6): 580–587.

17 Corlett, S. and Mavin, S. (2018). Reflexivity and researcher positionality. In: *SAGE Handbook of Qualitative Business and Management Research Methods: History and Traditions* (ed. C. Cassell, A.L. Cunliffe, and G. Grandy), 377–398.

18 Charmaz, K., Denzin, NK., and Lincoln, YS. (2000). Grounded theory: objectivist and constructivist methods. In: *Handbook of Qualitative Research*, 2e, 509–536. SAGE Publications.

19 Ajjawi, R., Rees, C., and Monrouxe, L.V. (2015). Learning clinical skills during bedside teaching encounters in general practice: a video-observational study with insights from activity theory. *Journal of Workplace Learning* 27 (4): 298–314.

20 Morris, C., Reid, A.M., Ledger, A., and Teodorczuk, A. (2021). Expansive learning in medical education: putting change laboratory to work. *Medical Teacher* 43 (1): 38–43.

21 Reid, A.M., Ledger, A., Kilminster, S., and Fuller, R. (2015). Can the tools of activity theory help us in advancing understanding and organisational change in undergraduate medical education? *Advances in Health Sciences Education* 20 (3): 655–668.

5 Involving stakeholders

Katherine A. Moreau, Catherine M. Giroux, and Kaylee Eady

Learning objectives

By the end of this chapter, you should be able to:
- Define stakeholder involvement in clinical education research.
- Explain why stakeholders should be involved.
- Identify the types of stakeholders who may be involved.
- Implement strategies for involving stakeholders.

Introduction

There are many reasons to actively involve stakeholders in clinical education research. Numerous terms describe the phenomenon of involving lay people in research, including patient and public involvement (PPI), patient engagement, participatory research, and integrated knowledge translation (iKT) [1–4]. We have chosen to use the term 'stakeholder' in this chapter since it reflects those who have a vested interest in the outcomes of a clinical education study [5] and may include patients, caregivers, learners, educators, community members, clinicians, curriculum developers, and policy or decision makers. Diverse organisations (e.g. funders, governments, advocacy, and academic organisations) encourage or require researchers to involve stakeholders in all aspects of the research process, including the identification of research priorities [6–9]. Stakeholders have experiential knowledge and can contribute unique insights to research. Researchers and stakeholders can collaboratively ensure that research is responsive to all individuals and groups impacted by it. In this chapter, we draw on evidence from PPI in clinical and health research as well as participatory programme evaluation. We also adhere to the notion of 'nothing about us, without us', which advocates for actively involving stakeholders in research that affects them [10].

Who are the stakeholders?

Stakeholders are people or organisations with a concern or interest in ensuring the success of an organisation or system [11]. Within clinical education, the system usually refers to the successful education of future or current healthcare professionals. Examples of typical stakeholders are provided in Table 5.1. It is worth reflecting on your research topic/question and considering who might have a stake and whose input would be most valuable.

Why involve stakeholders?

Involving stakeholders in your research can be beneficial for you, your research process, society, and stakeholders themselves.

Stakeholder involvement supports effective research

By involving stakeholders in the research development process, you can address topics and research approaches that you might not otherwise consider. They provide insights into the needs and experiences of future participants and knowledge users, thus informing novel research questions and agendas [12, 13]. Their perspectives enhance research teams since they can ask questions that you might otherwise overlook (i.e. clarifying the methodology or purpose of the study). Often, stakeholders hold an insider perspective, meaning that they have a

---

Starting Research in Clinical Education, First Edition. Edited by Eliot L. Rees, Alison Ledger, and Kim A. Walker.
© 2024 The Association for the Study of Medical Education (ASME). Published 2024 by John Wiley & Sons Ltd.
Companion website: www.wiley.com/go/clinicaleducation

Table 5.1 Examples of potential stakeholders

Individuals	Organisations
Learners	Educational organisations
Patients	Healthcare organisations
Caregivers	Regulatory bodies
Healthcare professionals	Funding bodies
Educators	Policy makers
Curriculum developers	
Course/programme leaders	
Community members	

working knowledge of the study context [14, 15]. This knowledge may facilitate the creation of appropriate data collection tools as well as increase recruitment and retention since you can tailor the study design and materials to the targeted participants' needs [3]. For example, the stakeholders in one study helped inform the timing and location of data collection to accommodate the needs of participants, based on their knowledge of the community of interest to the study. As a result, the research team achieved a higher response rate than expected [16]. In addition to informing the study design and data collection tools, stakeholders can also make recommendations for how to adapt or simplify language to improve accessibility, uptake, and the dissemination of findings [12].

Stakeholder involvement leads to use of the findings

Since research is often publicly funded, involving stakeholders has societal benefits. Stakeholders are well positioned to move findings into practice [17]. They have strong understandings of the research problem, context, and environment in which the findings are relevant as well as any barriers and facilitators to the use of findings [17]. Stakeholders are also well positioned to know what interventions may work to help share the knowledge generated with those who have the power to use it. Engaging in a process of iKT requires researchers and stakeholders (i.e. knowledge users) to make joint decisions that shape the research questions, interpret the study findings, and craft messaging around the results [17]. In this way, researchers and stakeholders work collaboratively to ensure that research findings are timely, relevant, and applicable to those who will need to use them [17, 18]. As an example, Hoddinott et al. described collaborating with patients as advisors on how best to disseminate findings beyond an academic audience [18]. The patients involved wrote reports, created blogs, and summarised findings creatively, demonstrating an in-depth knowledge of

their condition and of online sources of knowledge exchange with which the researchers were less familiar. For more information on disseminating the findings of research projects, see Chapter 28.

Stakeholder involvement facilitates capacity building

Stakeholder involvement creates an active partnership and can help reframe whose expertise is valued [13]. Historically, the research community has assumed that clinicians and researchers are most capable at prioritising research needs. However, input from stakeholders may show that other research priorities are more pressing and beneficial to the stakeholders themselves [13, 19].

Stakeholders may also gain new skills, attitudes, thought processes, and behaviours because of their involvement in a study [20, 21]. Process use – a programme evaluation concept relating to stakeholder involvement – can apply equally to clinical education research [20]. There are six types of processes that we can adapt to the research context:

1 Facilitating stakeholders' understanding of the topic.
2 Supporting and reinforcing the study intervention.
3 Increasing stakeholders' engagement, research, and critical-thinking skills.
4 Facilitating research and organisational development.
5 Infusing research thinking into the organisation's culture.
6 Promoting instrumentation effects (i.e. what gets measured gets done) and thus keeping stakeholders focused on research priorities [20].

By being involved in research processes, stakeholders can enter the research culture and learn how to consider things through a research lens. They can also use the skills (e.g. methodological and facilitation skills) they develop to build research capacity in their organisations, which has long-term benefits for both the stakeholders and their organisations.

What can stakeholder involvement look like?

Stakeholders may play various roles with varying degrees of involvement on a research project. They may form focus groups, pilot test study materials, speak at conferences, engage in stakeholder workshops, sit on advisory boards or long-standing committees, participate in single-day events, and collaborate on or lead all phases of a research study [22]. They may also be involved in the peer review of study findings. For example, the *British Medical Journal* invites patients or caregivers of those living with long-term conditions to peer review articles related to their conditions, as a way to increase the patient-centredness and relevance of its research, education, and scholarly comment articles [23]. In another example, medical students and faculty members from the Northern Ontario School of Medicine (NOSM) in Canada partner with Indigenous communities who have expressed an interest in exploring health-related research questions to collaborate in addressing the community-identified research priorities [24]. This collaboration is community-led to ensure that the research is culturally appropriate and community controlled, in keeping with the institution's social accountability mandate [24]. Both of these examples help illustrate how involvement occurs on a continuum ranging from low to high degrees of involvement [13]. Table 5.2 provides an overview of stakeholders' roles in clinical education research.

Stakeholder involvement can help to measure whether educational or research interventions achieve their objectives (i.e. stakeholders can help to measure quality and empowerment). Researchers can draw on existing guiding frameworks (e.g. the Public and Patient Engagement Evaluation Tool [PPEET], Cochrane's Six-Step Stakeholder Engagement Framework) to inform their involvement of stakeholders and to categorise, describe, and evaluate the involvement process and outcomes [13, 26, 27]. Given the diversity of engagement opportunities, clear guidance on how to categorise and describe stakeholder involvement is important for facilitating the evaluation of the involvement process, including the short, intermediate, and long-term outcomes of the involvement. Careful evaluation and dissemination of the stakeholder involvement strategies used across different research contexts and study types can help the field of clinical education cultivate an evidence-informed approach to involving stakeholders in research.

How can you identify stakeholders?

Depending on the topic, you may identify several stakeholders. Since it is not always feasible to actively involve all stakeholders, you can ask yourself the following questions:
- Which stakeholders do I want to work with and why?

Table 5.2 Stakeholders' roles in clinical education research

Role	Overview	Degree of involvement
Stakeholders as consultants	Researchers use strategies that primarily seek to gather information from stakeholders (e.g. through focus groups, town halls/community forums, advisory panels, email) for their use [13, 25]	Passive; decisions are made by researchers at all phases of the research process
Stakeholders as collaborators	Researchers and stakeholders establish and sustain an ongoing partnership in the research process. How stakeholders are involved in each research phase will vary across studies, but stakeholders play a role from early planning to dissemination and are often co-investigators [4, 13]	Active or passive; varies by study or team
Stakeholder-controlled research	Stakeholders lead the research process. Researchers are only involved at the request of the stakeholders, or when stakeholder organisations commission research on a topic from researchers [13]	Active; decisions are made by stakeholders at all phases of the research process

- Who can help me make important decisions about my study and gain access to potential participants?
- Who is most impacted by my research processes and my eventual study findings?
- Who will use or promote the use of my study findings? [5].

If there are still too many stakeholders, we recommend focusing on the involvement of those who have the power to use or influence the use of your study findings to change or improve clinical education practice [5]. Alternatively, you can limit involvement to primary stakeholders (i.e. those who stand to gain or lose something directly from your study) rather than secondary stakeholders (i.e. those who are indirectly affected, either positively or negatively, by your study). Not every identified stakeholder can or will want to be involved in each study phase and they may change throughout the study. It is also helpful to consider those who may wish to become co-investigators or collaborators throughout the duration of a research study. Moreover, community or patient outreach and advocacy groups, both internal and external to the research teams' organisations, may be a helpful starting point for identifying selected individuals.

When considering which stakeholders to include, you should also consider issues related to equity, diversity, and inclusion. The literature highlights that, often, the stakeholders involved in studies are atypical and represent those who are affluent, confident, and financially able to contribute [18]. However, when identifying who to involve, you should consider meaningfully involving individuals from a variety of backgrounds and experiences as well as those who identify as women, Indigenous Peoples, visible minorities/racialised persons, persons with disabilities, and LGBTQ+. Ultimately, the aim is to involve people who represent the demographic of those affected by the study topic while also remembering they are experts in their own experiences and the experiences of one person may not transfer to the experiences of a group, even if they share similar characteristics (e.g. socioeconomic status, ethnicity, and health conditions) [18, 28, 29].

Considerations when involving stakeholders

A key to engaging stakeholders is prioritising and cultivating meaningful relationships with them. This process of relationship building takes time as well as expertise on the part of the researchers and is important for establishing trust so that they feel comfortable expressing their views and concerns [18, 19, 30]. For example, Frerichs et al. conducted a study exploring stakeholders' perspectives on creating and maintaining trust in community–academic partnerships [31]. They found that community members valued co-learning and collaborative approaches to build trusting partnerships more than researchers did. The authors recommended that researchers employ strategies like jigsaws, think-pair-shares, and the use of project management software to effectively involve stakeholders and meaningfully build trust through collaboration [31]. Moreover, some stakeholders or stakeholder groups have, understandably, developed mistrust of research or healthcare institutions due to previous negative experiences or historical wrongdoings [22, 31, 32]. Recognising that relationship-building efforts may be hampered by the

research environment is important (e.g. stakeholders feeling uncomfortable entering into research or healthcare institutions, holding meetings during the typical workday when it is inconvenient for stakeholders with caregiving needs). Researchers looking to engage with stakeholders must consider what factors may unintentionally influence their engagement efforts and take steps to mitigate them (e.g. meeting in a neutral space, like a coffee shop, at a time convenient for them) [22, 29].

Logistics

Researchers and stakeholders may face logistical issues when collaborating in research. You may find it challenging to recruit stakeholders, coordinate schedules, and sustain stakeholder involvement throughout the study [12, 19, 33]. They may struggle to navigate the logistics of their involvement (e.g. coordinating other responsibilities, geographic distances, managing health conditions) [19, 34]. To illustrate these logistical tensions, Poland et al. attempted but were unable to recruit stakeholders with dementia as co-investigators [10]. Challenges included health professionals' and caregivers' assumptions that the cognitive capabilities of the person with dementia would limit their potential contribution. Moreover, caregivers also raised physical concerns about mobility and accessibility considerations that would hinder the participation of stakeholders with dementia as co-investigators [10]. A lack of clear guidance, policies, or procedures for involving stakeholders in clinical education research may create confusing and inconsistent expectations, which can vary from study to study.

Resources and support

Stakeholder involvement in research can also be resource intensive [12]. The time required for building relationships between everyone may be hindered by tight study timelines. Sufficient resources are required for recruitment and relationship building, especially with those stakeholders who come from underrepresented populations where you may need to actively engage the community to build rapport and trust prior to holding research-related discussions [18]. Time is also required to ensure that all team members have a shared understanding of study priorities [25]. Funding is another key resource constraint. Clinical education research currently has few funding opportunities – and even fewer focused specifically on stakeholder involvement [35]. Research involving stakeholders may face challenges related to funding and credibility owing to the use of research methods that differ from those traditionally used in clinical research [36]. Additionally, if stakeholders are only involved in researcher-driven studies once funding has been secured, they may miss valuable opportunities to contribute to research design [25]. Moreover, involving stakeholders in the study development and grant application phases can pose challenges for researchers who may not have funding to compensate stakeholders for their work if grants are unsuccessful [25].

Power differentials and tokenism

Issues of power and privilege are important considerations. Clinicians and researchers have traditionally held more power than patients and other stakeholder groups, leading to the latter groups' contributions being devalued or considered less credible due to negative assumptions, prejudices, or discrimination [32]. Involving stakeholders should be an active and collaborative process. It is important to create a space where they feel comfortable expressing their views, concerns, and experiences. Without meeting these preconditions, stakeholders may be wary to share due to the perceived risks (i.e. embarrassment, lack of safety, and financial implications) [30]. For example, as Flynn et al. illustrated, selected stakeholders, especially adolescents, may struggle to collaborate with researchers because it is an unfamiliar dynamic for them. There is a societal norm that adults 'know best', and thus, the adolescent stakeholders in their study were unable to freely share their thoughts and recommendations [19]. Tokenism – to give the appearance of involvement – is another challenge for you to be aware of. Increasingly, stakeholder involvement is a requirement for funding competitions or to align with institutional research policies [12]. Often, they are left feeling like they have been involved merely for the purposes of 'checking a box' rather than to authentically contribute to the study [37].

Similarity of involved stakeholders

Representing the diversity of stakeholders' perspectives and experiences in research is a key consideration. Often stakeholders are selected based on their abilities to understand and collaborate in research, rather than on the authenticity of their experiences as they relate to the study [38]. Thus, there is always a risk that they will be a relatively similar group, especially since those who are more confident and financially secure are more likely to volunteer to participate [18]. Moreover, researchers often draw on stakeholders from organisational pools or funding panels mainly consisting of white, educated people [18, 29, 36]. This practice is problematic since it can further marginalise the experiences of populations who are particularly underrepresented in research

and who also have unequal access to health care and education like visible minorities, persons with disabilities, and LGBTQ+ persons [36]. There are concerns stakeholders become familiar with working practices, receive research training and they may become 'professionalised', losing their lay perspectives in favour of aligning with those of the researchers [18, 36].

Strategies for involving stakeholders

You can use several strategies to involve stakeholders in your research. Rather than adopting these strategies uncritically, you should adapt them to the contexts and needs of both the stakeholders and your research [39].

Provide any necessary training

Research team members can complete training on how to involve stakeholders in research from their organisations or from an external organisation. Diverse workbooks, training modules, and planning tools are available online from organisations whose mandates centre on involving stakeholders in health research broadly (e.g. The Patient Centred Outcomes Research Institute's training modules, the National Institute of Health and Care Research (NIHR) INVOLVE resource kits, Arthritis Research Canada, and the University of British Columbia's Patient Engagement in Research plan workbook) [40–42]. These offerings target researchers looking to involve stakeholders and focus on collaborative planning and meaningful engagement; they also provide training to stakeholders who are interested in learning more about the research process. You should consider providing stakeholders with appropriate training to support them in developing an understanding of the research process and any preliminary research skills required, based on the individual and study's needs and goals [3]. This may be more necessary for those from patient and public groups than those from academic or professional organisations.

Communicate roles, goals, and expectations

Clear communication of roles, goals, and expectations on the part of both researchers and stakeholders is essential. To ensure effective engagement you should:

- Clearly communicate the purpose of the research, the rationale for stakeholders' involvement, and the potential impact of their involvement both initially and throughout the study [3, 30].
- Collaboratively define stakeholders' involvement early on to ensure a shared understanding of team member responsibilities.

- Discuss stakeholders' needs, experience, and skills in relation to the research context, with the understanding that their roles may evolve over time as their needs change, studies take shape, and discussions progress [33, 37].
- Be flexible with work arrangements, including the format and timing of research activities, to ensure that involvement is accessible to all.
- Clearly define and openly discuss your own role and expectations.

Provide compensation

Compensation is an important consideration. Underrepresented groups often undertake unpaid emotional labour, especially when sharing their personal health or social experiences for educational purposes [32]. You should consider compensating stakeholders for their time and expertise and reimbursing them for research-related expenses, wherever possible [3]. Types of expenses can vary widely depending on individuals' personal situations and the expectations of them. These expenses should be openly addressed in early discussions, and any limitations to reimbursement (e.g. funding limits) should be communicated clearly.

Engage in relational practices

To develop and sustain meaningful, collaborative partnerships, you need to foster positive relationships with stakeholders from the outset. This is particularly important with stakeholders who have historically been excluded from research, underrepresented in research, included only as research subjects, and/or involved only in a tokenistic fashion. Regular conversations between researchers and stakeholders and the use of plain language to build a common understanding amongst all team members are effective strategies for cultivating collaborative relationships [37]. Further, you need to establish and sustain reciprocal and safe research environments where stakeholders can feel comfortable to share their perspectives [30, 31]. Hoffman et al. [30] recommend involving a facilitator, with no stake in the research, to support such an environment. They summarise the foundational principles supporting stakeholder involvement in research. These principles include

- *Respect and equity*. Diversity, authenticity, integrity, and confidentiality.
- *Trust*. Transparency and honesty.
- *Empowerment*. Shared decision-making and ownership, flexibility, and institutional support [37].

Contributing to a culture of stakeholder involvement

Proper resources, guidance, and support can enable you to involve stakeholders in your research. An organisational approach to involvement could facilitate access to, as well as build and sustain relationships with, individuals and local or national groups [43] which may help you in your project. Your organisation should aim to embed stakeholder involvement throughout their research activities which can lead to increased funding, increased training opportunities, and the creation of new roles or committees [43]. Committees responsible for overseeing stakeholder involvement activities are an essential resource for organisations to incorporate into their practice [30]. Contributing to an organisational culture of stakeholder involvement can facilitate shared learning across research teams, departments/faculties, disciplines, and organisations [41].

Summary

In this chapter we have explored what it means to actively involve stakeholders in clinical education research. We have provided examples of the types of stakeholders, explained why and how you should involve them, and explored key considerations for those looking to undertake stakeholder involvement. With time, we hope that such involvement in clinical education research will become the norm and something that others reflect and publish on.

Top tips

- Involve stakeholders early in the research process and collaboratively define roles and expectations.
- Establish regular bidirectional communication using agreed media and language that is accessible to all.
- Take into account stakeholders' other commitments when planning meetings and activities.
- Provide stakeholders with the information required to make a useful contribution.

Common pitfalls

- Omitting crucial stakeholders whose involvement is essential to conduct your research and achieve impact.
- Neglecting the importance of building meaningful relationships with stakeholders. Relationships are key in achieving research success.
- Forgetting to check in with stakeholders through the lifecycle of your project. You should evaluate the stakeholder involvement process regularly.

Ethical issues

- It is crucial to recognise the contribution of stakeholders to your research. This may be in the form of acknowledgements, co-authorship of outputs, or financial compensation.
- All members of the research team, including stakeholders, should agree on ground rules including any confidentiality requirements.
- There is the potential for power differentials to influence stakeholder relationships and contributions to the project. Discussing these upfront and remaining open and honest can mitigate future problems.

References

1 Nguyen, T., Graham, I.D., Mrklas, K.J. et al. (2020). How does integrated knowledge translation (IKT) compare to other collaborative research approaches to generating and translating knowledge? Learning from experts in the field. *Health Research Policy and Systems* 18 (1): 35.

2 Jull, J., Giles, A., and Graham, I.D. (2017). Community-based participatory research and integrated knowledge translation: advancing the co-creation of knowledge. *Implementation Science* 12: 150–159.

3 Bate, J., Ranasinghe, N., Ling, R. et al. (2016). Public and patient involvement in paediatric research. *Archives of Disease in Childhood. Education and Practice Edition* 101 (3): 158–161.

4 Forsythe, L.P., Carman, K.L., Szydlowski, V. et al. (2019). Patient engagement in research: early findings from the Patient-Centered Outcomes Research Institute. *Health Affairs (Millwood)* 38 (3): 359–367.

5 Alkin, M. and Vo, A. (2017). *Evaluation Essentials: From A to Z*. New York, NY: Guilford Press.

6 Hanson, F. and Hanson, R. (2017). Reflections from a patient and carer on involvement in research and integrating care in the health system. *International Journal of Integrated Care* 17: 1–3.

7 Telford, R., Boote, J., and Cooper, C. (2004). What does it mean to involve consumers successfully in NHS research? A consensus study. *Health Expect.* 7: 209–220.

8 Domecq, P., Prutsky, G., Elraiyah, T. et al. (2014). Patient engagement in research: a systematic review. *BMC Health Services Research* 14: 1–9.

9 Canadian Institutes of Health Research (2018). Strategy for patient-oriented research – patient engagement framework 2018. http://www.cihr-irsc.gc.ca/e/48413.html (accessed 2 May 2023).

10 Poland, F., Charlesworth, G., Leung, P., and Birt, L. (2019). Embedding patient and public involvement: managing tacit and explicit expectations. *Health Expectations* 22 (6): 1231–1239.

11 Stakeholder, N. (2022). *OED Online*. Oxford University Press Web. 21 November 2022.

12 Brett, J., Staniszewska, S., Mockford, C. et al. (2014). Mapping the impact of patient and public involvement on health and social care research: a systematic review. *Health Expectations* 17 (5): 637–650.

13 Boote, J., Telford, R., and Cooper, C. (2002). Consumer involvement in health research: a review and research agenda. *Health Policy* 61: 213–236.

14 Morse, J. (2010). How different is qualitative health research from qualitative research? Do we have a subdiscipline? *Qualitative Health Research* 20 (11): 1459–1464.

15 Babbie, E. (2008). *The Basics of Social Research*. Belmont, CA: Thompson Wadsworth.

16 Shen, S., Doyle-Thomas, K.A.R., Beesley, L. et al. (2017). How and why should we engage parents as co-researchers in health research? A scoping review of current practices. *Health Expectations* 20 (4): 543–554.

17 Canadian Institute of Health Research (2015). A guide to researcher and knowledge-user collaboration in health research. https://cihr-irsc.gc.ca/e/44954.html (accessed 2 May 2023).

18 Hoddinott, P., Pollock, A., O'Cathain, A. et al. (2018). How to incorporate patient and public perspectives into the design and conduct of research. *F1000Research* 7: 752.

19 Flynn, R., Walton, S., and Scott, S.D. (2019). Engaging children and families in pediatric health research: a scoping review. *Research Involvement and Engagement* 5: 32.

20 Patton, M.Q. (2007). Process use as a usefulism. *New Directions for Evaluation* 2007 (116): 99–112.

21 Patton, M.Q. (1997). *Utilization-Focused Evaluation: The New Century Text*, 3e. SAGE Publications.

22 Rowland, P. and Johannesen, J. (2020). Patient engagement and compassionate care. In: *Without Compassion, There Is No Healthcare: Leading with Care in a Technological Age* (ed. B. Hodges, G. Paech, and J. Bennett), 59–77. Montreal, QC: McGill University Press.

23 British Medical Journal (2022). Guidance for BMJ patient and public reviewers. https://www.bmj.com/about-bmj/resources-reviewers/guidance-patient-reviewers (accessed 2 May 2023).

24 Maar, M., Boesch, L., and Tobe, S. (2018). Enhancing indigenous health research capacity in northern Ontario through distributed community engaged medical education at NOSM: a qualitative evaluation of the community engagement through research pilot program. *Canadian Medical Education Journal.* 9 (1): e21–e32.

25 Jackson, T., Pinnock, H., Liew, S.M. et al. (2020). Patient and public involvement in research: from tokenistic box ticking to valued team members. *BMC Medicine* 18 (1): 79.

26 McMaster University (2022). Faculty of health sciences: Public & patient engagement: Public and patient engagement evaluation tool. https://ppe.mcmaster.ca/our-products/public-patient-engagement-evaluation-tool#:~:text=The%20Public%20and%20Patient%20

Engagement,(e.g.%2C%20health%20research (accessed 2 May 2023).

27 Tomlinson E, Parker R. (2021). Six-step stakeholder engagement framework: Cochrane collaboration. https://training.cochrane.org/sites/training.cochrane.org/files/public/uploads/Six%20Step%20Stakeholder%20Engagement%20Framework.pdf (accessed 2 May 2023)

28 Lefkowitz, A., Vizza, J., and Kuper, A. (2022). Patients as experts in the illness experience: implications for the ethics of patient involvement in health professions education. *Journal of Evaluation in Clinical Practice* 28 (5): 794–800.

29 Rowland, P. and Kumagai, A.K. (2018). Dilemmas of representation: patient engagement in health professions education. *Academic Medicine* 93 (6): 869–873.

30 Hoffman, A., Montgomery, R., Aubry, W., and Tunis, S.R. (2010). How best to engage patients, doctors, and other stakeholders in designing comparative effectiveness studies. *Health Affairs (Millwood).* 29 (10): 1834–1841.

31 Frerichs, L., Kim, M., Gaurav, D. et al. (2017). Stakeholder perspectives on creating and maintaining trust in community-academic research partnerships. *Health Education and Behaviour.* 44 (1): 182–191.

32 Paton, M., Naidu, T., Wyatt, T. et al. (2020). Dismantling the master's house: new ways of knowing for equity and social justice in health professions education. *Advances in Health Sciences Education: Theory and Practice* 25: 1107–1126.

33 Manafo, E., Petermann, L., Mason-Lai, P., and Vandall-Walker, V. (2018). Patient engagement in Canada: a scoping review of the 'how' and 'what' of patient engagement in health research. *Health Research Policy and Systems* 16 (1): 5.

34 Liabo, K., Boddy, K., Bortoli, S. et al. (2020). Public involvement in health research: what does 'good' look like in practice? *Research Involvement and Engagement* 6: 11.

35 Institute of Medicine,Greiner, A. and Knebel, E. (2003). *Health Professions Education: A Bridge to Quality.* Washington, DC: The National Academies Press.

36 Green, G. (2016). Power to the people: to what extent has public involvement in applied health research achieved this? *Research Involvement and Engagement* 2: 28.

37 Harrison, J.D., Auerbach, A.D., Anderson, W. et al. (2019). Patient stakeholder engagement in research: a narrative review to describe foundational principles and best practice activities. *Health Expectations* 22 (3): 307–316.

38 Martineau, J.T., Minyaoui, A., and Boivin, A. (2020). Partnering with patients in healthcare research: a scoping review of ethical issues, challenges, and recommendations for practice. *BMC Medical Ethics* 21 (1): 34.

39 Biddle, M.S.Y., Gibson, A., and Evans, D. (2021). Attitudes and approaches to patient and public involvement across Europe: a systematic review. *Health & Social Care in the Community* 29 (1): 18–27.

40 Patient-centred Outcomes Research Institute (2022). Research fundamentals: Preparing you to successfully contribute to research. https://www.pcori.org/engagement/research-fundamentals (accessed 2 May 2023).

41 National Institute for Health and Care Research (NIHR) Involve. (2022). Developing training and support 2022. www.invo.org.uk/resource-centre/training-resource (accessed 2 May 2023).

42 Clayton, H., Hoens, A.M., Backman, C.L., et al. (2018). Workbook to guide the development of a patient engagement in research (PEIR) plan. https://www.arthritisresearch.ca/wp-content/uploads/2018/06/PEIR-Plan-Guide.pdf (accessed 2 May 2023).

43 Turner, G., Aiyegbusi, O.L., Price, G. et al. (2020). Moving beyond project-specific patient and public involvement in research. *Journal of the Royal Society of Medicine* 113 (1): 16–23.

6 Sampling and recruiting participants

Jennifer Cleland, Kirsty Alexander, and Amudha Poobalan

Learning objectives

By the end of this chapter, you should be able to:
- Distinguish between a population and a sample.
- Explain the importance of appropriate and adequate sampling in quantitative and qualitative research.
- Recognise the various types of quantitative sampling and the importance of balancing rigour and practicality.

- Discuss the various types of qualitative sampling and the principles of sample size estimation in qualitative research.
- Choose from common recruitment approaches for quantitative and qualitative research projects.

Introduction

In an ideal world, you may wish to gather information from every individual in your population, that is, the group of interest. This is difficult to achieve because it is time consuming, expensive, and actually unnecessary. Instead, it is standard practice to use a sample, to examine part of the population to represent the whole. Sampling means that you only study part of a larger group in order to draw meaningful conclusions.

How you go about sampling is very important and will depend on a variety of factors, such as your research questions, what you are studying, how you are studying it (the research design), and the context. Sampling considerations are important in both quantitative and qualitative research, when considering a target population/group and when drawing a sample that will either allow generalisation and precision or transferability and depth (see Chapter 3). Because goals and needs vary, there is no single, correct way to sample. There are, however, appropriate (and inappropriate) ways to sample depending on the nature of the study and research question.

In this chapter, we consider sampling in quantitative research followed by qualitative research, using clinical education examples and scenarios. We also discuss potential sampling challenges and how to mitigate these in real world scenarios without compromising research quality and integrity. Issues associated with recruitment are discussed at the end of the chapter.

Sampling in quantitative research

In quantitative research, sample size and sampling considerations are usually (but not always – see later) made with the goal of generalising findings and inferences from a representative sample to the larger population from which the sample was drawn. Sampling is the process by which a sub-set of the population (the sample) is selected to represent the characteristics of the larger group.

The selection of an appropriate representative sample is crucial. For example, let us assume you want to do a study about overall student satisfaction with a particular part of the curriculum. You know from the data held by the school that 40% of the class are male, 60% female. Your sample needs to reflect this – if you have 60% males and 40% females in your sample, it will not accurately reflect the composition of the class (the population). If your data is not collected from a representative sample (sampling bias), then you cannot draw conclusions about the whole population. Sampling bias can be further illustrated with another example of collecting student feedback. Where giving feedback is voluntary, only those with strong views are likely

Starting Research in Clinical Education, First Edition. Edited by Eliot L. Rees, Alison Ledger, and Kim A. Walker.
© 2024 The Association for the Study of Medical Education (ASME). Published 2024 by John Wiley & Sons Ltd.
Companion website: www.wiley.com/go/clinicaleducation

to complete or return feedback forms. Furthermore, if feedback is sought via distribution of paper forms, only those attending the class will be able to participate. Those who have not attended class may represent a different subgroup of students, so your data may be less reliable and accurate.

No sample is perfect, but there are sampling techniques that help maximise the representativeness of the sample.

Random sampling – the gold standard?

Random, or probability, sampling consists of selecting enough, representative participants at random from a population to ensure that results are indicative of the population. Random selection implies that each member of the population as a whole or of sub-groups of the population has an equal chance of being selected. This allows you to study a relatively small proportion of the population and gain results that are likely to represent the population more broadly. This makes research studies possible that would otherwise be infeasible.

If you do not use random sampling, your study might be biased towards particular sub-groups in the population. For example, if we wanted to understand student beliefs about the use of 3D technology in anatomy, and we proposed to survey students via email, it would be very important which students we sent the survey to, and which students responded. For example, less technically adept students may be less likely to respond to emails thus biasing our sample. If we only sent the survey to medical students in one medical school, or one geographic location, or one-year group, then our results would not reflect the beliefs of medical students more broadly. Even if we sent the survey to every medical student in our country and only 10% responded, might there be reasons that the other 90% did not respond that would influence their beliefs about technology integration (such as not having an email address)?

For randomisation to work for achieving generalisation, it must be done appropriately for your research question, context, and population. Education researchers commonly employ one of four random-sampling strategies: simple, stratified, proportional, and cluster sampling (see Table 6.1).

Each of these approaches has strengths and limitations. For example, simple random sampling selects participants from the target population without consideration for sub-groups, categories, or differences between the participants. However, this allows researchers to show that their results are representative of the population broadly while giving them limited power to answer more nuanced questions

Table 6.1 Four common random-sampling strategies with examples

Approach	Example	Sample
Simple	Survey a random sample of trainees from a country-level list of trainees based on a sample size calculation	1000 trainees selected by random number generation
Stratified	Survey trainees from each type of training locality/region	500 trainees from urban locations 200 trainees from rural locations and so on
Proportional	Survey a representative number of trainees from each region based on the trainee population in each region	150 trainees from Region x 100 from Region y 500 from Region z and so on
Cluster	Survey all trainees from a particular cluster (e.g. randomly selected region)	All 300 trainees from Region A All 300 trainees from Region D All 400 trainees from Region G

about sub-groups. For example, if there are 'difficult to access' groups amongst your population, unless you plan to sample them separately, your results may not be representative of these 'difficult to access' groups. However, if that consideration is not pertinent to your research question and/or context, then simple randomisation might be appropriate. For simple random sampling, (i) obtain as complete list as possible of the population, (ii) assign a random sequential order to each participant in the population (assign participants ID numbers), (iii) decide the sample size number needed (using a sample size calculation: see later), and (iv) select the sample by running a random number generator. Participants then have an equal and fair chance of being selected.

Another variant of random sampling technique is called 'systematic random sampling', where the researchers select the sample using a sampling interval. For example, if you have a list of 5000 adults and you require a representative sample of 50, select every 100th case. In this technique, you need to make sure that the original list is randomly ordered to start with – and the starting point of the sample selection should also be determined randomly.

Stratified sampling selects participants from different groups, levels, or strata in the population so that results will account for important variation in the population. In order to do this, you need to first identify the strata that differentiate participants from one another and then sample an appropriate number of participants from each stratum. By equally representing the specific characteristics, this sampling technique allows for the sample to reflect the diversity of the larger population and prevents findings for smaller groups in the population being ignored due to lack of representation. For example, if you wanted to study satisfaction with training and suspected that this might differ based on location of training (urban/rural), then doing a simple random sample would risk most of your data coming from residents in urban regions if higher numbers of residents are based in urban settings. To manage this, you might intentionally sample by strata so each locality is proportionally represented. This would allow you to compare results between groups. If the strata are identified appropriately, this technique produces samples that are more representative of the population than a simple random sample.

Proportional stratified random sampling is a refinement of stratified sampling which selects participants from different groups, levels, or strata in the population, but in addition does so at a rate proportional to their overall representation in the population. This allows for the sample to reflect key characteristics of the population at large that could have been lost through simple random sampling and allows results to be comparable between subgroups and generalisable to the entire population. For instance, if you wanted to survey health professionals on their experiences with work–life balance, you could reasonably assume that gender would be an important factor that would influence results. Then your sample needs a similar gender breakdown to that of the whole population for the results to be valid. Proportional stratified random sampling is superior to simple random sampling when key strata are identifiable at the outset because it can help to minimise sampling errors that are always possible with simple randomisation (in this example, accidentally overrepresenting men).

Cluster sampling selects participants from naturally occurring groups or clusters of the population for analysis. This allows you to focus your efforts on one or more clusters (like specific nursing schools) and generalise your results to the entire population of these schools. For cluster sampling to work, the clusters should be similar to the larger population in terms of matching its characteristics. You need to first identify clusters that might be appropriate for analysis and then to randomly select which cluster(s) to study. For instance, and thinking of the UK context, you might want to study if the views of student support, or careers advice, differ across the clusters of new versus traditional medical schools, or research-intensive versus other medical schools.

Which approach is best, or most appropriate, depends on your research question and population of interest. Moreover, and crucially, randomisation is only appropriate if generalisation is the goal in quantitative research and you are working within a post-positivist paradigm (see Chapter 3). The notion of conceptual generalisability, or transferability, is the parallel in qualitative research (see later).

Sampling decisions and their effects on generalisability

In most clinical education research, participants are usually not selected via randomisation because they are already an existing sample or because they are representative in some way given the topic under study. Such convenience sampling (see Table 6.2) is often the only type of sampling possible. The issue is that there is no precise way of generalising from a convenience sample to a population. For example, in a context where there are two nursing schools in the same city, students from nursing school A may be very different from those of nursing school B because the two schools attract different applicants. Any results from school A cannot necessarily be generalised to school B.

However, the primary purpose of the research may not only be to generalise but to better understand relationships that may exist. For example, suppose you are investigating the relationship between undergraduate performance and career destination. Imagine that the only available sample is the alumni from your single school. The study is completed, and the results indicate a moderate relationship: Nursing students who have higher performance tend to have different postgraduate pathways than those with lower grades. Should we then ignore the findings or suggest that the results are not valid or credible? That would seem excessively cautious. It is more reasonable to interpret the results as valid for nursing students similar to those studied, such as those from the same country/ education and training system. The decision is not to dismiss the findings but to be cautious in interpreting the results, limiting them to the type of participants in the sample. As more and more research amasses with different convenience samples, patterns become clearer. Several areas of clinical education research have progressed via many accumulative studies using convenience samples.

It is important to be as precise as possible in reporting sampling procedures. If some type of probability sampling procedure was used, it will inevitably be described in a paper. Explicit reporting of a non-randomised sample approach is less common. However, if a non-randomised sample was used, it should be obvious in the methodology section of the article (usually under 'Participants'). The following descriptions are typical (and drawn from some of our own papers): 'The sample population was drawn from xx final year medical students undertaking their first clinical placement of the academic year at xx Hospital' [1]; 'Study participants included all Year 1 undergraduate medical students at the five Scottish medical schools' [2] and 'We followed up a group of students who entered into medical school at the Universities of x and y in 2007 from their first year to graduation in their fifth year' [3].

So, how many is enough?

In quantitative research, you can decide on the number of participants using a power calculation. Power is the probability of detecting a real effect. Sample size calculations are complex, but practical advice is available from various sources ([4, 5], see also: https://www.qualtrics.com/uk/experience-management/research/determine-sample-size).

These sources give more details of the sample size problem and explain the four inter-relating factors which affect its solution: significance level, statistical power, analysis procedure, and effect size. They also provide practical guidance for carrying out power calculations for your own research questions.

If you do not have enough people in your sample to find a difference (i.e. your study is underpowered), conducting the study would be unethical because it would have a high chance of producing misleading results. If the results are negative (e.g. a randomised controlled trial that found no difference between team-based learning and lectures in respect of examination performance), then the question will always remain whether the lack of effect was due to insufficient numbers rather than anything to do with the intervention. Unfortunately, compared to clinical research, it is rare for a description of the power calculation to be provided in the methods section of papers in education research. This means conclusions are drawn inappropriately and poor-quality research abounds, influencing later studies.

Sampling in qualitative research

While quantitative researchers use complex mathematical formula to decide on a sample, which accurately represents a broader population, qualitative researchers choose samples which make it possible to study issues in depth. Qualitative researchers make a series of decisions not only about how many individuals (or documents, observations, media sources, or other qualitative media) to include in a study and how to select these sources but also about how much data to collect from each source, as well as the conditions under which this selection will take place.

As a result, just like many other aspects of qualitative research, deciding on a sample relies on researcher interpretations, experience, and tacit knowledge [6]. This means it can be difficult for those newly entering the field and who are yet to gain experience in making sampling judgements. Moreover, a reliance on implicit understandings can also mean that the process of deciding sample size in qualitative research can appear to lack rigour – indeed qualitative research has been criticised for giving little or no justification for the sample sizes that are actually used in research [7]. This means that you may be unsure how much data you need.

In this section we, therefore, discuss guidelines, models, and commonly accepted norms for creating a sample, to make this process more transparent and approachable.

Mapping the sample to the study

Qualitative research aims to develop knowledge about how individuals and groups produce, experience, and interpret their worlds [8]. Consequently, the objects of study are often complex social or cultural phenomena, group interactions, meaning-making, attitudes, and values [9] (see Chapter 3). It is therefore first essential to be clear in your mind what the fundamentals of your study are, and secondly to understand how your sample will enable you to achieve these. Some starting questions are

- What is your research aim and paradigm? Most qualitative research is undertaken from an ontological perspective that does not aim to generalise, but rather obtain insight into a specific phenomenon (see Chapter 3). However, post-positivist qualitative studies do exist and may require a large, random sample [10] and require a different approach to purposive sampling than is described in this chapter.
- What is your study population and are there sub-populations within this? Will you directly compare sub-populations or case studies? How similar or different do you predict the experiences recounted to be? See [6] for a useful discussion of how to think about your population and estimate a reasonable size for each (sub)group.

- How lengthy and rich is your data source likely to be? For example, a narrative interview that asks a physiotherapy trainee to recount their trajectory through training may be longer than one where you ask them to discuss a specific incident.
- What is your analytic approach? The overall purpose and level of detailed inquiry required by your approach will impact the required sample size. For example, Creswell [11] suggests twice to three times the number of participants for grounded theory research in comparison to phenomenological analysis (see below for further discussion).
- What are your own limits? The expected number of participants will be very different for a master's thesis or internal evaluation, in comparison to a PhD thesis or piece of publishable research. Ensure that the size is aligned to your purpose, time, and budget, all of which will differ depending on whether you are working on your own or as part of a large team.

So, how much is enough?

Given the complexity of the phenomena under study in qualitative research, sources should be 'information-rich' cases [12] containing detailed ('thick') descriptions, which allow as much relevant data about the phenomena to be gathered as possible [8]. It may, therefore, be tempting to collect high volumes of data, aiming to capture every aspect of your topic from every angle. There are, however, several practical restraints to consider. The first is that the amount of data must be manageable to permit a high-quality analysis, necessitating 'close observation, careful documentation and thoughtful analysis' [13]. Too much data can overwhelm and make it difficult for you to undertake a deep analysis that remains sensitive to cases and subgroups [14]. Second, data collection requires prolonged contact with participants, which takes researcher time and potentially more cost, for example, for transcription. In general, quality is more important than quantity. Third, data saturation, the point at which no new information is observed in the data from the completion of additional interviews or cases [15], is a common justification for the use of a particular sample size in qualitative research [16]. Saturation means that, if data collection and analysis were to continue, this would not lead to new relevant information [17]. Saturation can be determined as: 'code saturation' (when no new relevant issues or topics are identified); and 'meaning saturation' (when no new relevant insights, perspectives, or angles are identified) [16]. However, it is important to acknowledge that there

are debates in the literature about these concepts of saturation and whether these are actually consistent with the values and assumptions of thematic analysis (arguably the most common form of primary analysis in qualitative clinical education research, see Chapter 18). Other authors have suggested striving for theoretical sufficiency [18], the point where you have gained sufficient understanding for your purposes, rather than striving for 'no new understandings', as with data saturation.

Moreover, the concepts of saturation provide little guidance for estimating actual sample sizes prior to data collection. Indeed, many qualitative researchers state when to stop data collection cannot be determined (wholly) in advance of analysis (e.g. [19]). However, in reality, often decisions about the sample need to be taken in advance for practical reasons, such as applying for ethics permission and estimating the costs and time required for your study.

Assessing the norms for research similar to your own can be a useful starting point (see [13] for a summary). Some guidance is provided in Box 6.1. See also Malterud et al. [20] for a model based on 'information power' to estimate sample size by focussing on particulars of your study.

As illustrated above, samples in qualitative research tend to be substantially smaller than in

---

BOX 6.1   Guidance for estimating qualitative sample sizes.

Thematic analysis of data from homogenous participants.
  Typically around 20–30 interviews where resources allow for this

Large in-depth constructivist study. Around 50 interviews [14]

Phenomenological research. 10 interviews [10]

Grounded theory. Around 15–30 people [10, 11]

For studies utilising focus groups: 3–5 groups of 6–10 individuals [21]

Case study designs. Typically 3–5 cases [11]

An ethnography. Approximately 100–200 units of observation [22]

An autoethnography. One person or a number of people if comparing personal stories [23]

Notes

A study that compares sub-populations is much more likely to require greater numbers of participants.

A novice researcher may need a slightly larger sample to identify nuanced theoretical aspects than someone more experienced [20].

quantitative studies to permit a sufficiently in-depth analysis. Another key difference is that qualitative samples are almost always purposive: the sample is specifically chosen because the researcher believes these sources will provide rich information with thick descriptions of the phenomena under study. This makes practical sense when one is attempting to deeply understand the experiences of a particular group (not measure their experience nor generalise their experiences to others).

Five common qualitative sampling strategies are described in Table 6.2.

It is still important to remember the objectives of your study at this stage. Different sampling strategies have the potential to yield different samples.

Table 6.2 Common purposive sampling strategies with examples

Approach	Example	Sample
Informant	Interview students representing minority ethnic groups	10 students from each of the target groups
Extreme case and intensity	Interview students representing the majority and minority groups	5 students from each of the target groups = 10 students
Quota	Interview the same number of students from each target ethnic group	2 students × 5 different ethnic groups = 10 students
Snowball	Interview a student representing a target ethnic group, then ask them to help you to identify additional students in the target group, and so forth	1 student from the target group + 2 of that student's friends + 7 of their friends = 10 students
Opportunistic or emergent sampling (often referred to as convenience sampling)	Where the researcher takes advantage of events and opportunities to collect relevant data	Going up to students in the medical school café and asking them if they will be willing to participate in your study
Maximal variation sampling	A sample is made up of extremes or is chosen to ensure a wide variety of participants. The goal of this type of sampling is to gain an understanding of a certain topic from a wide variety of angles	Current students from the target group, plus students who are further on in the curriculum (but still have the other characteristics of the target group), other key stakeholders such as tutors

For example, snowball sampling may be ideal if you are intending a sample with strong commonalities and shared experiences, however, not if you are intending to explore a range of experiences. Opportunistic sampling may allow flexibility to capture up-to-date data on recent or impromptu developments, however, may be biased to extreme cases or the voices of those who are eager to participate. You may wish to start with one sampling strategy, and then switch to another, to help address emerging imbalances in the sample and this can be done if this is within the bounds of your ethical approval. Like sample size, sample composition, and the proposed methods of achieving this should be considered in advance. If there is a possibility you may need to change your sampling strategy, we recommend explaining contingency plans in your original ethical review application to avoid additional paperwork down the line (see Chapter 7).

As with quantitative research, qualitative research sample size decisions and sampling strategies should be transparently reported (typically in the methods section of your paper, thesis or presentation), to boost the trustworthiness of your research (see Table 6.3). Table 6.3 describes some common reporting weaknesses related to sampling.

Recruitment

Once the sample and sample size (i.e. who you want in your study and the number of participants needed) are determined, you need a plan for recruiting participants into the study. There are certain considerations at this stage.

Who approaches potential participants?
Consider your sample to decide on the most appropriate method to recruit. To attract sufficient participant numbers, it is usual to utilise several avenues to recruit, for example: social media, invitation email, newsletter entry, posters, in person at a lecture or meeting, or advertising during professional development events. It may be, however, that it is very difficult for you to contact your participant group directly without help from an insider, or gatekeeper. For example, a hospital psychiatry department is very unlikely to share the contact details of their trainees with you due to data protection regulations, but they might offer to send an email on your behalf or allow you to come to a teaching session to introduce the study. A gatekeeper is 'someone who has the authority to grant or deny access to potential participants and/or the ability to facilitate such access' [24]. As such, they can be crucial to your study's success. At a minimum, it is good practice to inform gatekeepers

Table 6.3 Common sampling reporting weaknesses and how to avoid them

Reporting weakness	Quantitative solution	Qualitative solution
Population/group is not well defined	Avoid vague descriptions such as 'trainees' (what year of training?) or 'high-performing students' (what does 'high' mean?) Demographic characteristics, such as age, gender, socioeconomic status, ability, and grade level, should be indicated, as well as any unique characteristics, for example, enrolled in a particular class, on placement in a particular specialty	Aim to give sufficient detail about aspects most pertinent to the study (e.g. in a study about work/life balance, which participants had dependents and the hours they spent each week on caring responsibilities as well as more generic characteristics such as gender)
Sampling method is not clearly described	Explicitly indicate the specific type of sampling procedure, such as simple random, stratified, cluster, and report sampling methods and provide sufficient detail. If you have used a stratified sampling procedure, the characteristics of each stratum should be included	Report all sampling approaches (convenience, snowball, extreme, etc.) and recruitment methods, along with the potential impact of these methods on the study. Limitations of these methods should be explained, such as the omission of a relevant perspective
Sample size is not sufficiently justified	Undertake a power calculation to justify the sample size. This will help you to demonstrate the probability of detecting an effect, if true differences exist	Critically reflect on whether you aim and expect to reach saturation, and whether it is appropriate to claim saturation when reporting your research. Researchers often fall back on references to data collection being halted when 'saturation was being reached', without a clear explanation of what type of saturation was sought, nor how and by whom this phenomenon was identified or confirmed

of the study, alert them to any risks and assure them of the level of anonymity for participants and the institution [24]. However, do follow the ethics guidance and procedures of your context when considering how best to recruit participants.

It is then important to consider who is going to approach potential participants. If the researcher (or an assisting stakeholder or gatekeeper) is in a position of power over the potential participants (e.g. the course lead or the Head of Assessment), people may find it hard to say 'no' if they do not want to take part. If the recruiter is a peer (as may be the case with student-led research), potential participants may also find it hard to refuse. In addition, if recruiting minority groups for a study (e.g. students with poorer scores or from specific ethnic groups), be sensitive as to how the participants are recruited and treated. Recruitment should always encompass respect, compassion, and cultural sensitivity [25]. See Chapter 7 for further discussion of these ethical considerations in recruitment.

Participant information

In Chapter 7, ethical issues around preparing information for participants will be discussed in detail. Here we discuss some of the basics of encouraging potential participants to engage in your study.

When preparing participant information sheets, it is also important to consider how to attract participants to your study and maximise your sample. Why should anyone participate? In addition to the clear information about the study, you should explain to participants why they might want to take part. For example, you might want to clearly outline the problem your study aims to tackle and why their contribution will be useful. When articulating your study title, you may also want to strike a balance between clarity about the research topics and something eye-catching, especially when you are studying busy health professionals or students. Some individuals may be motivated to participate to feel they are contributing to productive research, some because they wish to know the results of your study, or because they wish to hear the opinions of others in a focus group. Others may be encouraged by extrinsic incentives such as a certificate of participation for their professional development portfolio, complimentary refreshments or lunch, or a small monetary reward. While only a minority (8%) of clinical education studies recruiting trainees as participants offer tangible incentives, these do appear to be correlated with higher study quality and citation counts [26]. Expectations surrounding incentives to participate vary substantially across cultural contexts, so ensure you are in line with local expectations. In addition, remember that different incentives may cause different individuals to participate in your study and create sampling bias. For example, some participants may feel unable to justify participating if their travel costs and/or time is not reimbursed, whereas this may be unimportant for those in more affluent financial circumstances. Similarly, a $10 voucher might encourage participants who would not have completed a survey otherwise, however, they may not be motivated to complete it honestly.

Summary

This chapter has shared guidance on diverse approaches to sampling and recruitment, whilst encouraging you to think critically about the best decisions for your own study. Our main advice is to be clear about your research goal and use this goal to make decisions about sampling and recruitment. To avoid common pitfalls and flaws in your research, spend time thinking about sampling and recruitment before you start your study.

Top tips

- When deciding your sample, consider factors such as your research aim and paradigm, population of interest, type of data, and planned analysis methods. Your own time and resources are also important to consider.
- Look to published examples and seek advice from supervisors, peers, or collaborators who have worked within similar time and resource constraints.
- Demonstrate the worth and trustworthiness of your study to gatekeepers and other stakeholders, so they will help you to access participants. Time spent identifying and talking to individuals and organisations who may promote your study and invite participation is time well spent.
- Consider what could motivate people to volunteer for your study and make these benefits clear in the information you provide for participants.
- Describe your sampling strategy precisely and position your discussion appropriately. Do not claim generalisability or state sweeping implications if your sample is not representative of the whole population.

Common pitfalls

- Failing to clearly define the population of interest for your research. Specificity is key.
- Defaulting to convenience sampling without considering other options. The easiest option is not always the most appropriate.
- Inaction when recruitment is difficult and slow. Talk to supervisors or collaborators if you feel additional recruitment strategies may be required.
- Inadequate explanations of sampling size and methods when reporting studies. Readers need these details to judge the quality and implications of your research.

Ethical issues

- If your study is insufficiently powered, there is a risk of producing misleading results. Seek guidance from experienced researchers to ensure your research can make a valid contribution.
- Strike a balance between motivating participation and avoiding coercion. Consider whether incentives are appropriate and make the benefits of participating in your study clear.
- Reflect on power dynamics if recruiting participants from your own organisation. An administrative contact may be more appropriate for sending recruitment materials.

References

1 Thomas, I., Nicol, L., Regan, L. et al. (2014). Medical students driven to distraction. Improving patient safety teaching through the use of a simulated ward round experience: a prospective control study. *BMJ Quality and Safety*. https://doi.org/10.1136/bmjqs-2014-003272.

2 Cleland, J.A., Johnston, P., French, F.H., and Needham, G. (2012). Associations between medical school and career preferences in Year 1 medical students in Scotland. *Medical Education* 46: 473–484.

3 Husbands, A., Mathieson, A., Dowell, J. et al. (2014). Predictive validity of the UK clinical aptitude test in the final years of medical school: a prospective cohort study. *BMC Medical Education* 14: 88.

4 Cohen, J. (1988). *Statistical Power Analysis for the Behavioral Sciences*, 2e. Hillsdale, NJ: Lawrence Erlbaum Associates.

5 Stansfield, R.B. and Gruppen, L. (2022). Power analyses: planning, conducting and evaluating education

research. In: *Researching Medical Education*, 2e (ed. J. Cleland and S. Durning), 43–48. Oxford: Wiley.

6 Van Rijnsoever, F.J. (2017). (I can't get no) saturation: a simulation and guidelines for sample sizes in qualitative research. *PLoS One* 12 (7): e0181689.

7 Marshall, B., Cardon, P., Poddar, A., and Fontenot, R. (2013). Does sample size matter in qualitative research?: a review of qualitative interviews in IS research. *Journal of Computer Information Systems* 54 (1): 11–22.

8 Miles, M.B., Huberman, A.M., and Saldaña, J.M. (2013). *Qualitative Data Analysis: A Methods Sourcebook*, 3e. SAGE Publications.

9 Ng, S., Lingard, L., and Kennedy, T.J. (2014). Qualitative research in medical education: methodologies and methods. In: *Understanding Medical Education: Evidence, Theory and Practice*, 2e (ed. T. Swanwick), 371–384. Chichester: Wiley-Blackwell.

10 Creswell, J.W. (2002). *Educational Research: Planning, Conducting, and Evaluating Qualitative and Quantitative Research*. Upper Saddle River, NJ: Pearson Education.

11 Creswell, J.W. (1998). *Qualitative Inquiry and Research Design: Choosing Among Five Traditions*. Thousand Oaks, CA: SAGE Publications.

12 Patton, M.Q. (1990). *Qualitative Research and Education Methods*, 2e. Newbury Park, CA: SAGE Publications.

13 Omona, J. (2013). Sampling in qualitative research: improving the quality of research outcomes in higher education. *Makerere Journal of Higher Education* 4 (2): 169–185.

14 Sandelowski, M. (1995). Sample size in qualitative research. *Research in Nursing & Health* 18: 179–183.

15 Guest, G., Bunce, A., and Johnson, L. (2006). How many interviews are enough? An experiment with data saturation and variability. *Field Methods* 18: 59–82.

16 Vasileiou, K., Barnett, J., Thorpe, S., and Young, T. (2018). Characterising and justifying sample size sufficiency in interview-based studies: systematic analysis of qualitative health research over a 15-year period. *BMC Medical Research Methodology* 18 (1): 1–18.

17 Bryman, A. (2013). *Social Research Methods*, 3e. Oxford: Oxford University Press.

18 Dey, I. (1999). *Grounding Grounded Theory*. San Francisco, CA: Academic Press.

19 Braun, V. and Clarke, V. (2019). Reflecting on reflexive thematic analysis. *Qualitative Research in Sport, Exercise and Health* 11 (4): 589–597.

20 Malterud, K., Volkert, D.S., and Guassora, A.D. (2016). Sample size in qualitative interview studies: guided by information power. *Qualitative Health Research* 26 (13): 1753–1760.

21 Morgan, D.L. (1997). *Focus Groups as Qualitative Research. Qualitative Research Methods Series, 16.* Thousand Oaks, CA: SAGE Publications.

22 Morse, J.M. (1994). Designing funded qualitative research. In: *Handbook of Qualitative Research* (ed. N.K. Denzin and Y.S. Lincoln), 220–235. Thousand Oaks, CA: SAGE Publications.

23 Adams, T.E., Ellis, C., and Jones, S.H. (2017). Auto-ethnography. In: *The International Encyclopedia of Communication Research Methods*. (Eds. Matthes, J., Davis, C.S., and Potter, R.F.), Oxford: Wiley

24 King, N. and Horrocks, C. (2010). *Interviews in Qualitative Research*. London: SAGE Publications.

25 Savin-Baden, M. and Howell Major, C. (2013). *Qualitative Research: The Essential Guide to Theory and Practice*. Oxon: Routledge.

26 Stovel, R.G., Ginsburg, S., Stroud, L. et al. (2018). Incentives for recruiting trainee participants in medical education research. *Medical Teacher* 40 (2): 181–187.

7 Conducting ethical research

Anne-Marie Reid and Susan Jamieson

Learning objectives

By the end of this chapter, you should be able to:
- Explain the importance of an ethical approach to research.
- Distinguish between ethics and governance and explain why both are important.
- Recognise stages in the research process where ethics need to be considered.
- Identify typical requirements for ethical approval processes.
- Address common ethical dilemmas.

Introduction

This chapter will explain what is meant by ethics in research and why it is important to adopt an ethical approach. We will identify the differences between ethics and governance of research and outline why they are important considerations in any study. Many new researchers plan their studies and feel overwhelmed once they realise that gaining ethical approval is a precursor to data gathering in empirical research, and that it may be a time-consuming process. This chapter aims to demystify the ethical considerations, provide guidance on the type of documentation required, and support you in avoiding common pitfalls.

We start by providing an overview of the ethical principles underlying research, then give a brief historical perspective on their importance and place this in the context of clinical education. As different ethical concerns may arise at different stages in your study, we will consider these with reference to Tracy's framework [1]. This framework describes procedural ethics (gaining ethical approval from the relevant ethics committee), situational ethics (considerations regarding the type of research setting and participants involved), relational ethics (the relationship between the researcher and participants and how this might impact on the study) and exiting ethics (ending the relationship with participants and dissemination of findings). We will guide you through each of these stages towards good ethical conduct for the benefit of your future participants and the quality of your research.

By the end of the chapter, you should therefore not only feel more confident in meeting the requirements for gaining ethical approval, but more importantly, understand ethics as a consideration throughout the research process. The chapter will explore the value of adopting an ethical and reflexive approach to your studies and will signpost further sources of advice and support.

Ethical principles in research

Ethics concerns our moral behaviour and how this follows the rules by which we live as part of a society with other people. These rules are derived from deontology, which dictates whether actions are for good or for bad, as derived from the philosopher Kant [2]. When applied to research involving human participants, four key principles underpin this: beneficence, non-maleficence, respect for autonomy, and equity [3]. In essence, these can be summarised, respectively, as doing good, avoiding harm, respecting the independence of others, and treating all fairly, with consideration of individual characteristics such as age or disability. Principlism, the approach of applying the aforementioned four ethical principles, is common in healthcare and related research, though it has been subject to criticism [4] and alternative ethical frameworks exist [5]. Nevertheless, these four

---

Starting Research in Clinical Education, First Edition. Edited by Eliot L. Rees, Alison Ledger, and Kim A. Walker.
© 2024 The Association for the Study of Medical Education (ASME). Published 2024 by John Wiley & Sons Ltd.
Companion website: www.wiley.com/go/clinicaleducation

principles of ethical behaviour provide a useful framework for clinical education researchers to guide thinking and behaviour. To understand why these principles are important, and the circumstances under which they came to be fundamental to undertaking research with human participants, it is helpful to explain this within a historical context.

Brief historical perspective

The first recorded reference to ethical approaches in medicine is in the Hippocratic Oath (Hippocrates, fifth century BCE), whereby doctors are required to commit themselves to doing good for their patients, making patients their first concern, maintaining the upmost respect for life, and avoiding harm. Despite this, shocking examples of harmful research on humans without their voluntary consent and with the involvement of doctors in the process has come to light in recent times.

For example, Porton Down in the United Kingdom, a chemical warfare research installation, built in 1916, is known to have tested nerve gas agents on hundreds of military personnel without voluntary consent, causing illness and, in some cases, fatalities. Scientists and doctors were involved in this testing which continued over a number of decades. Similarly, under Nazism, the cruel and lethal experiments performed by doctors and scientists in the concentration camps came to light during the Nuremberg War Crimes trials following the second World War. The shock of discovering the role of doctors in this led to the Declaration of Geneva in 1948 (revised 2016 [6]), designed to guide the conduct of doctors, whilst the Nuremberg Code of 1947 was designed to set standards for medical research [7].

The Nuremberg Code first introduced the idea of gaining voluntary, informed consent for participation in medical research and emphasised that research should be undertaken for the good of society. The Declaration of Geneva was developed from this and is the oath now taken by doctors requiring them to put the patient's health and well-being first, respect the autonomy and dignity of patients, keep secrets disclosed by patients and maintain the utmost respect for human life.

Despite these important developments, research on humans in the absence of informed consent has continued to come to light. In the infamous 'Tuskegee experiment' in the United States (1932–1972), the Public Health service allowed syphilis in a poor, rural black population to progress untreated so that the development of the disease could be documented [8]. Other examples include the involvement of orphans in an experiment to investigate

diagnostic tests for tuberculin in an orphanage in the United States. This involved injecting tuberculin solution into various parts of the body, resulting in pain and suffering for many of the children and, in some cases, long-term damage [9].

Relevance to research in clinical education

These historical examples may seem far removed from the education research that you conduct or would like to undertake. Indeed, the need to gain ethical approval for research in clinical education is relatively recent and has required codes of practice developed more specifically for this purpose. These include codes developed by the American Educational Research Association [10], the British Educational Research Association [11], and the Netherlands Code of Conduct for Research Integrity [12].

The language of these codes is in line with the ethical principles outlined above and reinforces the importance of seeing ethical approval in research not as a 'hurdle to be surmounted' [13], but as a tool to guide your thinking and behaviour; from designing your study, through all stages of conducting your research, to exiting the study and disseminating the findings. The potential harm to participants in clinical education research may not be of the magnitude identified in the above historical examples, but clinical education research may still have a significant psychological impact on participants or risk wasting the time of clinicians and others participating in the research. Later in the chapter, we will signpost you to some case studies which illustrate these points.

The remainder of the chapter is presented in accordance with Tracy's framework [1], introducing procedural, situational, relational, and exiting ethics in turn (see Figure 7.1).

Procedural ethics

Procedural ethics is often at the forefront of new clinical education researchers' concerns. It involves gaining approval, that is, getting the 'go ahead' for your research based on documented assurances of how you will uphold ethical principles in protecting participants throughout the process. Gaining ethical approval may seem a hindrance that gets in the way of embarking on the exciting stage of data collection, but is justifying what you hope to achieve at an early stage in the process.

For research studies based on a university campus, or undertaken by a researcher completing a higher degree, local departmental Research Ethics

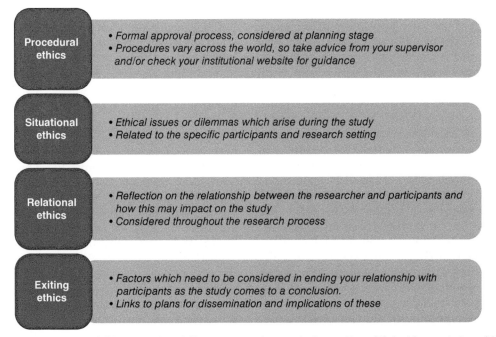

Figure 7.1 Aspects of Tracy's [1] framework at different stages of research. *Source*: Tracy [1] / with permission of SAGE Publications.

Committees (RECs) or Institutional Review Boards (IRBs) review applications based on submission of appropriate documentation. The documentation required, together with guidance on how to complete it, is normally available through links on the university website. In cases where healthcare settings such as hospitals or primary care clinics are the context for the research, advice needs to be sought on the specific approvals needed, and the documentation required.

In the United Kingdom, for example, where National Health Service (NHS) patients, staff, or premises are involved in research, approval has to be sought through the Health Research Authority (HRA) approval process [14]. Not all such cases of research will require ethical approval through an NHS research ethics committee, but in order to determine this, you are advised to check the HRA website for further guidance. Even where NHS ethical approval is not required for clinical education research, NHS 'R&D' (research-and-development) approval may be needed to fulfil governance requirements. Other countries may have equivalent regional or national arrangements.

Research governance refers to the standards of practice and structures in place at an organisational level to monitor and improve research and to ensure that the public is safeguarded. In a university, the work of the ethics committee is overseen through the governance structures at the university level, as

responsibility for breaches of ethical conduct ultimately lies with the organisation. One of the other areas relating to research governance concerns the legal requirements for the use of data provided by others and the assurances given on how this is protected. In the United Kingdom and elsewhere in Europe, this is determined through the General Data Protection Regulation [15] and similar legislation applies in other countries.

The relevant permissions, procedures involved, and the documentation required may vary to some extent according to the country you are in and the body responsible for overseeing research. Typical requirements for ethical approval and research governance purposes will be illustrated in the next section, with reference to the type of information which is normally required and the assurances which need to be given.

Documentation required
The ethics application will require the personal contact details of all the people undertaking and supervising the research. A summary of the study in accessible language is needed to allow a judgement to be made on any ethical issues arising from the study by people who are not experts in the field. Indeed, many ethics committees have patient/public representation to provide a sense-check on how a member of the public may view the research from the perspective of the potential for public good or

harm to participants. Justification is needed for the involvement of potential participants in the study, with special consideration given to anyone who may be deemed vulnerable, such as a young person under the age of 18 years, or a person who lacks capacity to give informed consent (e.g. individuals with intellectual disabilities or cognitive impairment). If your study is likely to involve such persons, then due consideration needs to be given as to how informed consent may be obtained, and it is advisable to seek early guidance from the appropriate ethics committee.

For participants to be able to provide informed consent, they need to understand the purpose of the study, why they have been chosen to participate, what they will be required to do, how long participation is likely to take, and any benefits or risks involved. This information is normally provided in a Participant Information Sheet which is given in advance to participants and allows them to seek any clarification before they decide whether or not to take part. Participants who consent will either sign a consent form which is kept as a record or give verbal consent which is recorded. The consent form requests permission for the data collection, storage of data, and use of data (in an anonymised form or otherwise) to inform the findings and dissemination through assessed work (e.g. dissertations or theses), research reports, presentations, or scholarly articles (see examples on companion website).

The ethics application form will ask for detail on your recruitment protocol, which should be designed to ensure that participants do not feel compelled to participate. Where possible, use a gatekeeper (a third party not directly involved with the research) to send out your recruitment email or flier. Removing the direct link between the researcher and potential participants reduces the likelihood of coercion. The ethics application form will also ask if the potential participants have any dependent relationship with the researcher(s). This may not seem relevant when you are a student conducting research with peers, but in fact it requires some consideration. For example, might there be some pressure for a peer to take part in your study due to an existing friendship? If so, this could be considered as coercion. If you are a more senior student and hoping to recruit participants from more junior years of your course then, again, you need to be careful that they do not feel under any pressure to participate. The same applies to members of staff wishing to recruit their students as participants. This is because there is a power dynamic involved in research relationships and this will be explored in more detail below. Dependent relationships are not

necessarily a barrier to gaining ethical approval, but the ethics committee will expect you to demonstrate you have given these due consideration and will implement strategies to mitigate against coercion, such as using a gatekeeper to recruit participants.

Considerations in procedural ethics

As you prepare the ethics application, you will need to anticipate potential ethical issues and consider how you might mitigate against these. Common ethical considerations are introduced below.

Explicit versus implicit consent

We have already mentioned the importance of gaining informed consent for data collection, but it is worth emphasising that you should always receive explicit informed consent. What we mean by this is that the participants should sign their name, or check a box, or give verbal agreement to the effect that they consent to a specific part of the research process. Indeed, consent forms may ask prospective participants to separately give their agreement to different aspects of the research; for example, a participant might agree to one form of data collection (an audio-recorded interview) but not another (a video-recorded interview). Sometimes researchers consider the return of completed paper surveys or submitted online surveys as implied consent, but this is not good ethical practice, because there can be no assumption that the consent is informed. We recommend that participants confirm their consent before starting a survey.

It is also key to remember that participants have the right to withdraw at any time, and this must be communicated clearly. However, in some circumstances, this may be limited to a specific duration, to compromise between respecting participants' autonomy and wasting resource (the researchers' time). For example, participants may be given two weeks to withdraw their data before analysis commences.

De-identifying data: ensuring confidentiality, maintaining privacy

Consistent with the principle of non-maleficence, it is important to ensure participants' confidentiality, that is, to ensure their privacy is protected. One aspect of this is de-identifying any data that is collected. One way of doing this is to anonymise the data; this means that the raw data cannot be linked back to any participant, whether via an identifying name or number; or via demographic data (age, qualifications, etc.) or specific references in direct quotations (which could make it possible to guess who participants are, particularly in small samples).

In this last case, specific names used by participants may need to be replaced by a generic term. For example, if a participant specifically identifies 'ward X' or 'Y medical school', these would be replaced with generic text such as 'a surgical ward' or 'an undergraduate medical school'.

Sometimes, it is important for you to be able to link data to the specific participants who provided it. For example, in quantitative research requiring correlations between different data sets, you would need to be able to link related data points (e.g. particular students' performance pre- and post-intervention). In a qualitative study involving interviews with trainees/residents on different placement rotations, you may want to ensure that you organise and analyse the data related to a specific rotation. In situations like these, each participant may be given a numerical identifier, such as P1 for 'participant 1'. If the research question requires the data to be sorted according to gender, for example, the identifier may include letters and numbers that help indicate participants self-identifying as female (F1, F2), male (M1, M2), unspecified (U1, U2), and so on. The list of identifiers given to individual participants is generally termed the code, or the key, and to ensure confidentiality it is often accessible by just a single individual on the research team.

Another method of de-identifying data, often used in qualitative research, is pseudonymisation, whereby the participant is given a fictitious name (pseudonym); a common technique is to assign pseudonyms beginning with each letter of the alphabet in turn. One issue worth considering is the possible need for a group pseudonym in certain contexts. In one of our resources on the companion website, a former master's student describes the issue she faced when studying the perceptions of different ethnic groups in relation to the hidden curriculum. Alumni of one ethnicity sometimes made statements about alumni of another ethnicity, and after consultation with experienced clinical education researchers about the best way to approach presenting the raw data, the decision was made to give each ethnic group a pseudonym, to avoid perpetuating stereotypes.

Online data collection

Ensure the confidentiality of participants during and following online data collection. Other areas requiring attention include conducting interviews in password-protected online 'venues' (institutionally approved meeting platforms), adopting methods for secure transfer or sharing of audio- and video files (e.g. a OneDrive account shared only by the research team), ensuring sufficient secure long-term storage space for audio- or video recordings, and checking ownership of data, since some software actually accords ownership to the manufacturer.

In the context of researching online forums, Roberts [16] discussed the status of posting online content and distinguishes between research participants whose confidentiality must be maintained, and authors, whose posts must be attributed. In an article provocatively entitled 'Fabrication as an ethical practice', Markham suggests the use of 'composite accounts' [17] to minimise inadvertent breach of confidentiality.

Data management

Since the advent of the GDPR [15] and similar data protection legislation, there may be a requirement in some contexts (e.g. the United Kingdom, EU) to provide participants with a privacy notice and to draw up a Data Protection Impact Assessment and a Data Management Plan. These documents encourage you to engage with the practicalities of ensuring confidentiality and the secure transfer, sharing, and storage of data. Whilst these are generally considered an aspect of research governance, there is clearly an overlap with ethical concerns, and ethics committees may require copies of these forms. Our advice is to contact your organisation's ethics committee or research governance office (or equivalent) to seek guidance about local requirements.

Guidance on compliance with ethical principles

Those new to clinical education research may sometimes be unsure how to explain the measures they are taking to ensure compliance with ethical principles. Some institutions have their own templates. See companion website for example wording which may help you to prepare your own ethics application form.

It is important to build in sufficient time for the application process since it takes several weeks or even months for your application to be reviewed. In our experience, it is not unusual for an ethics application form to require minor amendments, and this may add to the time before data collection can commence. However, as with revisions required for journal articles to be accepted, revisions required for ethics application forms potentially serve to make the research better quality.

Tracy makes clear that ethical research is not all about completing the application form for ethical approval before the study can take place (procedural ethics) [1]. Two types of ethical thinking that take place during the study are situational ethics and relational ethics.

Situational ethics

Situational ethics has otherwise been called micro-ethics [18] and refers to ethical issues or dilemmas that arise during the conduct of the research. Reid et al. [13] described several ethical dilemmas where the requirements of research projects potentially conflicted with their professional roles or responsibilities, whether as an academic, researcher, or clinician. For example, academics who were gatekeepers to student cohorts felt pressure to facilitate access to prospective research participants. In doctoral research on medical trainees' clinical decision-making, Smith occasionally had to step out of the researcher role, to provide clinical input for junior staff [13].

Insider research

If you are undertaking research projects with students or trainees in your own academic or healthcare context, you may face the particular challenge of undertaking insider research. This is the phenomenon whereby you are 'inside' the specific context, in the sense that you have privileged knowledge of that context. This does not mean to say that you necessarily work in the specific organisation in which the participants are based, but you may be a member of the same profession or general field. This brings advantages, such as knowing whom to approach for access to prospective research participants; or being able to more easily understand the language used by participants or their educational experiences. However, it also brings the possibility of bias, and it raises potential ethical issues.

When working within a post-positivist paradigm, you avoid bias by keeping yourself at a distance from the study and remaining objective to avoid influencing the outcomes. In a constructivist paradigm, where qualitative enquiry is undertaken as an insider researcher, it is important to question your own personal interests and the extent to which data gathering and interpretation may be influenced by these [19].

Relational ethics

Insider researchers must pay particular attention to relational ethics, which are ethical issues pertaining to the power relationship between researchers and participants. Walsh [20] argued that medical (and by extension other healthcare) students may be considered vulnerable in the sense that they may feel obliged to participate in research. Others question this, but identify that medical students who are invited to participate in research may experience undue influence [21], which is defined as 'offering an excessive reward to ensure compliance' [22]. Consistent with this, the British Educational Research Association and others advise against offering incentives to participants [11]. However, some researchers elect to give a token of appreciation; perhaps a voucher of low monetary value, believing this is not in itself enough to induce participation in a study. Stovel et al. [23] investigated the use of tangible incentives (money, monetary equivalents, or food) versus intangible incentives (non-measurable personal benefit, such as experiencing a novel educational intervention) in 215 medical education research articles from 2008. They found under-reporting of intangible incentives and advocated explicit reporting on these, as well as on tangible incentives.

The possibility for conflicts of interest is generally a domain in the ethics application form and the possibility of such conflicts must be anticipated and should be addressed in the study design, with specific measures in place to prevent coercion or undue influence. Commonly, to prevent (perceptions of) coercion, recruitment to a study is facilitated by an independent party who is not deemed to have power over the participants. Additionally, any funders supporting the research are identified for transparency.

It is worth remembering that coercion need not necessarily be teacher-to-student, or senior-to-junior; in addition to our earlier example of recruitment of peers for student-led research, another possible source of coercion in qualitative research is the use of snowball sampling (whereby initial participants recruit other potential participants). Snowball sampling can be a very useful method to identify individuals who may know about sensitive topics. For example, one of us supervised student projects that involved students exploring perceptions of cheating amongst peers. Snowball sampling proved to be a useful way of identifying participants when initial recruitment to the study was low, bearing in mind avoidance of coercion in the process. Use of snowball sampling illustrates the tension that may exist between ethical research conduct and pragmatic methodological decisions, especially in high-stakes situations such as master's or doctoral projects, or time-limited funded research.

External stakeholders

Another aspect of relational ethics is the existence of external stakeholders in the research setting. For example, where clinical education research is carried out in a clinical environment, we need to consider stakeholders such as patients, carers, family members, and members of various health professions, any or all of whom could be present. The notion of external stakeholders also relates back to situational ethics. This was exemplified by Smith (in Reid et al.) mentioned earlier in the chapter. As a Specialty Registrar in Trauma and Orthopaedics conducting a study with junior doctors for her PhD, she found that as a more senior clinician she had to step out of her researcher role at times to prioritise support for junior colleagues where patient safety was at risk [13].

One interesting ethical issue is whether consent should be required from patients who are present in the clinical setting, when they are not active participants in the research. Two opposing perspectives are proposed by a Canadian and a British research group conducting education research in their respective clinical settings. In each case, the relevant ethics review boards considered that as the focus was on teaching and learning, consent was not required from patients. Piquette et al. agreed that as patients were not the primary focus of their ethnographic study their consent was not required [24]. In contrast, Bezemer et al. felt the team should nevertheless obtain consent from patients present in the setting at the time [25]. In all cases, local advice needs to be sought.

What can help you to acknowledge situational and relational ethics? One answer is that you should employ reflexivity and be explicit about this when writing up the work [13]. Reflexivity refers to the impact that the researcher has on the research, and vice versa. For example, you might reflect on any impact you may have had on recruitment and how you mitigated against this. For more on reflexivity, see Chapters 3 and 14.

Exiting ethics and beyond

Ethical conduct of research continues after the research data has been collected and analysed. You also need to adhere to exiting ethics [1], which refers to ethical considerations as you end the study and seek to disseminate your work. Considerations include: responsibilities to participants, responsibilities concerning the data, and various considerations surrounding dissemination.

Exiting responsibilities

Your responsibilities to participants include ensuring that their anonymity/pseudonymity, confidentiality, and privacy continue to be upheld, consistent with the ethical approval obtained and with data protection legislation in your context; and that you provide participants with a summary of your findings where you have undertaken to do so. You may

also have an obligation to provide a summary of your findings to the ethics committee. Regarding data, you have a responsibility to store the data securely for the duration specified by your institution and/or relevant legislation. In the case of UK universities, this can be for up to 10 years. Often a project is undertaken in one context but also must comply with ethical requirements in another context (e.g. when a master's student conducts research in their local context but must also gain approval of the university that will accredit their degree). In this case, if the two institutions specify different durations for data storage, we advise storing data for the longer duration.

Ethics surrounding dissemination

Key ethical considerations when exiting the study relate to dissemination of research. Here, we simply touch on these issues since they are discussed further in Chapters 27–29. However, it is worth remembering that ethics around dissemination apply to other forms of dissemination, including conference presentations or workshops. Although the International Committee of Medical Journal Editors (ICMJE) has specified criteria for authorship [26], the topic is still one of concern [27, 28]. Six main issues to consider are honorary or gift authorship, ghost authorship, authorship order, 'salami slicing', plagiarism, and cultural perspectives on authorship.

Honorary or gift authorship is where someone who does not meet the criteria for authorship [26] is nevertheless included as an author. Ghost authorship is the converse situation, where someone who does merit inclusion as an author is omitted [26]. Authorship order [29] is an ethical issue because in specific disciplines the order in which your name is placed implies the size of contribution; moreover, since citations may only refer to the first (or first three) authors, order of authorship may impact an individual's research profile. If you are a new clinical education researcher, authorship order may be a difficult topic to raise, but we encourage having these conversations early in the research process. Salami slicing refers to multiple publications from essentially the same data, which inflates the publication record of the authors concerned, and also the number of publications on the topic. (Note that it is acceptable to publish aspects of the same study separately, such as the quantitative and qualitative findings from a larger-scale study.) Plagiarism is the use of another author's work without proper attribution. The principle of attributing source material applies to text, images, and other formats. In many contexts, plagiarism is regarded as research and/or academic misconduct, and it is taken seriously by professional bodies and regulators. It is popularly held that plagiarism represents a western cultural perspective, whereas in other cultures, it is regarded as good practice to reiterate the words of an authority. However, Simon has queried whether this is a stereotype [30]. Further ethical issues surrounding dissemination include minimising publication bias, by avoidance of 'salami-slicing' and by publication of 'negative' findings (results that do not agree with an initial hypothesis). Finally, where possible you should facilitate open access, making the full text of your publication freely available on the web, without infringing copyright. The librarian or Research Governance team in your organisation will be best placed to advise you about open-access possibilities.

Summary

Clinical education research should be conducted in an ethical manner throughout the research process. Ethical research includes paying attention to procedural, situational, relational, and exiting ethics. For clinical education researchers, it means applying the familiar ethical principles of beneficence, non-maleficence, respect for autonomy, and equity to research in a non-clinical, educational setting; or to education situations within the clinical setting. Through awareness of possible ethical issues, the design of research and completion of the ethical application form can be carried out in such a way as to anticipate and mitigate against ethical issues during the research study and beyond. This will take time in the short term, but ultimately this will develop your research practice and support the production of quality research.

Top tips

- Start thinking about potential ethical issues and ethics requirements as soon as you start to plan your study.
- Seek advice from supervisors and your local research ethics committee or institutional review board.
- Recognise the ethical review application as an opportunity to think through the whole research process. Early, detailed ethical considerations will alert you to any design flaws and save your time in the long term.
- Think carefully about how you will manage role conflict, for example, conducting interviews with fellow students. It may be useful to remind the participant that you are in your researcher role and may ask questions to which they may think you already know the answer.

Common pitfalls

- Being too prescriptive about your participants and study methods in your ethical review documentation. If you have problems recruiting by your chosen method, it is helpful to have a Plan B, which is included in your ethics form.
- Providing slightly different versions on different parts of ethical review documentation and recruitment materials. Read over carefully to ensure consistency.
- Specifying fieldwork dates on ethical applications that do not allow for potential delays. Indicate dates that allow sufficient time for the approval process to be completed and for unexpected research problems.
- Using personal contacts when your recruitment strategy is not working. Discuss alternative strategies with your supervisor/collaborators and submit an amendment to your ethics application if needed, to minimise the risk of coercion.

References

1 Tracy, S.J. (2010). Qualitative quality: eight "big-tent" criteria for excellent qualitative research. *Qualitative Inquiry* 16 (10): 837–851.

2 Solomon, R.C. (2005). *Introducing Philosophy*, 8e, 7. New York: Oxford University Press.

3 Beauchamp, T. and Childress, J. (1985). *Principles of Biomedical Ethics*, 4e. Oxford: Oxford University Press.

4 Hammersley, M. (2015). On ethical principles for social research. *International Journal of Social Research Methodology* 18 (4): 433–449.

5 Eikelboom, J.I., Ten Cate, O.T., Jaarsma, D. et al. (2012). A framework for the ethics review of education research. *Medical Education* 46 (8): 731–733.

6 World Medical Association (2017). WMA declaration of Geneva. https://www.wma.net/policies-post/wma-declaration-of-geneva (accessed 2 May 2023).

7 British Medical Journal (1996). The Nuremberg code (1947). *British Medical Journal* 313 (7070). https://www.bmj.com/content/313/7070/1448.1

8 McVean, A. (2019). *40 Years of Human Experimentation in America: The Tuskegee Study*. Office for Science and Society 30 December 2020. https://www.mcgill.ca/oss/article/history/40-years-human-experimentation-america-tuskegee-study.

9 Lederer, S. and Davis, A.B. (1995). Subjected to science: human experimentation in America before the Second World War. *History: Reviews of New Books* 24 (1): 13.

10 American Educational Research Association (2011). AERA code of ethics: American Educational Research

Association approved by the AERA Council February 2011. *Educational Researcher* 40 (3): 145–156.

11 British Educational Research Association (2018). *Ethical Guidelines for Educational Research*, 4e. London: BERA.

12 KNAW; NFU; NWO; TO2-federatie; Vereniging Hogescholen; VSNU, Nederlandse gedragscode wetenschappelijke integriteit. DANS 2018.

13 Reid, A.M., Brown, J.M., Smith, J.M. et al. (2018). Ethical dilemmas and reflexivity in qualitative research. *Perspectives on Medical Education* 7 (2): 69–75.

14 Health Research Authority (2020). Accessing study support and advice services. https://www.hra.nhs.uk/planning-and-improving-research/research-planning/access-study-support-advice-services (accessed 6 May 2023).

15 UK Government (2018). Data Protection Act. www.legislation.gov.uk/ukpga/2018/12/contents/enacted (accessed 6 May 2023).

16 Roberts, L.D. (2015). Ethical issues in conducting qualitative research in online communities. *Qualitative Research in Psychology* 12 (3): 314–325.

17 Markham, A. (2012). Fabrication as ethical practice: qualitative inquiry in ambiguous internet contexts. *Information, Communication & Society* 15 (3): 334–353.

18 Guillemin, M. and Gillam, L. (2004). Ethics, reflexivity, and "ethically important moments" in research. *Qualitative Inquiry* 10 (2): 261–280.

19 Varpio, L., O'Brien, B., Rees, C.E. et al. (2021). The applicability of generalisability and bias to health professions education's research. *Medical Education* 55 (2): 167–173.

20 Walsh, K. (2014). Medical education research: is participation fair? *Perspectives on Medical Education* 3 (5): 379–382.

21 van den Broek, W.S., Wouters, R.H., and van Delden, J.H. (2015). In response to 'medical education research: is participation fair?'. *Perspectives on Medical Education* 4 (3): 158–159.

22 Bartholomay, E.M. and Sifers, S.K. (2016). Student perception of pressure in faculty-led research. *Learning and Individual Differences* 50: 302–307.

23 Stovel, R.G., Ginsburg, S., Stroud, L. et al. (2018). Incentives for recruiting trainee participants in medical education research. *Medical Teacher* 40 (2): 181–187.

24 Piquette, D., Moulton, C.A., and LeBlanc, V.R. (2015). Balancing care and teaching during clinical activities: 2 contexts, 2 strategies. *Journal of Critical Care* 30 (4): 678–684.

25 Bezemer, J., Cope, A., Kress, G., and Kneebone, R. (2014). Holding the scalpel: achieving surgical care in a learning environment. *Journal of Contemporary Ethnography* 43 (1): 38–63.

26 International Committee of Medical Journal Editors. (2019). Recommendations for the conduct, reporting, editing, and publication of scholarly work in medical journals. http://www.icmje.org/recommendations (accessed 6 May 2023).

27 Artino, A.R. Jr., Driessen, E.W., and Maggio, L.A. (2019). Ethical shades of gray: international frequency of scientific misconduct and questionable research practices in health professions education. *Academic Medicine: Journal of the Association of American Medical Colleges* 94 (1): 76–84.

28 Ten Cate, O. (2022). The ethics of health professions education research: protecting the integrity of science, research subjects, and authorship. *Academic Medicine: Journal of the Association of American Medical Colleges* 97 (1): 13–17..

29 Maggio, L.A., Artino, A.R. Jr., Watling, C.J. et al. (2019). Exploring researchers' perspectives on authorship decision making. *Medical Education* 53 (12): 1253–1262.

30 Simon, D.J. (2019). Cross-cultural differences in plagiarism: fact or fiction. *Duquesne Law Review* 57: 73.

PART II

Evidence synthesis and mixed methods

Eliot L. Rees

This part of the book discusses evidence syntheses (types of literature reviews) and mixed methods research. These have been grouped together because both draw on a broad range of primary data collection methods (many of which are discussed in Parts III and IV).

Chapters 8 and 9 discuss evidence syntheses. Evidence syntheses have become extremely popular in clinical education research. With the enormous wealth of primary research published each year, robust reviews which aggregate and synthesise the findings are valuable to both educators and researchers. There are a number of potential advantages for you doing a high-quality evidence synthesis project as well:

- They give you an opportunity to claim a stake to a topic you might then do further primary research on.
- You will become intimately familiar with the literature on the topic and will therefore be able to identify the areas most ripe for future research.
- Evidence syntheses are often desirable to journals, in part because they usually become highly cited.
- You will develop skills in reviewing and critically appraising research.
- You do not usually need ethical approval, so if you are on a tight timeline this may be helpful.
- You do not need to rely on recruiting participants to your study which can sometimes be challenging.

Chapter 8 introduces evidence synthesis and discusses a range of different review types and how to pick one that aligns with your research question. This chapter explores how different review types can involve different approaches to data synthesis. Chapter 9 then talks through the different stages common to each review to enable you to develop a robust review protocol. Chapter 10 discusses realist research, which is a newer approach in clinical education which focuses on the relationship between context, mechanisms, and outcomes in educational interventions. This can be used for both secondary research (realist syntheses) and primary research (realist evaluations).

This part then moves on to consider mixed methods research. Chapter 11 introduces mixed methods research in general and discusses a range of approaches and when they might be suitable. The last two chapters in this part then offer two types of research that lend themselves well to mixed methods. Chapter 12 describes action research, which can be used when making transformative changes to education programmes and undertaking critical reflection. Chapter 13 introduces online data collection which can use a range of social media and novel online tools to harvest a variety of data for research.

Within this part you will find guidance on how to resolve the philosophical tensions of using both qualitative and quantitative methods in your research. Consider how your methods align with your beliefs and the types of knowledge you aim to produce with your research project. Thoughtful planning will mean that the sum of the project is greater than its constituent parts.

Starting Research in Clinical Education, First Edition. Edited by Eliot L. Rees, Alison Ledger, and Kim A. Walker.
© 2024 The Association for the Study of Medical Education (ASME). Published 2024 by John Wiley & Sons Ltd.
Companion website: www.wiley.com/go/clinicaleducation

8 Evidence syntheses: choosing an approach

Catherine M. Giroux, Susanne Mak, Rebecca Ataman, and Aliki Thomas

---

Learning objectives

By the end of this chapter, you should be able to:
- Define the term *evidence synthesis*.
- Identify common approaches to evidence synthesis used in clinical education.
- Select the appropriate evidence synthesis approach for addressing your research question.

Introduction

In this chapter, we define and describe the characteristics of evidence syntheses within the context of clinical education research. Specifically, we address the questions of what evidence syntheses are, why we use them, and when each approach is appropriate. Whilst numerous methods of evidence synthesis exist (e.g. meta-syntheses, meta-ethnographies, integrative reviews), this chapter will focus on those commonly used in clinical education, notably systematic reviews, scoping reviews, realist reviews, umbrella reviews, and narrative reviews [1, 2]. For more resources and information on conducting reviews including those not discussed in this chapter, please refer to the suggested references we have provided under the 'Further Reading' section.

What are evidence syntheses?

Evidence syntheses are reviews of the extant body of literature [1]. They consist of integrating the findings of individual studies and contextualising these findings within the larger body of knowledge on the subject [3]. Numerous approaches to synthesising evidence exist; systematic reviews may help to identify 'what' innovations work, while methods like realist reviews can provide a deeper understanding of why something works, for whom, and under what circumstances [2, 4]. The results of evidence syntheses are mainly used to contribute to the evidence base for implementing curricular innovations and can inform teaching, assessment, and policy decisions in clinical education [1, 5].

Evidence syntheses have become increasingly popular in clinical education research with an average of 46 reviews published annually between 1999 and 2019 and an increase of 2620% in the total number of reviews published during the same period [6]. It is not a new research method. Indeed, early examples date back to the 1900s; by the 1960s, they were commonly conducted in the social sciences, education, and psychology [7, 8]. In 1999, the Best Evidence in Medical Education (BEME) collaboration was established to facilitate syntheses that were inclusive of the study aims, designs, and outcomes unique to medical education research [9]. Notably, BEME aims to synthesise the available evidence into formats that can enable curriculum planners to make decisions about teaching and learning [10]. In clinical education especially, the focus on 'whether' education is effective often overlooks other useful questions such as 'how', 'why', 'when', and 'what' [11]. Thus, whilst early syntheses in clinical education consisted predominantly of systematic reviews, contemporary reviews (i.e. scoping reviews, realist reviews) increasingly address these more diverse research questions and educational contexts [6, 12].

Evidence syntheses in clinical education

Evidence syntheses can be used to guide practice, inform future reviews (i.e. one reason to conduct a scoping review is as a precursor to a systematic review)

Starting Research in Clinical Education, First Edition. Edited by Eliot L. Rees, Alison Ledger, and Kim A. Walker.
© 2024 The Association for the Study of Medical Education (ASME). Published 2024 by John Wiley & Sons Ltd.
Companion website: www.wiley.com/go/clinicaleducation

and subsequent empirical research, identify gaps, and map historical publication practices [13]. They can be a useful way for people doing research degrees to understand the topic area, identify research gaps, and justify the need for their research. A current evidence synthesis can also support a competitive funding proposal, through identifying research gaps and establishing a need for the proposed study. Still, they are not easy. They are not something that can be done on the 'side' and should not be mistaken for a simple course assignment. Systematic reviews, for example, are reported to take an average of 67.3 weeks to complete and publish, involve approximately five team members, including a librarian or information specialist, subject-matter experts, and synthesis methodologists [8, 14].

If you are interested in conducting an evidence synthesis, there are several features, potential benefits, and challenges you should consider. The underlying assumptions regarding the nature of knowledge are a key aspect that may set one approach apart from another [1, 12]. For example, quantitative systematic reviews are rooted in *post-positivism* (i.e. knowledge is external to the individual and can be verified through observation) whilst narrative reviews can be *constructivist* in nature, meaning that knowledge is viewed as being socially constructed [1]. Your stance about what constitutes knowledge influences the review question, the methodology you select (e.g. choosing whether a systematic or narrative review approach is most appropriate to address the review question), how you interpret data, and how the findings are transferred to other contexts [15, 16]. For these reasons, it is helpful to reflect on your team's composition and perspectives (i.e. positionality). Review teams are required to make decisions about what populations and languages to include in the review and what data to extract. These decisions will be explored in greater detail in Chapter 9. Inviting a diverse group of team members, including those most likely to benefit from – or be interested in – the results (i.e. stakeholders), can promote a greater richness of perspectives [5] (see Chapter 5).

Evidence syntheses allow clinical educators to shift from relying solely on experience-based opinion to considering and integrating the best available evidence into their educational practices [6]. Syntheses are central to knowledge translation and may contribute to bridging the gap between research and decision-making, especially in applied fields like clinical education [7, 13]. According to the Canadian Institutes of Health Research, knowledge translation is 'a dynamic and iterative process that includes the synthesis, dissemination, exchange,

and ethically-sound application of knowledge'. Syntheses provide the evidence base for other knowledge translation tools and products that support patient care such as policy briefs, patient decision aids, and clinical practice guidelines [7].

In the following sections, we provide an overview of common approaches to evidence synthesis. Specifically, we operationally define and provide an overview of why and for what purposes clinical education researchers should use each approach. Additionally, Table 8.1 and Box 8.1 demonstrate how different review types can align with different questions related to the topic of using online learning in clinical education.

Overview of evidence synthesis approaches

Systematic reviews

Systematic reviews are increasingly common and can be undertaken to determine whether current practices are informed by evidence [24]. Their focus on efficacy or effectiveness is valuable for ascertaining the potential impact of an intervention on a given outcome; however, it can create challenges for clinical education which often requires a broader contextual exploration of what works, for whom, and in what circumstances [10, 25]. Typically, systematic reviews help to inform decision-making, healthcare or educational delivery, and policy development [1, 24, 26]. They can directly inform – and even overturn – existing teaching and assessment practices based on the results of their effectiveness [27]. For example, in early 2020, Dedeilia et al. conducted a systematic review with the goal of identifying existing challenges for medical and surgical education due to the COVID-19 pandemic; they sought to establish educational methods that could effectively ensure educational continuity for medical students and junior physicians [28].

Systematic reviews are 'a review of a clearly formulated question that uses systematic and explicit methods to identify, select, and critically appraise relevant research, and to collect and analyse data from the studies that are included' [1, 3]. They include a clearly articulated and focused question, defined inclusion and exclusion criteria, a comprehensive search strategy, a systematic screening and selection process, an appraisal of study quality, and an analysis and synthesis of the extracted data [1, 3, 7, 24]. The specific analysis method chosen depends on the question(s) being asked but includes three main types, quantitative, qualitative, or mixed methods approaches [1, 3, 7].

Table 8.1 Comparison of evidence synthesis approaches

	Quantitative systematic reviews and meta-analyses	Qualitative or mixed methods systematic reviews	Scoping reviews	Umbrella reviews	Narrative reviews	Realist reviews
Potential research question	How effective is online learning compared to face-to-face learning in clinical education?	How and why is online learning an effective intervention compared to face-to-face learning in clinical education?	What is known about the ways in which online learning is delivered in clinical education?	How effective is online learning compared to face-to-face learning across educational research?	What are the benefits and challenges of using online learning in clinical education, as reported in existing published literature?	Why, how, in what contexts, for whom, and to what extent does online learning support clinical education?
Search type	Comprehensive	Comprehensive	Comprehensive	Comprehensive	Generally not comprehensive	Purposive, to reach theoretical saturation
Epistemology (i.e. how each review type views the nature of knowledge)	Knowledge is viewed as external to the individual (post-positivist)	Varies (may be post-positivist or constructivist) Knowledge may also be seen as *pragmatic*, meaning it is acquired through action and reflection, thus allowing researchers the use of multiple paradigms and methods to answer the research question [17]	Knowledge is typically viewed as being socially constructed (constructivist)	Knowledge is viewed as external to the individual (post-positivist)	Varies (can be post-positivist or constructivist)	Knowledge (generative causal explanations including context, mechanisms, and outcomes) is viewed as being incomplete but can be continuously improved (Pawson and Tilley's Realism)
Critical appraisal	Required	Required	Not required	Required	Not required	Not required
Team members	Generally multiple authors, including content experts, methodologists, and information specialists (i.e. librarians)	Generally multiple authors, including content experts, methodologists, and information specialists (i.e. librarians)	Generally multiple authors, including content experts, methodologists, information specialists (i.e. librarians), and community stakeholders	Generally multiple authors, including content experts, methodologists, and information specialists (i.e. librarians)	May be single author (i.e. expert in the field) but generally multiple authors	Generally multiple authors, including content experts, methodologists, information specialists (i.e. librarians), and community stakeholders
Reporting guidelines	PRISMA	PRISMA	PRISMA-ScR	Unavailable	Unavailable	RAMESES
Example articles in clinical education	[18]	[19]	[20]	[21]	[22]	[23]

BOX 8.1   Case study

Simon is a first year PhD student studying clinical education. He is in the process of deciding what his doctoral research will look like. Simon's experience of taking online classes has given him an appreciation for the benefits and challenges of online learning, sparking his interest in exploring the evidence associated with online learning in clinical education. Simon knows he likes working with literature and figures that conducting an evidence synthesis may be a good option for at least one of his studies.

Simon's PhD supervisor encourages him to start thinking about the research question for his study since this will inform his choice of evidence synthesis. Simon is not certain where to start but being the keen and analytical researcher that he is, he sits down and maps out several common synthesis approaches used in clinical education research and appropriate research questions that he could explore. Table 8.1 highlights Simon's comparison chart.

Simon plans to bring his comparison table to his next meeting with his PhD supervisor, where he intends to discuss the benefits and challenges of each approach in the context of his project. He also wants to get his supervisor's feedback to determine which questions (and thus, which evidence synthesis method or approach) will provide answers that will best advance scientific knowledge of online learning and provide meaningful, practical guidance to educators, curriculum designers, and other stakeholders. Simon knows that once he selects a research question and review design, he will need to invite team members to join his review. He will also need to check what reviews have already been published on his topic. He would like both methodological and content expert support and would also like to include a librarian with expertise in evidence syntheses to help develop and refine his searches. Simon thinks it might be helpful to talk with other PhD students who have completed evidence syntheses to learn more about the approaches they used and the methodological support they required. He looks forward to discussing his questions and ideas with his supervisor and starting to develop his review protocol.

Quantitative systematic reviews

Quantitative systematic reviews may be what you typically think of when you hear the term 'evidence synthesis'. They combine and compare the results of experimental research to draw conclusions about the efficacy or effectiveness of an intervention and usually include quantitative data like odds ratios [7]. Quantitative or mixed method systematic reviews can include a meta-analysis component. Meta-analysis refers to the use of statistical techniques to integrate the results of included studies [1, 7]. For example, Pei and Wu [18] conducted a systematic review and meta-analysis to explore whether online learning works better than in-person or face-to-face learning in undergraduate medical education. They drew on the Participants, Interventions, Comparisons, Outcomes (PICO) format to inform their inclusion criteria, thereby ensuring they were including similar studies that could be compared quantitatively. The authors evaluated the quality of the included studies using the Medical Education Research Study Quality Instrument (MERSQI) and quantitatively synthesised the findings from each study using statistics [29].

Systematic reviews using meta-analysis are often considered high level evidence since they draw on randomised controlled trials, which are seen to limit bias [24, 25]. However, this approach is not necessarily compatible with applied clinical education research. The controlled experiments that are necessary for meta-analysis can be challenging to conduct in educational contexts (i.e. it can be difficult to double blind researchers and participants) and can become ethically problematic in the case of withholding educational interventions, like specific academic accommodations or instructional content, from some learners [1, 10, 25]. Furthermore, even when controlled experiments exist, the wide variation in results often seen in clinical education can make it challenging to synthesise these studies using meta-analysis [25].

Organisations like the Cochrane and Campbell Collaborations and the Joanna Briggs Institute provide helpful guidance on how to plan, conduct, and report the findings of systematic reviews. As an example, the Cochrane Collaboration offers a handbook for researchers interested in conducting systematic reviews that outlines each step of the process whilst the Joanna Briggs Institute provides specific training courses and manuals for conducting evidence syntheses (see 'Further Reading' section). Still, it may prove difficult to rely on such guidelines, which are intended for biomedical research, since they privilege certain ways of knowing (e.g. controlled experiments) over others that are also prevalent in clinical education (e.g. qualitative or observational research) [30].

Qualitative systematic reviews

In contrast to the focus on efficacy and effectiveness in quantitative systematic reviews, qualitative systematic reviews focus on analysing human experiences and cultural and social phenomena [24, 26]. They can be important for exploring or explaining why interventions are (or are not) effective from the perspectives of the participants involved [24]. Qualitative research can help to generate evidence that explores practices and motivations, increases understanding of behaviour, develops interventions, provides insights into student or patient experiences, and can enhance our understanding of organisational and culture change [31]. These reviews summarise the findings of qualitative studies, often focusing on 'how' and 'why' questions; expert researchers interpret the findings to represent the meanings of the collected work and portray an interpretation of the phenomenon under study, recognising that no two researchers will have exactly the same interpretation [4, 31]. Thus, this process requires you to critically explore your subjectivity [4] (reflexivity, see Chapter 3).

In these reviews, you can aggregate the findings of included studies using qualitative research techniques [31]. This process was used in Carroll et al. [19] qualitative systematic review that aimed to explore UK healthcare professionals' experience of online learning. They identified clear inclusion criteria (i.e. study sample must consist of formally employed health professionals engaged in e-learning, with student experience recorded as an outcome). The authors appraised the quality of the included studies using the consolidated criteria for reporting qualitative research (COREQ), which is a 32-item checklist for reporting interviews and focus groups [32]. Finally, they used thematic analysis to generate a new thematic framework to describe and explain health professionals' experiences of online learning.

Mixed methods systematic reviews

Taking a mixed methods approach to systematic reviews allows you to combine the findings of quantitative intervention or effectiveness studies with qualitative studies that explore or seek to better understand phenomena or experiences [33, 34]. Since this can result in evidence that enhances or extends a uniquely qualitative or quantitative approach [3], mixed methods systematic reviews are helpful for holistically informing clinical, policy, and organisational decisions [33].

Mixed methods systematic reviews follow the same process as other systematic review types in terms of design, but they draw from mixed methods research approaches to integrate, analyse, and interpret the data from both quantitative and qualitative research [2, 33]. For example, McCutcheon et al. [35] undertook a mixed methods systematic review to explore the impact of both online and blended learning vs. face-to-face learning of clinical skills of undergraduate nursing students. They included experimental design studies (e.g. randomised controlled trials), observational studies, cohort studies, and surveys; they also included qualitative studies (e.g. case reports, action research) that described nursing students' perceptions on the impact or effect of online learning. The quality of both quantitative and qualitative studies was appraised using tools identified by the Joanna Briggs Institute (JBI-Meta-Analysis of Statistics Assessment and Review Instrument & JBI-Qualitative Assessment and Review Instrument) and analysed the findings using a narrative synthesis approach.

Scoping review

Scoping reviews are a form of evidence synthesis commonly used to map the breadth and depth of the existing information on a concept, topic, or field of study [36–38]. This methodology affords flexibility, enabling the research team to revisit and revise inclusion criteria using an iterative approach [15, 36, 38]. Their broad nature allows the research team to include diverse literature, extending beyond peer-reviewed articles. Consequently, scoping reviews can include non-peer reviewed literature such as position papers, websites, and unpublished dissertations, providing an extensive map of what has been previously studied and discussed [15, 36].

Scoping reviews are well-suited for subjects where there is sufficient and potentially diverse literature [39]. They may also be useful for lesser-known topics that are emerging in the literature [36, 39]. In all instances, these reviews aim to map what has been written – specifically relating to project scope, what has been learned previously, and possible future areas of scholarship [36, 39]. An interpretative lens is also needed when conducting scoping reviews: the research team must engage in reflexivity to produce nuanced findings that encompass both convergences and divergences of the included data [15, 39]. Several reasons for conducting a scoping review exist beyond mapping and describing the extant literature. These reasons may include: (1) determining primary concepts and definitions, (2) identifying the main characteristics of a concept, (3) pinpointing gaps in the existing evidence, (4) developing an understanding of how research was conducted on a topic, and (5) as a precursor to conducting a systematic review [36, 37].

Different stakeholder groups can drive scoping reviews, such as researchers who identify a knowledge gap or educators who have expressed a need for greater understanding on a topic. For instance, leaders of clinical education programmes may wish to conduct a scoping review to identify what programme aspects contribute to professional identity formation in rehabilitation professionals. Mak et al. mapped the literature on professional identity and professional identity formation in occupational therapy, physical therapy, and speech-language pathology. The findings of this review shed light on the descriptions and definitions of these concepts, their possible influences, and gaps in the literature with respect to the role of symbols and rituals in the professional identity formation of these rehabilitation professionals [40].

Realist reviews

Realist reviews are designed to synthesise the literature on why (i.e. mechanisms) and in what circumstances (i.e. context) an intervention works (i.e. outcome) [41]. Context refers to any feature of the physical or social environment that can trigger a mechanism. A mechanism, such as a decision-making process is a context-sensitive process that causes an intervention to work. An outcome can be any measure of intervention success or failure – intended or unintended, long- or short-term [41–43]. We can see context, mechanisms, and outcomes illustrated by Price and colleagues' explanation of how remediation programmes for practising doctors restore patient safety. In this example, the context included a doctor understanding the consequences of not changing their behaviour or improving their performance. This understanding triggered the mechanism, which consisted of the doctor evaluating the costs and benefits of the behaviour change. The result of this context and mechanism led to the doctor having the motivation to engage with remediation or change their goal [44].

Realist reviews are used when researchers wish to understand how, why, for whom, and in which contexts interventions work. They are appropriate when:

- Evidence for an intervention is available from diverse settings (e.g. from both high- and low-income country contexts) indicating diverse outcomes (e.g. showing that student self-efficacy varies by country income level), but why and how differences exist are poorly understood.
- Trying to understand intervention challenges (e.g. reviewing the literature to understand how to improve the delivery of an intervention).

- Stakeholders request the development of context-specific recommendations to improve an intervention.

In addition to containing context, mechanisms, and outcomes, the basic realist review question formula may also include the questions 'for whom', 'for what duration' and 'to what extent', amongst others [45].

The ultimate goal of a realist review is to generate causal explanations by linking together context, mechanisms, and outcomes into context-mechanism-outcome-configurations (CMOCs). These causal explanations are organised into a programme theory [41]. Since researchers must develop and refine a programme theory in this review type, realist reviews are considered to be 'theory-driven'. Not only can a programme theory advance our understanding of how an intervention works, but it can provide explicit recommendations to optimise the delivery of the intervention [41, 46]. Specifically, it can inform educators as to the expected outcomes given the use of an educational intervention in a certain context, as well as how that intervention can be expected to work.

Narrative reviews

Narrative reviews provide a summary of the existing published literature on a topic shaped by the perspective of the research team that conducted the review [1, 47, 48]. They have been described as 'simplistic', since the aim of conducting such a review is to determine what has been written about a subject without attempting to generalise its findings or add to the existing body of literature on the given topic [49]. Conversely, narrative reviews can also be seen as scholarly pieces of work that incorporate both critique and interpretation, providing a perspective with supporting evidence [47]. It is the elements of critique and interpretation, as well as the stance taken by the research team, that differentiate narrative reviews from preliminary literature reviews often used to summarise existing literature [47, 50].

Reasons for conducting a narrative review include developing an understanding of a topic, learning the terminology used, and identifying future directions for empirical research [1, 51]. Therefore, the exploratory nature of a narrative review may lend itself well to those who are new to an area of literature. They are often implemented by researchers, students, educators, and practitioners to obtain a broad perspective on a topic and subsequently to contribute to their knowledge base [51]. When writing a narrative review, authors often choose to include certain empirical studies to support their stance on a particular topic [1, 47, 51].

Narrative reviews often do not report on the methods used to conduct the review (e.g. search strategy, inclusion criteria, critical appraisal) [1, 51]. Benbassat [52] reported on the findings of a narrative review conducted to identify the characteristics of medical learning environments that negatively influence students' well-being. He briefly described the methods used to conduct his search strategy, including keywords and databases. However, there were other databases excluded from his search strategy, possibly leading to articles having been missed in his initial search which highlights the issues with this type of review.

It is important to note that there are different perspectives on whether to include methods or not in a narrative review. Some researchers have suggested that the lack of clarity on the methods and the particular stance taken by the author makes it difficult to reproduce the review and may introduce a risk of bias [1, 51]. Therefore, a group of authors have taken this a step further and proposed certain criteria to evaluate the quality of narrative reviews [53]. However, others have suggested this potential risk of bias must be weighed against the rationale of the research team for their choice of scholarly works to be included in the review [47].

Umbrella reviews

Umbrella reviews are designed to combine previously synthesised literature (i.e. to synthesise existing reviews). Whilst umbrella reviews could integrate any set of reviews that use the same methodology and standards [54], they most often synthesise the findings from systematic reviews containing either qualitative or quantitative information [55, 56]. Consequently, umbrella reviews commonly answer similar questions to those found in systematic reviews, including estimating, identifying, or comparing the topic under study. In clinical education, researchers could conduct an umbrella review to investigate the effectiveness of a series of educational interventions within a single group of learners, which can then guide educators' decisions on whether to implement the intervention(s) with their same identified group of learners [55]. For example, Onyura et al. conducted an umbrella review to identify the relationship between curricular designs (i.e. the overarching course or programme structure) and instructional designs (i.e. the specific tools or strategies employed by educators) commonly employed in undergraduate medical education, and learning outcomes [57].

Given the growth in published evidence syntheses, umbrella reviews are becoming more common [58]. Their broad, yet comprehensive nature allows authors to compare results and interpretations across included reviews, explore the reasons for their findings, and propose areas for future research and educational practice [55, 59–61]. Whereas most review types focus on analysing the results of single studies, umbrella reviews analyse the findings of multiple evidence syntheses (e.g. systematic reviews). Onyura et al. included and analysed the results of 36 systematic reviews – consisting of a total of approximately 1396 independent studies – on curricular and instructional design approaches [57]. Thus, the authors were able to draw conclusions based on a broad scope of evidence that could be used to inform educational practice and directions for future research.

Choosing the appropriate evidence synthesis approach

As with any scientific inquiry, the chosen research methods and data analysis techniques depend on the research question being asked. Chapter 9 explores the methodological and design considerations of evidence syntheses in greater detail. For now, we will focus on using the research question as a guide to select the most appropriate evidence synthesis approach. The following illustrative case study aims to provide a concrete example of a research topic that could be addressed using different types of evidence syntheses. In this example of using online learning in clinical education, you will see how the research question changes depending on the chosen synthesis approach. You will also notice differences in how each synthesis type addresses the nature of knowledge. Finally, we have provided exemplar reviews within clinical education to help contextualise what topics and questions may be addressed by each synthesis approach (Box 8.1).

Summary

In this chapter, we have defined the term 'evidence syntheses' and contextualised their use within the field of clinical education. We have also provided an overview of commonly used synthesis approaches, namely systematic reviews, scoping reviews, realist reviews, umbrella reviews, and narrative reviews. You should now have a better sense of each synthesis approach and their applications. Importantly, we have highlighted the alignment between the research question and the type of evidence synthesis selected. Each synthesis approach is uniquely suited to addressing specific questions. These research questions will inform the subsequent methods and design of your review. The next chapter will explore the process of designing evidence syntheses.

Top tips

- If you are planning a programme of research, start with an evidence synthesis. It will help you to familiarise yourself with the existing literature and claim a stake on a topic.
- Consider what type of question you are seeking to answer with your review and select a synthesis approach that aligns.
- Check what other reviews have been published on your topic of interest. If there has been a recent scoping review, it may be suitable to do a more focused review on a specific aspect of the topic.
- Where possible, build a team around you who can support you in undertaking an evidence synthesis. Your team could include your experienced supervisors, mentors, peers, and librarians.

Common pitfalls

- Thinking evidence syntheses are quick and easy. Removing the step of collecting new data does not make them a quick choice.
- Limiting your review to whether education 'works' (is effective). Asking 'how', 'why', 'when', and 'what' questions may allow you to better inform the work of educators and curriculum designers.

Ethical issues

- Evidence syntheses do not usually require ethical approval as you are not collecting any original data and therefore do not have human participants. This can make them a good choice for student projects where time is limited, although the work involved should not be underestimated.

Further reading

Cochrane Training (2022). Cochrane handbook for systematic reviews of interventions. https://training.cochrane.org/handbook/current (accessed 3 May 2023).

Knowledge Translation Program (2022). What review is right for you? https://whatreviewisrightforyou.knowledgetranslation.net/ (accessed 3 May 2023).

JBI Manual for Evidence Synthesis (2019). 8.1 Introduction to mixed methods reviews. https://jbi-global-wiki.refined.site/space/MANUAL/4689215/8.1+Introduction+to+mixed+methods+systematic+reviews (accessed 3 May 2023).

Sattar, R., Lawton, R., Panagioti, M., and Johnson, J. (2021). Meta-ethnography in healthcare research: a guide to using a meta-ethnographic approach for literature synthesis. *BMC Health Services Research* 21: 50.

Wolgemuth, J., Hicks, T., and Agosto, V. (2017). Unpacking assumptions in research synthesis: a critical construct synthesis approach. *Educational Research and Reviews* 46 (3): 131–139.

References

1 Maggio, L.A., Thomas, A., and Durning, S.J. (2019). Knowledge synthesis. In: *Understanding Medical Education: Evidence, Theory, and Practice*, 3e (ed. T. Swanwick, K. Forrest, and B.C. O'Brien), 457–469. Wiley Blackwell.

2 Kastner, M., Antony, J., Soobiah, C. et al. (2016). Conceptual recommendations for selecting the most appropriate knowledge synthesis method to answer research questions related to complex evidence. *Journal of Clinical Epidemiology* 73: 43–49.

3 Grimshaw JM (2010). A guide to knowledge synthesis: Canadian Institutes of Health Research. https://cihr-irsc.gc.ca/e/41382.html (accessed 2 May 2023).

4 Kelly, M., Dornan, T., and Yardley, S. (2014). New opportunities in health care education evidence synthesis. *Medical Education* 48 (10): 1029.

5 Maggio, L.A., Ninkov, A., Costello, J.A. et al. (2021). Knowledge syntheses in medical education: Meta-research examining author gender, geographic location, and institutional affiliation. *PLoS One* 16 (10): e0258925.

6 Maggio, L.A., Costello, J.A., Norton, C. et al. (2021). Knowledge syntheses in medical education: a bibliometric analysis. *Perspectives on Medical Education* 10 (2): 79–87.

7 Tricco, A.C., Tetzlaff, J., and Moher, D. (2011). The art and science of knowledge synthesis. *Journal of Clinical Epidemiology* 64 (1): 11–20.

8 Horsley, T. (2019). Tips for improving the writing and reporting quality of systematic, scoping, and narrative reviews. *The Journal of Continuing Education in the Health Professions* 39 (1): 54–57.

9 Gordon, M. and Gibbs, T. (2014). STORIES statement: publication standards for healthcare education evidence synthesis. *BMC Medicine* 12: 143–151.

10 Gordon, M., Carneiro, A.V., and Patricio, M.F. (2015). Enhancing the impact of BEME systematic reviews on educational practice. *Medical Teacher* 37 (8): 789–790.

11 Gordon, M., Vaz Carneiro, A., Patricio, M., and Gibbs, T. (2014). Missed opportunities in health care education evidence synthesis. *Medical Education* 48 (6): 644–645.

12 Gordon, M. (2016). Are we talking the same paradigm? Considering methodological choices in health education systematic review. *Medical Teacher* 38 (7): 746–750.

13 Horsley, T., Steinert, Y., Leslie, K. et al. (2020). The use of BEME reviews in the medical education literature. *Medical Teacher* 42 (10): 1171–1178.

14 Borah, R., Brown, A.W., Capers, P.L., and Kaiser, K.A. (2017). Analysis of the time and workers needed to conduct systematic reviews of medical interventions using data from the PROSPERO registry. *BMJ Open* 7 (2): e012545.

15 Thomas, A., Lubarsky, S., Varpio, L. et al. (2020). Scoping reviews in health professions education: challenges, considerations and lessons learned about epistemology and methodology. *Advances in Health Sciences Education: Theory and Practice* 25 (4): 989–1002.

16 Eva, K.W. (2008). On the limits of systematicity. *Medical Education* 42 (9): 852–853.

17 Biesta, G. (2009). How to use pragmatism pragmatically? Suggestions for the twenty-first century. *Education and Culture* 25 (2): 34–45.

18 Pei, L. and Wu, H. (2019). Does online learning work better than offline learning in undergraduate medical education? A systematic review and meta-analysis. *Medical Education Online* 21 (1): 1666538.

19 Carroll, C., Booth, A., Papaioannou, D. et al. (2009). UK healthcare professionals' experience of online learning techniques: a systematic review of qualitative data. *Journal of Continuing Education in the Health Professions* 29 (4): 235–241.

20 Tang, B., Coret, A., Qureshi, A. et al. (2018). Online lectures in undergraduate medical education: scoping review. *JMIR Medical Education* 4 (1): e11.

21 Ortega, M., Marchese, V., Zarro, M. et al. (2021). Digital and blended curriculum delivery in health professions education: an umbrella review with implications for doctor of physical therapy education programs. *The Physical Therapy Review* 27 (1): 4–24.

22 Cook, D.A. and Steinert, Y. (2013). Online learning for faculty development: a review of the literature. *Medical Teacher* 35 (11): 930–937.

23 Wong, G., Greenhalgh, T., and Pawson, R. (2010). Internet-based medical education: a realist review of what works, for whom, and in what circumstances. *BMC Medical Education* 10 (1): 12.

24 Munn, Z., Stern, C., Aromataris, E. et al. (2018). What kind of systematic review should I conduct? A proposed typology and guidance for systematic reviewers in the medical and health sciences. *BMC Medical Research Methodology* 18 (1): 5.

25 Reed, D., Price, E., Windish, D. et al. (2005). Challenges in systematic reviews of educational intervention studies. *Annals of Internal Medicine* 142 (12): 1080–1089.

26 Sharma, R., Gordon, M., Dharamsi, S., and Gibbs, T. (2015). Systematic reviews in medical education: a practical approach: AMEE guide 94. *Medical Teacher* 37 (2): 108–124.

27 Hammick, M., Dornan, T., and Steinert, Y. (2010). Conducting a best evidence systematic review. Part 1: from idea to data coding. BEME guide no. 13. *Medical Teacher* 32 (1): 3–15.

28 Dedeilia, A., Sotiropoulos, M.G., Hanrahan, J.G. et al. (2020). Medical and surgical education challenges and innovations in the COVID-19 era: a systematic review. *In Vivo* 34 (3 Suppl): 1603–1611.

29 Reed, D.A., Cook, D.A., Beckman, T.J. et al. (2007). Association between funding and quality of published medical education research. *Journal of the American Medical Association* 298: 1002–1009.

30 Gordon, M., Daniel, M., and Patricio, M. (2019). What do we mean by 'systematic' in health education systematic reviews and why it matters! *Medical Teacher* 41 (8): 956–957.

31 Pearson, A. (2004). Balancing the evidence: Incorporating the synthesis of qualitative data into systematic reviews. *JBI Reports* 2: 45–64.

32 Tong, A., Sainsbury, P., and Craig, J. (2007). Consolidated criteria for reporting qualitative research (COREQ): a 32-item checklist for interviews and focus groups. *International Journal for Quality in Health Care* 19 (6): 349–357.

33 Lizarondo, L., Stern, C., Carrier, J. et al. (2020). Chapter 8: mixed methods systematic reviews. In: *JBI Manual for Evidence Synthesis* (ed. E. Aromataris and Z. Munn). The Joanna Briggs Institute. https://synthesismanual.jbi.global. https://doi.org/10.46658/JBIMES-20-09.

34 Dixon-Woods, M., Agarwal, S., Jones, D. et al. (2005). Synthesising qualitative and quantitative evidence: a review of possible methods. *Journal of Health Services Research & Policy* 10 (1): 45–53.

35 McCutcheon, K., Lohan, M., Traynor, M., and Martin, D. (2014). A systematic review evaluating the impact of online or blended learning vs. face-to-face learning of clinical skills in undergraduate nurse education. *Journal of Advanced Nursing* 71 (2): 255–270.

36 Peters, M.D.J., Marnie, C., Colquhoun, H. et al. (2021). Scoping reviews: reinforcing and advancing the methodology and application. *Systematic Reviews* 10 (1): 263.

37 Peters, M.D.J., Marnie, C., Tricco, A.C. et al. (2020). Updated methodological guidance for the conduct of scoping reviews. *JBI Evidence Synthesis* 18 (10): 2119–2126.

38 Thomas, A., Lubarsky, S., Durning, S.J., and Young, M.E. (2017). Knowledge syntheses in medical education: demystifying scoping reviews. *Academic Medicine* 92 (2): 161–166.

39 Mak, S. and Thomas, A. (2022). An introduction to scoping reviews. *Journal of Graduate Medical Education* 14 (5): 561–564.

40 Mak, S., Hunt, M., Boruff, J. et al. (2022). Exploring professional identity in rehabilitation professions. *Advances in Health Sciences Education: Theory and Practice* 27 (3): 793–815.

41 Pawson, R. (2006). *Evidence-Based Policy: A Realist Perspective*. Thousand Oaks, CA: SAGE Publications 196 pp.

42 Pawson, R. and Tilley, N. (1997). *Realistic Evaluation*. London: SAGE Publications.

43 Pawson, R. (2013). *The Science of Evaluation: A Realist Manifesto*. London: SAGE Publications 240 pp.

44 Price, T., Wong, G., Withers, L. et al. (2021). Optimising the delivery of remediation programmes for doctors: a realist review. *Medical Education* 55 (9): 995–1110.

45 Wong, G., Greenhalgh, T., Westhorp, G. et al. (2013). RAMESES publication standards: realist syntheses. *BMC Medicine* 11: 21.

46 Merton, R. (1967). *On Sociological Theories of the Middle-Range. On Theoretical Sociology: Five Essays Old and New*, 39–72. New York: Free Press.

47 Greenhalgh, T., Thorne, S., and Malterud, K. (2018). Time to challenge the spurious hierarchy of systematic over narrative reviews? *European Journal of Clinical Investigation* 48 (6): e12931.

48 Thorne, S. (2018). Rediscovering the 'narrative' review. *Nursing Inquiry* 25 (3): e12257.

49 Paré, G., Trudel, M., Jaana, M., and Kitsiou, S. (2015). Synthesizing information systems knowledge: a typology of literature reviews. *Information Management* 52 (2): 183–199.

50 Bryne, J.A. (2016). Improving the peer review of narrative literature reviews. *Research Integrity and Peer Review* 1: 12.

51 Noble, H. and Smith, J. (2018). Reviewing the literature: choosing a review design. *Evidence Based Nursing* 21 (2): 39–41.

52 Benbassat, J. (2013). Undesirable features of the medical learning environment: a narrative review of the literature. *Advances in Health Sciences Education: Theory and Practice* 18 (3): 527–536.

53 Baethge, C., Goldbeck-Wood, S., and Mertens, S. (2019). SANRA- a scale for the quality assessment of narrative review articles. *Research Integrity and Peer Review* 4: 5.

54 Sutton, A., Clowes, M., Preston, L., and Booth, A. (2019). Meeting the review family: exploring review types and associated information retrieval requirements. *Health Information and Libraries Journal* 36 (3): 202–222.

55 Aromataris, E., Fernandez, R., Godfrey, C.M. et al. (2015). Summarizing systematic reviews: methodological development, conduct and reporting of an umbrella review approach. *International Journal of Evidence-Based Healthcare* 13 (3): 132–140.

56 Aromataris, E., Fernandez, R., Godfrey, C. et al. (2014). *Methodology for JBI Umbrella Reviews. Joanna Brigg's Institute Reviewer's Manual*. The Joanna Briggs Institute: Adelaide.

57 Onyura, B., Baker, L., Cameron, B. et al. (2016). Evidence for curricular and instructional design approaches in undergraduate medical education: an umbrella review. *Medical Teacher* 38 (2): 150–161.

58 Fusar-Poli, P. and Radua, J. (2018). Ten simple rules for conducting umbrella reviews. *Evidence-Based Mental Health* 21 (3): 95–100.

59 Hartling, L., Chisholm, A., Thomson, D., and Dryden, D.M. (2012). A descriptive analysis of overviews of reviews published between 2000 and 2011. *PLoS One* 7 (11): e49667.

60 Grant, M.J. and Booth, A. (2009). A typology of reviews: an analysis of 14 review types and associated methodologies. *Health Information and Libraries Journal* 26 (2): 91–108.

61 Pollock, M., Fernandes, R.M., Becker, L.A. et al. (2021). Chapter V: Overviews of reviews. In: *Cochrane Handbook for Systematic Reviews of Interventions Version 6.2 (updated February 2021)* (ed. J. Higgins, J. Thomas, J. Chandler, et al.). Cochrane.

9 Evidence synthesis: key steps and design considerations

Claire Duddy and Sophie Park

Learning objectives

By the end of this chapter, you should be able to:
- Assemble a team and develop a protocol for an evidence synthesis.
- Identify the key steps involved in an evidence synthesis and consider the implications of decisions taken at each step.

- Recognise the range of approaches to assessing quality in evidence syntheses and ways these can shape the nature of your review.
- Describe ways to integrate stakeholder knowledge and perspectives in the development and conduct of evidence syntheses.

Introduction

Having developed a research question and selected an appropriate review type to answer it (see Chapter 8), the next step is to develop a protocol for your evidence synthesis. This chapter will advise on the key design steps which involve a multitude of decisions about how the chosen approach will be implemented within your project. For example, how will relevant evidence be identified and selected for inclusion? Which data should be extracted, and how? How will the data be synthesised together? There are also important practical considerations. Do you have the necessary expertise to conduct the synthesis, or can you involve others to support you? Are there ways that you can involve stakeholders to strengthen your evidence synthesis project? What is achievable within the time and resources available for your review project?

The decisions you make at each step will shape the review and its findings. No evidence synthesis is perfect. Even with the most comprehensive search strategy, you will only ever be able to assemble a partial understanding of your topic, based on what has been researched, written up, and published so far. Sometimes, your contribution to knowledge in a topic area may be to demonstrate a gap in the literature. However, what is important is that you acknowledge your constraints and be explicit about the choices made throughout the

review project. This chapter aims to support you in this process.

Assembling a project team

Any evidence synthesis project is likely to involve assembling a project team with the necessary content and methodological expertise to conduct the research. However, the size of this project team will depend on the context in which the evidence synthesis is carried out. Some projects are undertaken by large teams of researchers with access to significant resources (expertise, time, and funding). However, many valuable evidence syntheses have been produced by much smaller teams. If you are a student, you may be undertaking most of the work involved in an evidence synthesis on your own. If this is you, we recommend that where possible, you seek the input of your supervisor(s) to help you to shape the overall design of the project and a librarian (information specialist) to help you to develop your search strategy. If you can, consider seeking a collaboration with a fellow student, supervisor, or early career researcher to support some processes, such as double (duplicate) screening of search results.

Depending on availability of resources, the review team is likely to have a number of common roles. First, a methodological expert (with experience in the review approach you have chosen) will guide

---

Starting Research in Clinical Education, First Edition. Edited by Eliot L. Rees, Alison Ledger, and Kim A. Walker.
© 2024 The Association for the Study of Medical Education (ASME). Published 2024 by John Wiley & Sons Ltd.
Companion website: www.wiley.com/go/clinicaleducation

decisions around review processes and analysis. An information specialist (e.g. librarian) will advise on or conduct literature searches. The team might also include members with content or experiential expertise, including researchers, practitioners, patients, or service users. These wider stakeholders can help you to shape relevant research questions, determine the scope of the project, support review processes and the analysis with perspectives based on lived experience, and inform your dissemination plans. Bansal et al. [1] realist review of medical education to develop person-centredness involved a four-person team with content experts, a methodologist, and information specialist, and was supported by a wider stakeholder group.

Terminology for stakeholder involvement can be diverse [2]. Whatever language you use to describe the involvement of patients, experts by experience, public contributors, policy-makers, practitioners, or anyone else, ensure you are clear about what you mean and be consistent throughout the project. This can also be a helpful process to discuss directly with your team members, helping to clarify early how roles and responsibilities might be negotiated (see Chapter 5).

It is also important from the outset to consider how the project findings might be disseminated or shared. To reach the right audience and give an evidence synthesis project the best chance of making a real impact on practice or policy, you should think about the most relevant networks you could tap into and routes to disseminate findings (see Chapter 28). Stakeholder involvement in outputs can often be most helpful if embedded into the project from the outset, for example discussing the strengths and limitations of research questions, inclusion criteria and data extraction sheets. Park et al. [3] included different stakeholders in their review team including medical students and academic GPs (from different United Kingdom institutions) who were responsible for organising GP placements. The team also included a patient representative, who was an actor experienced in portraying patient roles for medical education simulated teaching. These contributions helped to ensure a range of views, opportunities, and challenges that were considered at each step in the review process and analysis.

Planning an evidence synthesis

Developing a clear project plan – called a protocol – at the outset of an evidence synthesis will help to ensure that appropriate and realistic decisions are made at each step. Responsibilities for different aspects of the work can be allocated, and some timelines set. The extent to which each step can be pre-specified will depend to some extent on the chosen approach or method. A protocol can also improve 'rigour', ensuring your review systematically examines available evidence.

Some approaches (e.g. systematic reviews with meta-analyses) follow strict guidelines that require all procedures to be clearly defined and specified in advance [4]. More constructivist forms of evidence synthesis will build in more flexibility to allow exploratory or iterative (i.e. where the research question or methods may evolve in response to the data) work as the project progresses [5]. Many approaches are now associated with well-accepted standards for conduct and reporting (the EQUATOR network collates guidelines for many study designs, including reviews, see https://www.equator-network.org/reporting-guidelines), and we encourage you to follow these to produce a high-quality review. Whatever approach you choose, it is crucial that you describe and make explicit each of your decision-making steps. This ensures that the approach used is transparent, making visible the strengths and limitations of your review findings.

No matter what approach you choose, writing a protocol for an evidence synthesis provides an opportunity for you to begin familiarising yourself with your topic, the landscape of the literature to be reviewed, and your role within the project. You can register your evidence synthesis protocol at the outset of your project [6]. Evidence syntheses with a focus on clinical education can be registered with the Best Evidence Medical Education collaboration (https://bemecollaboration.org/Reviews+in+Progress), whilst the PROSPERO register (https://www.crd.york.ac.uk/prospero) covers a wide range of disciplines. Several clinical journals accept fuller versions of protocols for publication as standalone papers. For example, Kelly et al. [7] protocol outlines the steps that will be taken in a mixed methods review focused on generalism in clinical practice, defining the approach that will be taken to identify evidence, the eligibility criteria for studies to be included, and the planned approach to synthesise qualitative and quantitative data. Publishing a detailed protocol provides an opportunity to provide more detail on the planned methods for a project (but be aware these may attract a publication fee).

Registering or publishing a protocol lets you share your work before or whilst it is underway, helping to reduce duplication and potentially enabling collaboration with teams working on similar topics or ideas. When embarking on a potential evidence synthesis project, it is a good idea to begin by searching for any published reviews and protocols to help you to understand where your project will fit in. A published protocol is also intended to reduce reporting biases by allowing readers to compare published evidence syntheses with the original plans.

Key steps in evidence synthesis

An evidence synthesis protocol should include detail on each of the planned steps in the method. Approaches to evidence synthesis have evolved from a range of ontological and epistemological positions (see Chapter 3). They tend, nevertheless, to have some key steps in common (see Figure 9.1).

No matter what approach you adopt, all evidence syntheses require work to identify and gather potentially relevant literature, a process to sift through and select documents to be included, and to extract relevant data from those documents, and

finally, a coherent approach to assess and make sense of that data. At each stage, you will be responsible for making important decisions that will ultimately determine the findings of the evidence synthesis project and the knowledge it has produced.

Step 1: define the scope

Before beginning to search for evidence, you should consider and discuss with your team in detail what type of evidence is needed to answer your research question and what kind of documents will contain relevant data. For example, a systematic review to examine effectiveness of an intervention (e.g. a meta-analysis) would need to collect published results of randomised controlled trials that report the effectiveness of the intervention in question. Rees et al. [8] used such an approach to compare the effects of peer-teaching with faculty teaching in undergraduate medical education and found no statistically significant differences in knowledge or skills outcomes. However, a review that aims to synthesise evidence

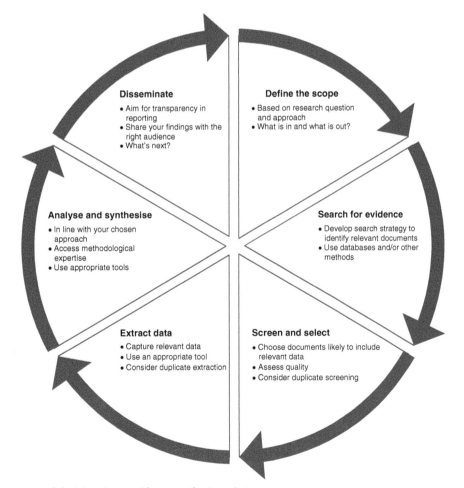

Figure 9.1 Key steps and decisions in an evidence synthesis project.

about experiences or perceptions might need to focus on identifying relevant qualitative research. For example, Krishnasamy et al. [9] conducted a meta-ethnography of qualitative research to explore how medical education affects empathy and compassion in medical students.

Some approaches to evidence synthesis involve strict criteria about the nature of the material that can be included in a review, but others are more open and may be inclusive of studies of multiple designs and other types of material, such as the 'grey literature' (conference presentations, dissertations, published and unpublished reports, government documents and other types of material). At this stage, informally exploring the wider literature by running simple searches on the web or in an academic search engine like Google Scholar can help you to develop your understanding of what is out there and whether or not your planned review is feasible.

It is also important to give careful thought to the specifics of what the evidence synthesis will include and what will be out of scope. Remember, no evidence synthesis can cover everything, you must carefully consider the priority, audience, and feasibility of each project. Tools like 'PICO' (Population, Intervention, Comparison, Outcome) or 'SPIDER' (Sample, Phenomenon of Interest, study Design, Evaluation, Research type) can help teams to structure a search strategy [10]. For example, a review might focus only on a key population of interest, such as final-year student midwives, or the team might decide it is more helpful to look broadly across a range of learner populations to learn from other disciplines and cultures, including data relating to undergraduate and postgraduate education, or clinical education as a whole. The overall approach chosen for the evidence synthesis may also influence these decisions. For some review types, firm decisions must be made about inclusion and exclusion criteria at the outset and set down in the protocol to be followed. Other approaches allow more flexibility and so these criteria may evolve in response to the data and the developing analysis as a review project progresses.

The decisions made about what is 'in' and what is 'out' will shape the rest of the project and define the scope of the knowledge claims that can be made based on its findings. For example, limiting the time period of literature included, the country of publication, the type of process or intervention examined, the particular perspective (e.g. patient, student, teacher, organisation), or context (clinical education as a whole, nursing, medical education, undergraduate, postgraduate, etc.) will all carry

important implications for the knowledge produced. It is often useful to draw on the collective wisdom of your supervisor(s), any wider project team members, and any other stakeholders with content expertise who can help you to determine coherent boundaries around the project and ensure that you are developing knowledge that will be useful in real practice.

Step 2: search for evidence

Once the decision has been made about what will be included (and just as importantly, excluded) in a review, the next step is designing a search strategy. The most common approach is to use several bibliographic databases, such as PubMed or CINAHL (see companion website for further details of databases and other resources that you might find useful). These bibliographic databases are searchable collections of references of published material within one or more academic disciplines. They vary in size and coverage and you should give careful consideration as to how many and which resources you will use, bearing in mind how comprehensive your review aims to be, but also the time and resources available [11]. It is useful to read about each database you plan to use, so you are aware of its strengths and any potential weaknesses in relation to what material it will include (and from where). Many databases are subscription-based and researchers usually gain access to search them via their institution or library, although some can be accessed and searched for free.

Searching itself involves developing a list of terms that describe the key parts of the research question and combining these together. For example, in a realist review of education strategies to develop learners' person centredness, Bansal et al. [1] combined a range of terms describing 'medical education' with terms describing 'person-centredness' to identify relevant documents. A good search strategy will include a range of terminology to describe each concept, not forgetting to consider potential synonyms, alternative spellings and word endings (e.g. educate, education, educator, and educators). At this stage, access to a librarian (information specialist) can be invaluable, if one is available. Librarians can advise on appropriate databases and in developing the search strategies themselves. Content experts in the research team and wider stakeholder group can also play a role. They are likely to be familiar with the language used in the relevant topic area and can suggest relevant search terms. The terms from each concept should be combined appropriately using Boolean operators such as 'OR' or 'AND'. It is beyond the scope of this chapter to go into detail about developing sets of search terms, but we recommend 'Further Reading' on this below [12–15].

Additional material may be identified via other methods, including reference searching or citation searching (following up the references of included studies, or searching for new studies that have cited them), 'handsearching' (nowadays on screen) key journals, or searching for, or directly contacting, the authors of key studies. These methods can help to improve comprehensiveness, potentially picking up studies missed by database searches, and demonstrating a robust approach to searching. They are also sometimes the most efficient methods of quickly gathering relevant material [16].

Step 3: screen and select documents

All searches, no matter how well designed, retrieve a mixture of relevant and irrelevant material. Therefore, there is a need to develop a process to 'sift' or screen documents to identify those that can contribute relevant data to your evidence synthesis. This process is often termed 'screening' and may involve several steps and more than one member of the review team. To help make the process more efficient, screening often begins with consideration of the title and/or abstract of each potentially relevant paper – those that are obviously out of scope can be discarded without reading them. Sometimes, the eligibility of a particular paper will not be clear from reading the title and abstract alone and so it is necessary to read the full text to ascertain if it meets the eligibility criteria and can contribute useful evidence to a review.

Devising a screening process usually involves clearly setting out the inclusion and exclusion criteria for the review, so that these can be applied consistently by the different members of the review team. You must also consider how many people will be involved in this process. In the medical literature, systematic reviews have tended to make efforts to be 'comprehensive', so enabling them to produce 'generalisable' findings. Traditionally, 'double screening' or 'duplicate screening' has been recommended as a quality control measure, helping to ensure that no relevant material slips through the net. However, the value of double screening has been questioned, both in terms of its added value and cost-effectiveness [17]. Screening everything in duplicate is a labour-intensive and time-consuming process. Some review approaches do not aim to be comprehensive, but instead aim for a 'good enough' or representative selection of relevant material, to suit their purpose or approach. When this is the case, double screening becomes less critical, and it

may be acceptable for only a portion of screening decisions to be made in duplicate, or for a researcher to work alone. New tools such as 'text mining' are increasingly used to support screening, bringing potentially key papers to the top of the 'pile' [18]. You should carefully consider what is expected and what is necessary for your project.

Inevitably, you will come across documents where some aspect of the study design or angle on the topic creates uncertainty about inclusion. These 'borderline' cases are an opportunity for your team to unpick and refine your inclusion criteria and how they are operationalised in the review – discussion of such papers can help you to really focus down on what your review aims to cover and contribute.

It is essential to set up good data management processes that enable you to keep track of the documents identified, considered and ultimately included or excluded from your review. At each stage, it is important to keep a record of screening decisions, as these numbers are typically reported as part of the descriptive results of a review, allowing readers to understand how the review team assembled the evidence included in the synthesis and which documents have contributed data to the analysis. These details are often presented both in narrative text and in a flow diagram, following the dominant Preferred Reporting Items for Systematic Reviews and Meta Analyses (PRISMA) publication standards [19].

Assessing quality

Many types of evidence synthesis include a step at which the quality or rigour of the included evidence is assessed in some way. The need for this assessment or 'critical appraisal' and the approach that should be adopted will vary depending on the approach to evidence synthesis you choose and on the type of study design (or other documents) included in your review.

As with other steps, some approaches to evidence synthesis require strict limitations to be placed on the inclusion of particular study designs or methods and have predefined approaches and tools in place to assess the quality of each included study. Many tools and checklists have been developed, which can help you to apply consistent standards to appraise the documents you include. Gilligan et al. [20] review of interventions to improve medical students' interpersonal communication included randomised and quasi-randomised controlled trials. They used the Cochrane Risk of Bias tool, to assess the reporting of key elements of study design. Two separate members of the review team independently assessed each included study. However,

Gordon et al. [21] adopted a different approach in their review of medical education responses to the COVID-19 pandemic, using the same risk of bias tool alongside other approaches to assess quality, with the aim of also evaluating how well each educational intervention or development was described.

Other approaches may judge 'quality' using different criteria or values. For example, some review types may include a judgement of relevance to the review question, whilst others might seek more in-depth analysis in the included studies (for example, the use of educational theory), or reflexivity. In some reviews, these assessments may be used to exclude material that does not meet a particular standard. More commonly, this material may be included, but the results of the quality evaluation are reported, and any implications for the review team's confidence in their findings are drawn out. You can also comment on common areas of methodological strength or weakness in the existing literature to draw recommendations for future research.

Ultimately, there is no right answer to how, when, and why to conduct a particular quality assessment. However, it is crucial for your team to consider possible options, to choose a method that suits your chosen approach to evidence synthesis and meets the needs of your project and to be able to explain how and why you have opted for a particular design.

Step 4: extract data

The outcome of the screening and selection process will result in a set of relevant documents that meet the review's eligibility criteria. All of these documents will have something to contribute to answer the research question, whether that is a measure of the effectiveness of an intervention, qualitative data that provides insight to understand experience, or clues that can support theory development. However, the set of included documents will also contain a raft of other information, necessitating careful attention to capture the relevant data that can be used in the evidence synthesis.

As ever, different processes are appropriate for different approaches, and your protocol should set out clearly how you plan to capture the relevant data contained within included documents. In a qualitative review or realist review, the aim may be to extract sections of relevant text. In this case, qualitative analysis software (e.g. NVivo) that facilitates coding may be the most appropriate tool. For other reviews, developing a 'data extraction form' to consistently capture a standard set of data from each included document

might be best. Piloting these processes with a subset of included papers can help to ensure that they work and provides the opportunity to make tweaks, as needed [22, 23].

As with the other steps, it is often helpful for more than one researcher to be involved, to help ensure rigour and consistency in this process. You should consider both what is expected and what is appropriate and feasible for your review project.

If working with stakeholder or Personal and Public Involvement (PPI) groups, sharing pilot data extraction sheets can generate helpful discussion about key areas to focus on and the terminology used to describe the data captured. No review can include everything (however tempting), so pragmatic decisions will need to be made about what will or will not appear in your data extraction form.

Once extracted, the data will become the equivalent of the empirical data collected in a primary research study. This will be the 'source' the review team must come back to again and again, as you analyse and re-analyse the emerging results. It is essential to ensure that the data extraction process developed is robust and meets the need of the evidence synthesis. In particular, you should ensure that your coding or forms capture enough information to understand the context in which something was claimed or described, so that the subsequent analysis can be as specific and accurate as possible.

Step 5: analyse and synthesise

Analysis and synthesis of the extracted data are the next step, the method of which should have been agreed as part of the protocol. Your methods will be informed by your research question(s) and your chosen synthesis approach (see Chapter 8). You will also need to plan who will conduct the analysis, and how, and consider the software or other tools that might support this work. The potential value of the wider review team and any wider stakeholder groups at this stage should also be considered in some detail – is there a role for these groups in supporting the analysis stage? Access to appropriate methodological expertise or training at this stage may be essential. For example, a statistician may be required to produce a meta-analysis, a realist methodologist to advise on the application of a realist logic to the data included in the review, or an economist to calculate cost-effectiveness.

The analysis process also entails writing. We often conceptualise 'analysis' and 'writing up' as finite, discrete stages of a project, but the act of writing and shaping the results, and addressing the synthesis findings to a particular audience are themselves part of the analytical process. Writing and re-writing the findings is a process of refinement and shaping the knowledge claims that will be made on the basis of the analysis. No single write up can include all of the analytical findings identified during an evidence synthesis, and all outputs that are produced will be 'partial' in some way. What is interesting to highlight within the data might change depending on current policy, practice, or personal priorities and constraints at a particular time.

As at other steps, the wider stakeholder group and PPI colleagues can help to support the approach taken, so that the final 'products' of the review are considered throughout the project. Review teams should discuss, debate, and examine the potential key messages and likely audiences for their findings, before and during writing. Depending on the available resources, review teams may be larger or smaller and might include a range of experiential or 'insider' knowledge (e.g. practitioners, public contributors, policy-makers). Plan when and how this range of perspectives might be important to include in the review process. All review teams have particular hopes and dreams for their evidence synthesis outputs. This is not wrong, but it is essential to make these visible to your evidence synthesis readers. So be clear about who is involved and how their involvement has shaped the review approach and in what ways. All evidence syntheses involve interpretation, which is inevitably a dialogic process of engaging with materials in relation to your own values and experiences. Making these values and experiences explicit is therefore important, so the reader can gauge how interpretations were made and how these have shaped the review in particular ways.

Step 6: dissemination

How your results are disseminated is as important to consider as the actual review. Some evidence syntheses have several different outputs, while others combine their findings into one report. It can be helpful to publish the protocol which can then be cited in a final report. This also alleviates any word count limitations by keeping the description of methods to a minimum in subsequent publications. The topic and scope of your review will to some extent determine the type of output. Some outputs provide a descriptive overview. Others explicitly focus on one 'pot' or subset of data. Some may orientate the write-up around a particular topic, others might focus more strongly on the method and the

ways in which this facilitated or limited the production of knowledge in the review project. You should consider carefully who to involve in writing. Including a variety of different perspectives in the authorship team can be a really good way to create cognitive dissonance within the writing process, helping to clarify and develop ideas prior to publication.

Presenting emerging results at conferences can be another helpful step in beginning to formulate ideas in relation to a particular audience or focus, as well as a means of sharing your results with research or practitioner communities. For example, in a review focused on the perspective of trainee pharmacists, presenting and discussing data or findings with a PPI group or policy-maker stakeholder group can prompt new thinking, making different connections or drawing on different data for different groups. Different types of stakeholders may ask different questions and reveal different perspectives, priorities, and gaps within the synthesis data.

The provision of executive summaries, visual resources, or social media, which provide key messages for different audience groups, can be very impactful [24] (see Chapter 28). This can help to raise awareness of the review findings and even enable them to inform future policy or practice.

Summary

Evidence syntheses should be well-planned and designed by the research team at the outset, in a similar way to a primary research project. Developing a clear protocol should be based around detailed consideration of the decisions that need to be made at each important stage of the project. This includes the approach that will be taken to search for and select the material that will be included in the review, to analyse and synthesise that material, and to ensure quality and rigour in those processes. The involvement of patient and public representatives and other stakeholders beyond the review team should also be considered at the outset, and clear roles and responsibilities allocated to researchers and stakeholder groups to help ensure the delivery of your research objectives. The chosen approach will affect the extent to which each step can be pre-specified, with some teams specifying every detail and others planning a degree of flexibility in line with their ontological perspectives. Finally, it is important that the protocol explains the rationale for the decisions and their possible implications.

Top tips

- Read published and registered protocols for evidence syntheses. This can help you to understand how different methods can be implemented.
- Recruit the right people to your project team and wider stakeholder groups. This can help you to ensure that you have access to appropriate content and methodological expertise.
- Consider what it is feasible to do well within the time and resources available to you. It will not be possible to answer all your research questions within a single review so you must focus, prioritise, and be realistic about timelines and workload.
- It is essential to set up good data management processes that enable you to keep track of the documents identified, considered, and ultimately included or excluded from your review.

Common pitfalls

- Lack of clarity on research questions and focus. Pinning these down can help you to make appropriate decisions about your overall approach and how it should be implemented.
- Mismatches between your approach and methods can create inefficiencies and prevent you from producing a high-quality output. Make sure your decisions about the design of the review project match its purpose, the approach you have chosen, and the available time and resources.
- Projects can be negatively impacted both by a scarcity of literature or by an overwhelming volume. Exploratory searches conducted at the outset of the project can help you to understand the extent and shape of the existing literature and determine whether there will be enough to work with, or whether you may need a narrower focus to ensure a project is feasible.

Ethical issues

- Most review projects do not currently require ethical approval as they involve working with secondary data that has already been published. You may, however, need to secure confirmation that your project is exempt from your institution or supervisor.

- Unlike involving participants in primary research, the involvement of stakeholders (including patients or members of the public) as evidence synthesis co-researchers will not require ethical approval. However, it is important for review teams to ensure the development of respectful, mutually beneficial relationships with these contributors.

Further reading

For step-by-step guidance on developing review projects using different approaches: BEME. Review Stages guidance.

Booth, A., Sutton, A., Clowes, M., and Martyn-St James, M. (2021). *Systematic Approaches to a Successful Literature Review*. London: SAGE Publications.

Gough, D., Oliver, S., and Thomas, J. (2017). *An Introduction to Systematic Reviews*. London: SAGE Publications.

Sandelowski, M. and Barroso, J. (2007). *Handbook for Synthesizing Qualitative Research*. New York: Springer Publishing Company.

References

1 Bansal, A., Greenley, S., Mitchell, C. et al. (2021). Optimising planned medical education strategies to develop learners' person-centredness: a realist review. *Medical Education* 56 (5): 489–503.

2 Abrams, R., Park, S., Wong, G. et al. (2021). Lost in reviews: looking for the involvement of stakeholders, patients, public and other non-researcher contributors in realist reviews. *Research Synthesis Methods* 12 (2): 239–247.

3 Park, S., Khan, N.F., Hampshire, M. et al. (2015). A BEME systematic review of UK undergraduate medical education in the general practice setting: BEME guide no. 32. *Medical Teacher* 37 (7): 611–630.

4 Cochrane Training. (2022). Cochrane Handbook for for Systematic Reviews of Interventions version 6.3 (updated February 2022). Cochrane. http://www.training.cochrane.org/handbook (accessed 3 May 2023)

5 Wong G., Westhorp G., Pawson R. and Greenhalgh T. (2013). Realist Synthesis: RAMESES Training Materials. http://www.ramesesproject.org/media/Realist_reviews_training_materials.pdf (accessed 3 May 2023).

6 Pieper, D. and Rombey, T. (2022). Where to prospectively register a systematic review. *Systematic Reviews* 11 (1): 8.

7 Kelly, M., Cheung, S., Keshavjee, M. et al. (2021). Characterising generalism in clinical practice: a systematic mixed studies review protocol. *BJGP Open*. 5 (4): BJGPO.2021.0029.

8 Rees, E.L., Quinn, P.J., Davies, B., and Fotheringham, V. (2016). How does peer teaching compare to faculty teaching? A systematic review and meta-analysis. *Medical Teacher* 38 (8): 829–837.

9 Krishnasamy, C., Ong, S.Y., Loo, M.E., and Thistlethwaite, J. (2019). How does medical education affect empathy and compassion in medical students? A meta-ethnography: BEME guide no. 57. *Medical Teacher* 41 (11): 1220–1231.

10 Cooke, A., Smith, D., and Booth, A. (2012). Beyond PICO: the SPIDER tool for qualitative evidence synthesis. *Qualitative Health Research* 22 (10): 1435–1443.

11 Eva, K.W. (2008). On the limits of systematicity. *Medical Education* 42 (9): 852–853.

12 Brunton, G., Stansfield, C., Caird, J., and Thomas, J. (2017). Finding relevant studies. In: *An Introduction to Systematic Reviews*, 2e (ed. D. Gough, S. Oliver, and J. Thomas). Los Angeles: SAGE Publications.

13 Booth, A., Sutton, A., Clowes, M., and Martyn-St James, M. (2022). Chapter 5: searching the literature. In: *Systematic Approaches to a Successful Literature Review*, 3e. SAGE Publications.

14 Sandelowski, M. and Barroso, J. (2007). *Searching for and Retrieving Qualitative Research Reports. Handbook for Synthesising Qualitative Research*. New York, NY: Springer Publishing Company, Inc.

15 Haig, A. and Dozier, M. (2003). BEME guide no. 3: systematic searching for evidence in medical education--part 2: constructing searches. *Medical Teacher* 25 (5): 463–484.

16 Greenhalgh, T. and Peacock, R. (2005). Effectiveness and efficiency of search methods in systematic reviews of complex evidence: audit of primary sources. *BMJ* 331 (7524): 1064–1065.

17 Shemilt, I., Khan, N., Park, S., and Thomas, J. (2016). Use of cost-effectiveness analysis to compare the efficiency of study identification methods in systematic reviews. *Systematic Reviews* 5 (1): 140.

18 Shemilt, I., Simon, A., Hollands, G.J. et al. (2014). Pinpointing needles in giant haystacks: use of text mining to reduce impractical screening workload in extremely large scoping reviews. *Research Synthesis Methods* 5 (1): 31–49.

19 Page, M.J., McKenzie, J.E., Bossuyt, P.M. et al. (2021). The PRISMA 2020 statement: an updated guideline for reporting systematic reviews. *BMJ* 372: n71.

20 Gilligan, C., Powell, M., Lynagh, M.C. et al. (2021). Interventions for improving medical students' interpersonal communication in medical consultations. *Cochrane Database of Systematic Reviews* 8 (2): CD012418.

21 Gordon, M., Patricio, M., Horne, L. et al. (2020). Developments in medical education in response to the COVID-19 pandemic: a rapid BEME systematic review: BEME guide no. 63. *Medical Teacher* 42 (11): 1202–1215.

22 Li, T., Higgins, J. P. T., and Deeks, J.J. (2022). Chapter 5: Collecting data. In: *Cochrane Handbook for Systematic Reviews of Interventions Version 63 (Updated February 2022)* (ed. J. Higgins, J. Thomas, J. Chandler, et al.). Cochrane.

23 Sutcliffe, K., Oliver, S., and Richardson, M. (2017). Describing and analysing studies. In: *An Introduction to Systematic Reviews*, 2e (ed. D. Gough, S. Oliver, and J. Thomas). Los Angeles: SAGE Publications.

24 Abrams R. (2019). NIHR School for Primary Care Research Blog. https://www.spcr.nihr.ac.uk/news/blog/is-there-a-doctor-in-the-house-lessons-from-a-public-engagement-event-at-the-bloomsbury-theatre (accessed 3 May 2023).

10 Realist research: unpicking the influence of context

Claire Duddy and Geoff Wong

Learning objectives

By the end of this chapter, you should be able to:
- Describe the key underpinning principles of realist research.
- Explain when a realist approach would be appropriate.
- Evaluate the implications of taking this approach for knowledge claims, project design, and dissemination.

- Comprehend the role of programme theory and principles of realist analysis.
- Describe the main stages of a realist review or realist evaluation.

Introduction

Earlier in this book, you were introduced to two research paradigms, post-positivism and constructivism (see Chapter 3). In this chapter, we will introduce another approach, *realism*. Realism sits somewhere between post-positivism and constructivism. Realist research seeks to understand how interventions work and the influence of context.

Though other approaches to realist research exist, this chapter concentrates on the approach originally devised by Pawson and Tilley [1], which has become increasingly popular with researchers and funding bodies, especially in the United Kingdom. In this chapter, we describe what realist research is, consider different approaches to realist research and when they might be appropriate, and discuss some important design considerations.

What is realist research?

Realist research is an approach to research that is based on a realist philosophy of science and understanding of the world (ontology). This understanding gives realists a distinctive starting point for their research: realists understand that the outcomes we observe in the world vary in different circumstances (called 'context' in realist terminology) and that the underlying causal forces that generate those outcomes (called 'mechanisms') are invisible and must be uncovered by research. Realist research, therefore, focuses on developing theoretical explanations for how and why things work, using either primary or secondary data to understand the relationships between important contexts, mechanisms, and outcomes. The focus is usually on explanation rather than judgement: realists seek to answer questions about 'how', 'why', 'for whom', 'to what extent' or 'in what circumstances', thus explaining the underlying causes of outcomes and going beyond an assessment of whether or not something happens or works.

The explanatory focus of realist research and its basis in a realist understanding of the world means the approach is particularly well-suited for those studying interventions or programmes that are complex and where outcomes depend on the contexts in which they are implemented. This strength underlies the growth of realist approaches in clinical education research, where complex interventions and context-dependent outcomes are the norms. Clinical education is a complex social world, calling for a research approach that can account for individual human actions, while taking into account all the wider contexts that can influence them. In this field, realist approaches offer you the opportunity to complement other research designs, adding new theoretical insights and

---

Starting Research in Clinical Education, First Edition. Edited by Eliot L. Rees, Alison Ledger, and Kim A. Walker.
© 2024 The Association for the Study of Medical Education (ASME). Published 2024 by John Wiley & Sons Ltd.
Companion website: www.wiley.com/go/clinicaleducation

understanding that can explain intervention successes and failures, and lead to practical, real-world recommendations for intervention and programme design and implementation [2].

It is important to recognise that realist research has its own language and terminology. To help clarify this, we have provided a table of definitions of common realist terminology (Table 10.1).

Table 10.1 Table of definitions of key realist terminology

Term	Definition	Illustrative example
Context	The conditions or circumstances in which mechanisms that generate observed outcomes are 'triggered' or activated In realist research, 'context' has a broad definition and may include material, social, psychological, organisational, economic, and many other influences – if they are understood by the researcher as affecting the operation of mechanisms [3]	You might identify aspects of individual learners' prior experiences or attitudes, features of the setting in which an educational intervention is delivered, or wider features of the curriculum or education policy as salient features of context
Context-mechanism-outcome configuration (CMOC)	A mental shortcut or thinking tool (heuristic) used to present a realist causal explanation for an outcome, presented as a relationship between some particular context(s) and mechanism(s)	In a context of learning through role modelling within hierarchical relationships (C), junior doctors passively comply with the prescribing habits and norms set by their seniors (O), because of fear of criticism (M) [4]
Demi-regularity	A semi-predictable pattern of outcomes that occurs in different settings One assumption made in realist research is that the outcomes we can observe are often patterned, although not necessarily invariably – i.e. they keep reoccurring in different settings, but not all the time	The recurrent observation in education that students will frequently ask their teachers if a topic area will be examined
Intervention (or programme)	An activity or set of activities introduced into an existing system with the aim of changing an outcome (avoiding an undesirable outcome or producing a desired one) The term is sometimes used interchangeably with 'programme', though this may sometimes refer to a larger-scale intervention(s) Interventions or programmes are usually introduced to improve something in response to identified problems	Objective Structured Clinical Examinations (OSCEs) were introduced to increase the consistency, validity, and reliability of clinical examinations
Mechanism	The underlying context-sensitive causal force that generates an outcome, often conceptualised as the response of an individual actor to important context(s)	In the prescribing example above, the mechanism that generates the observed outcome is the junior doctors' response to the hierarchical learning environment, summarised as 'fear of criticism' [4]
Outcome	Any outcome that is understood to be generated by a particular mechanism operating in a certain context This can include intended and unintended outcomes, and more proximal ('process') outcomes as well as the final intended outcomes of an intervention or process	In a topic exploring an educational intervention to improve an aspect of clinical practice, important outcomes may be identified at multiple steps, e.g. attendance, engagement, and learning may all be considered, as well as final outcomes related to clinical practice and any unintended consequences
Programme theory	A set of theoretical explanations about how a programme, intervention, or process is understood to work. Realist programme theories explain the processes by which outcomes of interest are thought to be generated, using causal explanations captured in the form of CMOCs In many realist projects, the final programme theory is provided in the form of a diagram or illustration that shows the relationship between the individual CMOCs developed during the analysis The final programme theory might highlight important contexts that affect many outcomes or illustrate how CMOCs are sequenced or connected to each other	In the prescribing example above, an 'overarching programme theory' is summarised in a diagram and narrative that consolidates the findings of the project [4] The overarching programme theory illustrates the complexity of the problem, identifying important contextual factors and key mechanisms that lead to a range of important outcomes

Table 10.1 (Continued)

Term	Definition	Illustrative example
Substantive theory	An established, formal theory drawn from any discipline that can be used to help understand the programme, intervention, or process under examination In the field of clinical education, education theories may be most pertinent to help understand how interventions or programmes 'work' (or not) See Chapter 4 for more discussion of how educational theories can be used in research	de Groot et al. [5] identified multiple educational theories that were used to support their analysis of patient-centredness in medical education, including situated learning and social learning theory

Primary and secondary realist research

Realist approaches can be applied to conduct both primary, empirical research and secondary review, evidence synthesis research. Primary (or empirical) realist research is typically termed 'realist evaluation', reflecting the origins of the approach in the evaluation tradition where it was developed to understand the workings of social interventions or programmes. Secondary realist research is termed 'realist review' or 'realist synthesis' and applies the same analytical approach to make sense of data extracted from documents that have already been published.

In both cases, realist approaches can encompass diverse types of data, generated by different methods or study designs. Both realist evaluation and realist review can be considered 'mixed methods' approaches in relation to data collection. Qualitative, quantitative, and mixed methods data can provide different insights and perspectives. Quantitative study designs can provide data that reveals common patterns of outcomes or associations (what realists might term 'demi-regularities'). Qualitative or mixed data might then be used to shed more light on when and how such patterns of outcomes are generated: this type of data can reveal details about important contexts and provide clues about the mechanisms that are at work wherever certain outcomes are observed. Whatever methods are chosen, it is essential that the data collection methods used are conducted rigorously; other chapters in this book provide valuable introductions to a wider range of primary research methods. Realist reviews can also include data produced in other ways, including insights from commentaries or grey literature, when it helps you to develop your understanding of what is going on.

It is your job to make sense of these diverse data sources, using them to assemble a more complete picture and understanding of a complex phenomenon or intervention. It is essential to keep the ultimate aim of the research in mind: the goal of this approach is to develop causal explanations for outcomes – to theorise about how, why, and when different outcomes occur. Such explanations are likely to be multiple and overlapping – complex interventions are messy – but the realist approach offers a way 'in' to start to unpack at least some of what is going on.

Realist research also often explicitly draws on existing theory to help to shape or support the analysis. For example, de Groot et al. [5] identified multiple educational theories that were used to support their analysis of patient-centredness in medical education, including situated learning and social learning theory. Existing substantive theory can play multiple roles in a realist project. At the outset, knowledge of existing theories can shape the research question or initial programme theory. For example, one realist evaluation project drew on sociocultural theories of workplace practices and experiential learning to develop their initial programme theory (termed 'conceptual framework') [6]. Such theories can also support different aspects of the analysis, providing clues about mechanisms or lending a focus to the project as a whole [7].

Could a realist approach help me?

Adopting a realist approach to your research project will inevitably involve an examination of both your purpose and the nature of your research topic. It is also important to consider the feasibility of the approach, especially in relation to the time and resources required, and the availability of methodological expertise to support the project. When deciding whether to use a realist approach, we suggest there are three fundamental questions to ask.

Are you researching a complex intervention or phenomenon?

One of the most common rationales for adopting a realist approach is the subject under study is in some sense 'complex', and therefore in need of an approach that can help to account for and understand this complexity. For realists, such complexity may have many facets, captured in Pawson's 'VICTORE' (volitions, implementation, context, time, outcomes, rivalry, emergence) framework [8], describing what makes a complex intervention 'complex'. This understanding of complexity emphasises the role of individuals who are involved in complex interventions. Those who deliver the intervention and those in receipt of it may vary in their responses and make important choices about their actions, which ultimately determine whether (and when, how, and why) the intervention 'works' or otherwise. Ultimately, these are the realist 'mechanisms' that realist researchers want to understand. However, the range of responses and choices is not without limits and this is where the role of context comes to the fore: different contexts constrain individuals' responses and choices when faced with an intervention. Identifying this interplay of context and mechanism is the crux of the realist endeavour, enabling researchers to pay attention both to the actions of individuals and to the wider circumstances that constrain and enable their behaviour. For example, when junior doctors prescribe antimicrobials, their decision on what to prescribe is more likely to be driven by what they think their senior colleagues would want them to prescribe rather than what might be recommended in local or national prescribing guidelines [4].

Does your research question or aim focus on explaining what is causing outcomes?

When undertaking any research project, the method(s) chosen must be able to provide the data needed to address the research questions. Therefore, a realist approach may be an appropriate choice whenever a research team has identified a need for new work to help answer more 'realist' research questions: how, why, when, for whom, in what circumstances, to what extent? In which contexts or by which mechanisms? Such a gap may have been identified by you, or others in the course of your reading or research. Existing systematic reviews or even informal scoping searches of the literature can often reveal the need for research with a more explanatory focus. Lefroy et al. [6] identified a focus on individual preparation for practice in the existing literature on newly qualified doctors and highlighted the gaps in existing knowledge about 'what works' in relation to apprenticeship or 'shadowing'

models of learning. This research team chose a realist evaluation approach to help them to make sense of success and failure in significant 'first experiences' for doctors as they transition to becoming qualified [6].

Is a realist approach feasible for your project?

As with all research, doing realist research rigorously can be labour and time intensive. Undertaking a realist project by yourself would be extremely challenging, and not something we would recommend. Research and the analysis in particular will benefit from working within a wider team, and, if possible, having access to a wider group of stakeholders who have an interest in how your project develops and the practical application of its findings (see Chapter 5). Realist analysis of both primary and secondary data requires researchers to become immersed in their data, in an iterative and in-depth process of analysis. There may be false starts and dead ends, and in unpacking different aspects of a topic, it can become difficult to maintain fixed boundaries around a research question. The RAMESES quality standards for realist reviews [9] and evaluations [10] suggest a process of 'progressive focusing' should be expected, allowing research teams the flexibility to prioritise different aspects of a research topic and work towards in-depth understanding of a smaller area, rather than a more broad and superficial understanding of a topic. Such focusing may respond to the data and emerging analysis itself. It may also reflect the needs of a research funder or commissioner, discussions within the project team, or the input of stakeholders, especially those representing groups who may be involved in developing or delivering an intervention, or those receiving it.

Access to advice, support, or training from someone with experience and expertise in realist methodology is highly recommended. Depending on your circumstances, you might: seek out PhD supervisors with a proven track record in supervising students using realist approaches, go on a training course, seek out or develop a peer-support group or ask questions on the RAMESES JISCMail list (www.jiscmail.ac.uk/RAMESES). Securing such expertise can help ensure your team maintains a clear focus on their purpose, be able to justify decisions taken throughout the research project, and ensure that realist analysis is conducted as it should be. Becoming an experienced and competent realist researcher takes time and practice. As in modern clinical practice, the old adage of 'see one, do one, teach one' is best avoided. The next section of this chapter provides an overview of what realist analysis looks like and involves – this is just a starting point and further reading is recommended below.

Programme theory and realist analysis

Realist research is often termed 'theory driven' or 'theory based'. Part of this term refers to the use of existing substantive theories to support realist analysis (as described above), but 'programme theory' is another type of theory that is a crucial part of any realist research project [11]. The term may be unfamiliar, but it simply refers to a description of how a programme or intervention is understood to work (or not). Such a description may be expressed in words, but it is typical to also see programme theories presented as diagrams that illustrate the important steps involved in the intervention under study (see Figure 10.1). Complex interventions usually have 'long implementation chains' – in other words, they can be broken down into a series of smaller steps and sequences, each of which must be taken, before the ultimate intended outcome of the intervention can be reached [8]. A programme theory might include theories about how an intervention is supposed to work (theories of change or action) and theories about how an intervention must be implemented in order for it to work (theories of implementation).

A realist programme theory is distinctive, in that it should aim to offer explanations for how each step is achieved (or not) by identifying and elucidating important contexts, mechanisms, outcomes – and relationships between these – at each step. For those following the approach developed by Pawson and Tilley, this usually involves using a heuristic known as a 'CMOC' or 'context-mechanism-outcome configuration' to structure how each causal explanation developed during analysis is expressed. Each CMOC is a theoretical causal explanation for how a particular outcome is produced in a particular context, underpinned by the data collected or reviewed in the project. An illustrative example is provided below – Figure 10.1 is reproduced from the RESTORE realist review project, which sought to understand remediation programmes for practicing doctors [12]. The final programme theory diagram illustrates the relationships between the individual CMOCs produced in this review.

All realist projects should begin and end with a programme theory. Part of the overall approach is a commitment to the accumulation and gradual improvement of knowledge [13]. As such, realists recognise that all projects begin *somewhere*, with some initial knowledge and understanding of the topic under investigation. An initial programme theory is therefore developed at the beginning, to try to capture what is already known and provide a starting point for you to 'test' (confirm, refute, or refine) that understanding as the project progresses. An initial programme theory may not necessarily be 'realist' in nature, that is, it may not specifically contain contexts, mechanisms, or outcomes. It might be a simple explanation of how an intervention or programme is assumed to 'work' or produce its outcomes. Articulating such an explanation at the outset of the project means that you can discuss areas of priority or potential focus and provide a framework for the analysis of data as the project progresses.

At the end of a project, a 'final' programme theory or, perhaps more accurately, a 'more refined' programme theory should be produced. There may not be a close resemblance to the initial starting point, but the refined theory should be realist in nature and so include, or be based upon, the development of evidence-based CMOCs. This end product represents a theoretical step forward, towards an improved understanding of the research question and the intervention or phenomenon under study. The findings of a realist project allow the research team and their key audiences to identify important contexts that may be changeable and the mechanisms that can and should be provoked to generate desirable outcomes. Typically, then, a final programme theory may form the basis for the development of recommendations or guidelines for policy or practice and intervention designs that directly address the salient contexts in which outcomes are generated or inform future research.

A brief overview of realist analysis

Realist research can draw on a multitude of types of data in analysis, whether this is collected in a realist evaluation project using various methods, or via the inclusion of multiple study designs and document types in a realist review. The process of analysis itself involves close examination and interpretation of the data available. Realist researchers use processes such as cross-case comparison, juxtaposing comparable and conflicting data to try to understand how similarities and differences in context affect outcomes. Multiple approaches to reasoning are applied: researchers must apply inductive logic to develop theories by examining the data; deductive logic to test the propositions set out in their

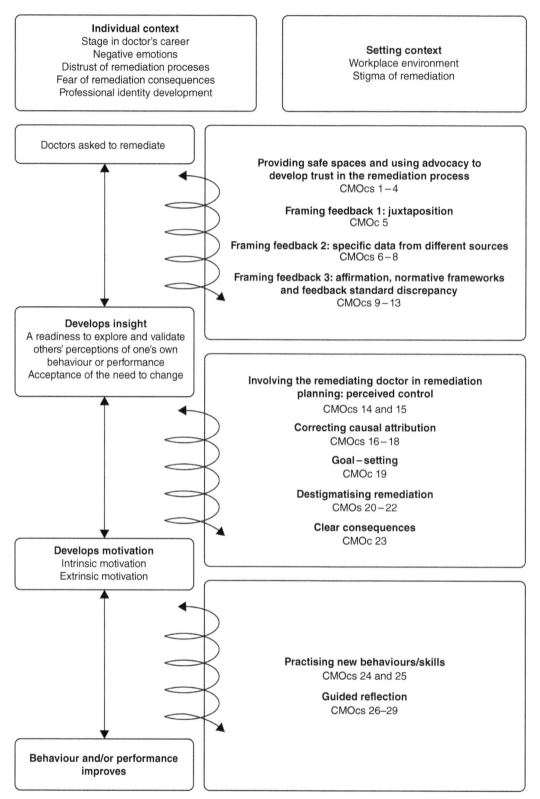

Figure 10.1 Programme theory of remediation. *Source*: [12]. http://creativecommons.org/licenses/by/4.0.

initial programme theory; and retroductive logic, to identify the invisible 'mechanisms' that are creating the outcomes or patterns found in the data [14].

The process is iterative and can be messy, involving multiple re-writings of the emerging CMOCs, refinement of the programme theory, and in-depth discussion in a project team or with wider stakeholders. These discussions are an essential step in shaping both the focus of the project and the analysis itself, as teams work together to move towards more plausible and complete interpretations of the data. This process can be seen in the case study of Robin in Box 10.1.

BOX 10.1   Case study of getting started in realist research.

Robin is a medical trainee and has noticed when working in different hospitals, she is treated differently by her seniors. Reflecting on the past three rotations, Robin suspects this may be because of the way the medical teams are organised. She noted that when she was working in a small team, seniors seem to be more interested in helping her to learn and in her welfare. In other teams, where Robin was one of a large number of trainees doing shifts at different times of the day and days of the week, no one seemed to take much interest in her. She wonders if this is because smaller teams are more reliant on trainees, so that supporting them is in everyone's interest.

Robin also has an interest in research and decides to explore this issue further. She begins by considering how she could best research the topic. The first step she takes is an exploratory search of the literature, to see what research has already been published, and she finds that this topic does not appear to be a well-researched area in medicine. Next, Robin decides to speak to people who might know something about the topic area. She approaches local medical educators, her current consultant, and educational supervisor to ask them what they think. One of them suggests this area is likely to be complex, and as Robin is trying to explain *why* this happens, she may want to consider using a realist approach.

Robin has not heard about this approach before, but with further enquiries and a bit of internet searching, managed to identify some open access materials on the RAMESES Project website (www.ramesesproject. org). Based on this, Robin believes that a realist review would be a useful first step to help her to build an initial understanding of the topic, based on existing research.

To build up her skills to do a realist review, Robin attends a course on realist reviews and realist evaluations. Based on what she learnt during the course, she formulates the following broad research question:

How, why, for whom and to what extent does a clinical team structure affect trainee learning and welfare?

Robin also develops a draft initial programme theory, identifying some important outcomes, and tentatively postulating some of the potentially relevant contexts and mechanisms involved in generating them:

When medical teams have a small number of trainees they work with regularly (context), the senior and more permanent members of the team are more likely to provide regular training to the trainees (outcome). They are also more likely to be supportive and act on any welfare concerns (outcome). This happens because of mutual dependence (mechanism), and an appreciation of the benefits to the team and its senior members that come from investing in their trainees (mechanism). Well-trained and happy trainees not only provide better care for patients (outcome) but can also be relied on to be 'a safe pair of hands' when the seniors are busy or on-call (outcome).

Robin realises she cannot do this research on her own. She sets about forming a project team, initially by approaching people she knows who she thinks might be interested, but also with the relevant content and methodological expertise, especially in realist research. With the help of this team and their contacts, she is also able to secure one day a week to work on the project, recruit a wider group of relevant stakeholders, and obtain the help of a librarian from a nearby university to help her to develop her search strategy. With this preparation, Robin is in a great position to start her realist project.

Involvement of stakeholders in realist projects

We have mentioned the roles that a stakeholder group might play in a realist project above. As in other research traditions (see Chapter 5), engagement with a group of relevant, interested people beyond your research team is common in realist research, and such groups can play a wide range of roles [15]. Stakeholder groups may be comprised of different types of people – the trick is to consider who may have relevant knowledge that could help you during your project. For example, if you are examining a particular educational intervention, you might consult with those involved in implementing it (e.g. trainers, teachers) as well as its intended or actual recipients (e.g. students). Both groups will have relevant 'lived experience' that can help you to inform your initial programme theory and your interpretation and understanding of the data you collect during your project. They are also likely to be able to alert you to implementation issues, which might affect any recommendations you develop based on your findings. It might also benefit from the involvement of those involved in developing policy or guidance, or other groups who have a stake in the outcomes – this might include patients or members of the public, who may ultimately be expected to receive the benefits of interventions in clinical education. For example, Papoutsi et al. [4] recruited patient representatives, carers, consultants, doctors-in-training at different stages, pharmacists, microbiologists, academics, and policy-makers – all groups with an important stake in improving junior doctors' antimicrobial prescribing decisions, but with potentially different perspectives on the nature of the problem under review.

Involving your stakeholders in the early stages of developing a project can help to ensure that your research question is both relevant and important in the real world and may help you to identify important areas of focus or to prioritise. In addition, having stakeholders who are representative of important audiences for your findings can help you to shape the project's outputs and dissemination. They can advise both on content, to help you to ensure that your key messages are communicated clearly, and on format, to ensure they are as relevant, attractive and accessible as possible.

Designing a realist research project

In many ways, designing a realist research project is not much different to designing any other research project. You begin by developing your idea and a specific research question(s) to be answered. It is important to remember the nature of typical 'realist' research questions and the purpose of adopting a realist approach. Typically, the approach will support questions with an explanatory focus and answer questions about how, why, when, for whom, in what circumstances, and to what extent an intervention works. As stated in the case study, consider

the team and other activities required to support you going forward.

You will need to give thought to your data sources. If you are conducting a realist evaluation, what kind of data will you need and how will you collect it? Realist evaluations typically employ mixed methods to gather multiple types of data. This might include, for example, routinely collected quantitative data, or a survey or questionnaire; it is also likely to include qualitative data collection, via interviews, focus groups, or focused observations. You can think creatively about data collection – there is no restriction on the type of data that be included, beyond the need to ensure that data that are relevant and needed to answer your research questions, and the constraints imposed by your resources and access to expertise in each data collection method (see other chapters in this book for more detail on different data collection methods).

For a realist review, data is typically gathered in the same way as for any other review or evidence synthesis, i.e. via searching the literature (see Chapter 9). However, bear in mind there may be some differences in data collection for a realist review, when compared with a conventional systematic review. There is no requirement for data collection to aim for exhaustiveness or comprehensiveness, and it is generally the case it will be more valuable to devote more project time to analysis than to searching and screening documents. As a result, you may choose to run more specific and focused search strategies, aiming to identify enough 'rich' documents containing relevant data for analysis. This approach means that supplementary or complementary searching approaches often grow in importance: additional material is likely to be identified via reference and citation searching, searching for studies related to those already included, or contacting authors or research groups [16, 17]. In addition, you should bear in mind that realist reviews do not typically restrict the inclusion of documents according to their study design. Document types that may be excluded from other types of review, including grey literature, commentary, and theory, may all be of value. As in any evidence synthesis, an experienced information specialist (librarian) can be an invaluable partner in helping to direct these activities.

You should discuss in advance when and how you and your team will analyse the data you gather. It is important to ensure that everyone involved shares an understanding of realist research and their role in the project. Important processes that form part of the analysis should be defined as much as possible in advance, while bearing in mind the iterative nature of realist projects. For example, for a realist review, you should specify the processes that will be used, and who will be involved in screening documents, extracting data, and analysis. You should also consider which tools you will use to support your research and share important materials with your team. For example, what software will you use to support quantitative and/or qualitative data analysis? What software will you use to organise and store references? How will you share and discuss emerging findings?

It is important to bear in mind the intended outputs and audiences for the research from the outset of a project. Where a realist research project has been commissioned by a specific organisation, this may be very clear, but where research may produce more general findings and recommendations, the likely routes for disseminating findings and getting them into practice might dictate some aspects of a project's focus and the presentation of findings.

All these decisions could be captured in a research protocol (see Chapter 9) – a published plan for a primary or secondary research project that describes the planned approach in some detail. Preparing a protocol has benefits for the research team, helping to ensure that everyone has the same understanding of important content and methodological concepts at play and clarifying the steps that will be undertaken throughout. It is equally important that each of the steps undertaken is well documented and recorded, to enable clear reporting later. There is a high expectation of transparency in the reporting of realist research – it is essential to be able to demonstrate how the realist analysis was performed and how the findings are based on the data collected. In other words, in any final publication or report of a realist project, the reader has to be able to clearly see how the raw data has informed the interpretations and inferences made within the programme theory.

Summary

Realist approaches to research offer a distinctive approach to data analysis that can help you to answer questions with an explanatory focus. Typically, a realist review or realist evaluation project will focus on answering questions about how, why, when, for whom, in what circumstances, and to what extent an intervention 'works'. In clinical education research, complexity abounds: many educational interventions can be understood as 'complex' in themselves, and they are inevitably introduced into complex environments. Adopting a realist research approach can help you to account for this and offer a way to explain how outcomes are affected by context and how and why things happen or 'work' (or not!).

Top tips

- Access to realist methodological expertise and training is essential, since it relies on a solid understanding of the approach. You should not 'see one, do one, teach one'.
- Both primary (realist evaluation) and secondary (realist review) projects share common features with non-realist research, although the approach to analysis is distinctive. You can draw on what you already know how to do when embarking on a realist project.
- Aspects of a realist research project can be planned in advance, but some elements of the work will develop iteratively and respond to identified data and the developing analysis. Build some flexibility into your plans and timelines to allow for this.
- Realist research is underpinned by a number of important assumptions that have implications for its execution. Researchers new to the approach must ensure that they have a good understanding of these at the start.

Common pitfalls

- Mixing up concepts like 'context' and 'mechanism' and struggling to develop CMOCs. Drawing on others' methodological expertise and experience can help you navigate challenges.
- Trying to do realist research on your own. The analysis in particular will benefit from working within a wider team, and, if possible, having access to a wider group of stakeholders.
- Different levels of understanding within a research team. Realist research is unfamiliar to many, and you may need to devote some time at the outset of a project to ensure everyone is in agreement and understands the nature of the approach and its strengths and weaknesses.

Ethical issues

- The ethical issues involved in realist research are no different from those involved in other approaches to research. Primary research (realist evaluation) will require ethical approval, but it is not likely to be needed for secondary research (realist review).
- The iterative nature of realist projects should be made clear to ethics committees, and you will need to find the right balance of pre-specifying your plans while maintaining some flexibility.

- Stakeholder involvement (where stakeholders are not *participants* in the research) is not likely to require ethical approval, but you should ensure that those engaged and involved are treated respectfully and enabled to contribute meaningfully.

Further reading

For guidance, quality and reporting standards for realist reviews and evaluations, see: The RAMESES Project. https://www.ramesesproject.org (accessed 21 May 2023).

For discussion of a wide range of methodological issues in realist research, see:Emmel, N., Greenhalgh, J., Manzano, A. et al. (ed.) (2018). *Doing Realist Research*. London: SAGE Publications.

The three main texts underpinning the 'Pawson and Tilley' branch of the realist family tree are: (a) Pawson, R. and Tilley, N. (1997). Realistic Evaluation. London: SAGE Publications (b) Pawson, R. (2006) Evidence-Based Policy: A Realist Perspective. London: SAGE Publications. (c) Pawson, R (2013) The Science of Evaluation: A Realist Manifesto. London: SAGE Publications.

References

1 Pawson, R. and Tilley, N. (1997). *Realistic Evaluation*. London: SAGE Publications.

2 Wong, G., Greenhalgh, T., Westhorp, G., and Pawson, R. (2012). Realist methods in medical education research: what are they and what can they contribute? *Medical Education* 46 (1): 89–96.

3 Greenhalgh, T., Pawson, R., Wong, G. et al. (2017). *What Realists Mean by Context; or Why Nothing Works Everywhere or for Everyone*. Oxford: The RAMESES II Project.

4 Papoutsi, C., Mattick, K., Pearson, M. et al. (2018). Interventions to improve antimicrobial prescribing of doctors in training (IMPACT): a realist review. *Health Services and Delivery Research* 6 (10): 1–136.

5 de Groot, E., Schönrock-Adema, J., Zwart, D. et al. (2020). Learning from patients about patient-centredness: a realist review: BEME guide no. 60. *Medical Teacher* 42 (4): 380–392.

6 Lefroy, J., Yardley, S., Kinston, R. et al. (2017). Qualitative research using realist evaluation to explain preparedness for doctors' memorable 'firsts'. *Medical Education* 51 (10): 1037–1048.

7 The RAMESES II Project (2017). "Theory" in realist evaluation. https://www.ramesesproject.org/media/RAMESES_II_Theory_in_realist_evaluation.pdf (accessed 5 May 2023).

8 Pawson, R. (2013). A complexity checklist. In: *The Science of Evaluation: A Realist Manifesto*, 33–46. London: SAGE Publications.

9 The RAMESES Project (2014). Quality standards for realist synthesis. http://www.ramesesproject.org/media/RS_qual_standards_researchers.pdf (accessed 3 May 2023).

10 The RAMESES II Project (2017). Quality standards for realist evaluation for evaluators and peer-reviewers. http://ramesesproject.org/media/RE_Quality_Standards_for_evaluators_and_peer_reviewers.pdf (accessed 3 May 2023).

11 Wong, G., Greenhalgh, T., Westhorp, G. et al. (2013). RAMESES publication standards: realist syntheses. *BMC Medicine* 11 (1): 21.

12 Price, T., Brennan, N., Wong, G. et al. (2021). Remediation programmes for practising doctors to restore patient safety: the RESTORE realist review. *Health Services and Delivery Research* 9: 11.

13 Pawson, R. (2013). Precursors and principles. In: *The Science of Evaluation: A Realist Manifesto*, 33–46. London: SAGE Publications.

14 The RAMESES II Project (2017). Retroduction in realist evaluation. https://www.ramesesproject.org/media/RAMESES_II_Retroduction.pdf (accessed 3 May 2023).

15 Abrams, R., Park, S., Wong, G. et al. (2021). Lost in reviews: looking for the involvement of stakeholders, patients, public and other non-researcher contributors in realist reviews. *Research Synthesis Methods* 12 (2): 239–247.

16 Booth, A., Wright, J., and Briscoe, S. (2018). *Scoping and Searching to Support Realist Approaches* (ed. N. Emmel, J. Greenhalgh, A. Manzano, et al.), 148–165. London: SAGE Publications.

17 Duddy, C. and Roberts, N. (2022). Identifying evidence for five realist reviews in primary health care: a comparison of search methods. *Research Synthesis Methods* 13 (2): 190–203.

11 Mixed methods research: the sum is greater than the parts

Catherine Scarff, Christy Noble, Koshila Kumar, and Wendy Hu

Learning objectives

By the end of this chapter, you should be able to:
- Identify research questions for which mixed methods research is appropriate.
- Discuss benefits, limitations, and challenges of mixed methods research.
- Outline options for designing, conducting, and reporting a mixed methods study.
- Identify the key quality criteria in a mixed methods study.

Introduction

Research problems and questions in clinical education are both messy and multifaceted, reflecting the real-life complexities of clinical practice. Examples of such complex questions include: Why do assessors fail-to-fail nursing students on clinical placements? How can validity evidence for a formative feedback tool be developed? Why are medical students disinterested in doing research? Do physiotherapy students apply the evidence-based practice principles they are taught at university? There are different philosophical traditions underpinning how such questions can be investigated. For example, clinical practice and much healthcare education and research have historically been viewed through a post-positivist lens, where knowledge is regarded as logical, objective, measurable, and amenable to prediction, control, and replication [1, 2]; researchers seek a single explanation to a problem and aim for generalisability. In contrast, in the social sciences such as anthropology, sociology, and some branches of psychology, knowledge is viewed as subjective, constructed, multifaceted and value laden; researchers seek to understand the perspectives or experiences of individuals or groups, whilst maintaining a close connection to how data are obtained, interpreted, and constructed. In short, quantitative methods are usually founded on a positivist stance, whilst qualitative usually in constructivism [3] (see Chapter 3).

From these philosophical standpoints, complex questions can be investigated using a single research method (i.e. qualitative or quantitative) or a mixture. In this chapter, we argue that a combination of research methods can answer questions more comprehensively by both extending theory and suggesting how findings could be put in practice. Mixed methods research seeks to integrate qualitative and quantitative methods and achieve the 'best of both worlds' and is thus well suited to the multifaceted questions posed within clinical education research. As mixed methods research explores quantitative aspects of research problems alongside qualitative ones, it offers an 'agnostic' position [4] that uses the most appropriate aspects of both research approaches to address the problem or question. A pragmatic stance which neither requires nor excludes particular research methods or their combination [5], and which can inform both the theory and practice of education, is well suited to educational research.

For clinicians, mixed methods research can be intuitively attractive due to strong similarities with patient assessment which also involves combining qualitative information (information from a referral letter, history taking) and quantitative data (laboratory investigation results) [6, 7]. Data collection may occur in one one time period (e.g. taking a glucose level at the same time as history from family when a patient has collapsed) or sequentially (e.g. taking a history then ordering investigations on a patient with non-acute abdominal pain) or over a period of time (e.g. revisiting the history over time, by different members of the treating team, with investigations conducted in stages, each informed by results from the previous, in a patient with a chronic illness).

Starting Research in Clinical Education, First Edition. Edited by Eliot L. Rees, Alison Ledger, and Kim A. Walker.
© 2024 The Association for the Study of Medical Education (ASME). Published 2024 by John Wiley & Sons Ltd.
Companion website: www.wiley.com/go/clinicaleducation

Both sets of data require their own interpretation but neither alone is sufficient. The different data must be integrated effectively to formulate an opinion on the patient's presenting problem at each consultation. Depending on the situation, one type of data (such as the history in a patient with mild headache in a community setting) may dominate or both may be equal. Patient assessments thus have scope for variation from the traditional sequence of history → physical examination → investigation. Similarly, the flexibility and adaptability of methods to suit the problem or question at hand characterises the mixed methods approach.

This chapter introduces mixed methods research with an overview of its use in clinical education. The chapter outlines areas to consider when planning and designing studies, including types of research questions which are appropriate for a mixed methods study, and methods for conducting and reporting mixed methods research. We discuss the benefits, limitations, and challenges of mixed methods research and provide tips on how to appraise the quality of a mixed methods study.

What is mixed methods research?

Mixed methods research is characterised by two essential elements: *mixture* and *integration* of different methods. In practice, using a mixture of research methods to answer a research question or address a problem means at least one qualitative and one quantitative method within the same study, based on a clear rationale for why both approaches are needed. Qualitative data (such as from focus groups, interviews, observation, see Part III) and quantitative data (such as from surveys, experiments, or measurements, see Part IV) yield different [8], but potentially complementary insights and perspectives on research questions.

Integration of the different methods [9] so that their combination better addresses the problem than one alone, can occur at different stages of a study and in several ways. There may be greater emphasis on either the qualitative or quantitative component, but there will always be both.

It is essential to recognise that integration is not simply the inclusion of quantitative and qualitative methods in the one study [10]. Studies where the different methods stand alone with no evidence of integration might be better described as multi methods research. Whilst the findings from each may align, combining them towards an integrated presentation or conclusion does not occur (see quality criteria for mixed methods research and [11]).

Both the qualitative and quantitative components of a mixed methods study must satisfy criteria for research quality as if they were each separate studies. One instance where this does not occur, for example, is where optional free text comments from an otherwise quantitative questionnaire are reported as the qualitative component of a 'mixed methods' study. We agree with other authors [12], this leads to superficial qualitative data that would not satisfy quality criteria for qualitative research. Such data can provide clues about participants' viewpoints and study directions, but do not directly address 'the "how?" and "why?" questions that are the core business of qualitative research' [12]. Best practice mixed methods research therefore comprises and combines good quality quantitative and qualitative research.

Why choose mixed methods research?

The fundamental reason for choosing a mixed methods approach is the complexity of the research question or problem to be explored. Mixed methods research is ideal where one type of data or research approach will not lead to sufficient insights or satisfactory answers, but their combination will enable complex phenomena, [6, 13] such as clinical learning environments to be better investigated. Mixed methods research is also suited for new challenging questions or problems [14] where little as yet is known. Greene et al. [15] identified five main purposes (see Table 11.1) for choosing mixed methods.

Creswell et al. [6] further suggest mixed methods research should be considered in order to explain or explore initial results, enhance quantitative findings with qualitative data, compare different cases, better engage participants such that meaningful outcomes and change may occur through the research, or evaluate programme implementation.

Table 11.1 Purpose of using a mixed method design [15]

Purpose	Explanation
Triangulation	Seeking corroboration of results from different methods
Complementarity	Gathering information from different methods
Developmental	Using one method to inform or develop another
Initiation	To see new perspectives or contradictory results
Expansion	To broaden enquiry through the use of other methods

Source: Adapted from Greene et al. [15].

Table 11.2 Considerations when planning a mixed methods study [7, 10]

Design	Resources
What is the purpose or aim of my study?	What expertise will be needed to meet this aim?
What is the structure and timing of data collection and analysis? Will they be sequential, parallel or convergent?	What timing(s) are possible? Do they match with the phenomenon to be researched? Are they practical?
What types of data are needed and how will they be collected? Which is the dominant method?	Can the research aim and questions be answered with different, accessible, data? What are the reasons for privileging one type of data, or keeping them equal?
How will the data be analysed and what inferences are drawn?	At what stage does the integration of the two methods occur? At what other time points and levels can – or should – integration occur?
Who is the target audience for the work?	In what forums and how will the results be presented?

Source: Adapted from Kajamaa et al. [7] and O'Brien and O'Sullivan [10].

In the next section, we provide examples of how different research aims may guide the choice of particular mixed methods research designs (see Table 11.2). You should carefully consider the purpose of your research [7, 15]; the types of evidence required to answer your question(s); and the resources available, prior to selecting a mixed methods approach.

How to plan and design a mixed methods project

The first consideration is to decide what research expertise is required. Working in a team may enable you to mitigate against time constraints in your project. For a student project, it may be just you and your supervisor(s). For other projects, the team may be larger. Regardless, you need time to understand and work with each other's different philosophical stances. Generally (though not always), quantitative methods are grounded in a post-positivist stance, and qualitative in constructivism (see Chapter 3). Cross over is possible, depending on the definition of paradigm held [16], but more often cross-disciplinary exchange and agreement is needed in a mixed methods study. You need to reconcile any epistemological differences amongst your team and consider the different ways each person may

work [7]. As a lead researcher, you will play a key role coordinating and to some extent integrating the philosophical views within the team to avoid members working in parallel silos. One view is that mixing methods amounts to a new paradigm; successful coordination may mean making differences explicit so that 'disharmony to reach unforeseen insight' [16] occurs. Everyone in the team should be open to explaining their stance, thus helping everyone to understand each other's perspective and readers to better understand the research. Perhaps Denscombe offers the best advice for reconciling differences [17], highlighting that 'it is not only allowable to mix methods from alternative and incompatible paradigms of research but it is also *desirable* to do so in order to provide answers that work – or, at least, that work better than those based on the use of just quantitative or just qualitative research'.

In summary, differences in philosophical stance and approach should be recognised, but united towards a shared research aim of using a mix which best answers the agreed research question [18].

The next task is to decide upon the practical aspects of the project. Table 11.2 aims to assist planning by posing the questions, considerations, and decisions you should make when embarking on a mixed methods study [7, 10].

How to choose your design

Given the flexibility and adaptability of mixed methods research, it is not surprising that there are varied and potentially confusing terms and typologies for mixed methods research designs. Two key considerations guide the choice, the intent of the integration, and whether this is to 'explain, explore, or converge' results [6]. As with clinical problems, design decisions may be made as findings emerge during the study rather than being fixed at the outset. That is, the design can follow a prescribed classification or it may be dynamic and responsive to a changing context or new findings [6]. As such, mixed methods research may be indistinguishable from action research (see Chapter 12). Some classifications also include the intended outcomes of mixed methods research in design considerations such as societal change (transformation) for an underserved or marginalised population [6].

Table 11.3 and the following section outlines common research designs and uses examples to illustrate some of their strengths and challenges, together with suggestions on when to choose the most appropriate design. If you are new to mixed methods research, it is probably easier to pick one design that resonates with your needs and follow the related set of literature. In summary, the key to a

Table 11.3 Mixed methods research design options. (from [6])

Design	When to use	Benefits	Challenges	Examples of mixed methods clinical education research studies
Convergent	When the intent is to combine or compare results of a qualitative and quantitative dataset. Where time is limited, but the team has the skills to do both together	An efficient and intuitive approach where both types of data are collected over the same time period. The qualitative and quantitative components often have equal priority	Often requires a team. May involve merging different types of data from samples which may differ in size and scope. Potential issues arise if results do not agree.	*Motivating medical students to do research: a mixed methods study using Self-Determination Theory* [19] Aims: to explore what motivates medical students to do research and to design more effective and evidence-based strategies to strengthen student interest in research during medical school. Context: undergraduate medical program in one Australian public university. Integration of findings: survey and interview findings were integrated informed by Self-Determination Theory.

Example:

Design	When to use	Benefits	Challenges	Examples of mixed methods clinical education research studies
Explanatory sequential	Where the intent is to explain initial quantitative results with qualitative data	Researcher deals with only one data set at a time. May suit problems which are more amenable to quantitative data collection and analysis. The qualitative part may strengthen the credibility of the quantitative findings by explaining how the quantified phenomenon comes about. One of the most straightforward to design and report on. A flexible approach, as the second phase emerges from the findings of first.	Takes more time than a convergent approach. Ethics approval may require amendments if the second phase differs from what was originally approved. Decisions are needed about which quantitative data to explain further and from whom (i.e. selection of the second sample)	*Changes in physiotherapy students' knowledge and perceptions of EBP from first year to graduation: A mixed methods study* [20] Aim: to explore physiotherapy student Evidence-Based Practice (EBP) outcomes (self-reported knowledge, attitudes and behaviours, and actual knowledge), from 'baseline' (prior to any training) to 'graduation' (after completion of all training). Context: undergraduate physiotherapy program in one Australia public university. Integration of findings: quantitative and qualitative findings presented separately; merged results also presented outlining divergent, congruent, and unique findings.

Example:

Table 11.3 (Continued)

Design	When to use	Benefits	Challenges	Examples of mixed methods clinical education research studies
Exploratory sequential	When a phenomenon is explored qualitatively and results used to inform the development of a quantitative instrument or tool. Testing of the tool occurs in a subsequent phase. Identifies new questions arising from qualitative data.	May suit problems which are more amenable to qualitative data collection and analysis, and/or where a tool to test questions on a larger sample is required. Is an emergent approach, as second phase depends on findings of first. The quantitative part may enhance acceptability of the qualitative findings by indicating the size of the qualitative phenomenon or a measurable outcome. Could lead to a new instrument.	Requires more time, and expertise including potential development of a new instrument. The ethics approval may need amendments after the qualitative phase is completed. Decisions about samples for each component and which qualitative data to use for the exploratory phase are required.	*Moving forward: Barriers and enablers to failure to fail – A mixed methods meta-integration* [21] Aims: to explore assessors' experiences of failure-to-fail of nursing students within work-integrated learning in an Australian context. Context: assessment of nursing students in work integrated learning context. Integration of findings: data were integrated throughout the study. Findings from the three separate parts – an initial literature review, followed by interviews and focus groups and then a survey – were analysed and reported elsewhere, and in this paper a meta-integration using Invitational theory was presented.

Example:

Source: Creswell and Plano Clark [6] / with permission of SAGE Publications.

successful project comes from thinking things through, planning, and justifying the choices made, taking into account the experience and resources available to you and your team.

In addition to the purpose of the proposed study, Table 11.3 highlights factors such as the time and expertise required [6, 7]. For those new to mixed methods research, a convergent option, where qualitative and quantitative components have similar priority, is probably the most feasible. In contrast, one component often dominates in sequential designs appealing more to those with greater expertise in one approach [6]. Sequential designs also require integration between the two waves of data collection and at the end of the study, and you may need to shift paradigms between study phases. This change of gears may feel jarring and awkward until the findings are successfully resolved, making this design a more complex and lengthy undertaking.

Other more complex applications of mixed methods designs such as mixed methods experimental or intervention design, mixed methods evaluation design, and the mixed methods case study design [6] can occur based on the purpose of the study and considerations outlined in Table 11.2.

When and how to integrate?

Integrating the qualitative and quantitative study components is the defining quality of mixed methods research. It is key to comprehensively addressing a complex research problem and producing findings which extend beyond 'simply adding together the results of separate qualitative and quantitative studies' [22]. Integration nevertheless can be a challenge to achieve effectively and with meaning.

Integration can occur at multiple points in a study; for example, in data collection, during data interpretation, and when reporting findings [23, 24]. Integration can also mean using results to inform the design or analysis of another part of the study at the same time, or in sequence [25]. A theory can also be used to integrate qualitative and quantitative components of a study together (e.g. as in Moran-Ellis et al. [24]).

Fetters et al. [23] suggest possibilities for integration, with methods such as connecting, where data sets connect to each other through sampling techniques; building, where one data set informs the data collection of another; merging, where two data sets are brought together for analysis; and embedding, where data collection and analysis join at several points. Other options include triangulation, where results are considered in relation to where they agree, disagree, or provide complementary information [9]; or by following a thread, where a theme from one component is traced across other components [9]; or with matrices, which may involve qualitising (turning quantitative findings into qualitative) or quantitising (turning qualitative findings into quantitative) data [25], to facilitate the direct comparison of different data from the same participants [26].

Table 11.3 provides some examples of mixed methods integration techniques. Both Rosenkranz [19] and Hughes [21] used theory to inform integration, whilst McEvoy et al. [20] merged their qualitative and quantitative data analysis to identify divergent, congruent, and unique findings.

How to report mixed methods research

A key challenge when reporting your project is how to adequately describe two methods and two sets of results, as well as the integration method and subsequent findings within journal word limits or other communications such as conference proceedings. Fortunately, more journals which specialise in mixed methods research are emerging and online supplemental reporting can be an option. Many journals have enhanced word limits for qualitative studies and extend this to mixed methods research. Examples used by authors include tables, diagrams, and flowcharts to explain the sequence and type of methods used and to present integrated findings, such as through matrices.

Quality criteria for mixed methods research

As mixed methods research has evolved and gained wider acceptance, thinking about how to assess its quality has progressed. Appraising each part of a study using accepted tools for qualitative and quantitative research has been suggested, but increasingly mixed methods specific criteria are used [27] so, integration can be appraised. Concepts such as inference quality, which focuses on quality of design and rigor in interpretation (as described by Tashakkori and Teddlie in [27]), and legitimation, which describes the 'trustworthiness' of data and its interpretation [18] have been proposed. As with all study designs, coherence between the purpose of the study, its conceptual framework, and the choices made about design, methods, and presentation of findings [10], study limitations and relationship to literature [28] should be considered when appraising quality.

O'Cathain et al. have devised the Good Reporting of A Mixed Methods Study (GRAMMS) [11] guideline for appraising mixed methods research which outlines areas researchers should report on:

1 Justification for using mixed methods with reference to the research problem.
2 Description of the design, with an emphasis of the purpose, priority of methods, sequence, and integration of methods.
3 Description of each method including sampling, data collection, and analysis.
4 Where and how integration has occurred and who conducted it.
5 Outline of the limitations of the study.
6 Rationale for the insights gained from mixing or integrating methods.

Other quality appraisal tools such as the scoring system proposed by Pluye et al. [29] can be applied to assess the quality of mixed study literature reviews and mixed methods research in general.

Benefits and challenges

Table 11.3 outlines some benefits and challenges of different mixed methods research designs. When well designed, mixed methods research offers potential benefits such as being a more efficient use of data, suiting the complexity and messiness of 'real-life' clinical education problems [4], and extending understanding beyond those of a single perspective [30]. It can be used for many areas of research and is not limited to certain contexts – it 'seems applicable to a wide variety of disciplines in the social, behavioural and health sciences' [6]. Mixing methods can improve the integrity and application of outcomes [14] by highlighting how they can be used in practice. This is reflected in its frequent use in programme evaluation, implementation science, and translational research.

The flexibility of mixed methods research confers advantages since using a mixture of methods can help counteract the particular disadvantages of each [6]. It can encourage researchers to develop skills in different research methods [6]. It can promote collaboration between researchers of different backgrounds and with diverse philosophical views and further 'allow for opportunities to develop new research questions or theories' [14] and set new research agendas [30]. Mixed methods research may be more persuasive due to the integration of findings from different methods and multiple perspectives leading to a more complete picture of the phenomenon being studied [13].

However, this type of research also presents challenges. You or your team will need to possess skills in both quantitative and qualitative methods and how to effectively integrate the two [6]. You will require greater time and resources to collect and analyse two types of data [6] and time requirements can be underestimated [14]. For example, quantitative researchers may be accustomed to spending more time on developing and implementing a survey instrument, whereas qualitative researchers can rapidly collect large amounts of data and need to allocate considerable time for data analysis.

As a comparatively new method, the acceptability and publication of mixed methods research have its own challenges [22]. 'Turf wars' over research paradigms mean that '[m]ixing requires expertise and resilience, amongst clashing expectations and cultures with other medical research' [4]. Splitting up work and publishing parts separately can lead to incoherent or conflicting results which are not resolved when components are reported separately. Transparent reporting that includes justifications for design choices and claims will help avoid such outcomes [28].

Summary

Mixed methods research offers a powerful way of untangling complex research problems and questions in clinical education that contributes to more meaningful and practical outcomes for clinical educators and scholars. It is becoming more acceptable and prevalent in clinical education research and understanding the benefits (and challenges) may lead you to produce impactful research.

Top tips

- Work as a team. Gather the skills needed, use available resources including expertise and time effectively, and learn from each other including in relation to different philosophical views to expand ideas.
- Agree on the research aims and revisit them regularly when communicating with supervisors / team members. This is especially important if individuals work on different parts of the study, so everyone retains the overall vision of the work.
- Mixed methods research 'speaks' [7] differently to different audiences. Consider what rationale and depth of explanation needs to be provided for each audience.
- Explicitly describe where and how integration occurs in the study as it may not be readily apparent.
- Use diagrams, flowcharts, and tables to clearly and efficiently communicate what can be a complex study design to readers and reviewers. This may also assist with word limits.
- Use images or graphics to both do and report integrated data analysis.

Common pitfalls

- Use of 'design by convenience' based on already available quantitative and qualitative data. Think through and ensure your design choices can be articulated and justified.
- Lack of integration, meaning a study is multi-methods rather than truly mixed methods. Use appropriate terms when reporting your study.
- Engaging in 'paradigm wars'. Avoid this by working on collaborative relationships and being open to epistemological differences, emerging practices, and controversies. Aim to be clear and transparent in reporting, using simple language.

Ethical issues

- Ensure effective communication occurs between members of the research team and that all have the opportunity to speak and be heard.
- Double, repeated, or sequential data collection may be burdensome on participants. Make instruments as brief as possible, offer compensation, and schedule convenient data collection times.
- In sequential mixed methods research, you may need to update your ethics application as your design evolves.

References

1 Irby, D.M. (1990). Shifting paradigms of research in medical education. *Academic Medicine* 65 (10): 622–623.

2 Kuper, A. and D'Eon, M. (2011). Rethinking the basis of medical knowledge. *Medical Education* 45 (1): 36–43.

3 Carter, S.M. and Little, M. (2007). Justifying knowledge, justifying method, taking action: epistemologies, methodologies, and methods in qualitative research. *Qualitative Health Research* 17 (10): 1316–1328.

4 Maudsley, G. (2011). Mixing it but not mixed-up: mixed methods research in medical education (a critical narrative review). *Medical Teacher* 33 (2): e92–e104.

5 Feilzer, M.Y. (2010). Doing mixed methods research pragmatically: implications for the rediscovery of pragmatism as a research paradigm. *Journal of Mixed Methods Research* 4 (1): 6–16.

6 Creswell, J.W. and Plano Clark, V.L. (2018). *Designing and Conducting Mixed Methods Research*, 3e. Los Angeles: SAGE Publications. 492 pp.

7 Kajamaa, A., Mattick, K., and de la Croix, A. (2020). How to . . . do mixed-methods research. *The Clinical Teacher* 17 (3): 267–271.

8 Johnson, R.B., Onwuegbuzie, A.J., and Turner, L.A. (2007). Toward a definition of mixed methods research. *Journal of Mixed Methods Research* 1 (2): 112–133.

9 O'Cathain, A., Murphy, E., and Nicholl, J. (2010). Three techniques for integrating data in mixed methods studies. *BMJ* 341 (7783): 1147–1150.

10 O'Brien, B.C. and O'Sullivan, P.S. (2017). Mixed methods in health professions education scholarship. *Journal of Graduate Medical Education* 9 (2): 253–254.

11 O'Cathain, A., Murphy, E., and Nicholl, J. (2008). The quality of mixed methods studies in health services research. *Journal of Health Services Research & Policy* 13 (2): 92–98.

12 LaDonna, K.A., Taylor, T., and Lingard, L. (2018). Why open-ended survey questions are unlikely to support rigorous qualitative insights. *Academic Medicine* 93 (3): 347–349.

13 McKim, C.A. (2017). The value of mixed methods research: a mixed methods study. *Journal of Mixed Methods Research* 11 (2): 202–222.

14 Schifferdecker, K.E. and Reed, V.A. (2009). Using mixed methods research in medical education: basic guidelines for researchers. *Medical Education* 43 (7): 637–644.

15 Greene, J.C., Carcelli, V.J., and Graham, W.F. (1989). Toward a conceptual framework for mixed-method evaluation designs. *Educational Evaluation and Policy Analysis* 11 (3): 255–274.

16 Ghiara, V. (2020). Disambiguating the role of paradigms in mixed methods research. *Journal of Mixed Methods Research* 14 (1): 11–25.

17 Denscombe, M. (2014). *The Good Research Guide: For Small-Scale Social Research Projects*, 5e. Maidenhead: McGraw-Hill, Open University Press.

18 Johnson, R.B. and Onwuegbuzie, A.J. (2004). Mixed methods research: a research paradigm whose time has come. *Educational Research* 33 (7): 14–26.

19 Rosenkranz, S.K., Wang, S., and Hu, W. (2015). Motivating medical students to do research: a mixed methods study using self-determination theory. *BMC Medical Education* 15 (1): 1–13.

20 McEvoy, M.P., Lewis, L.K., and Luker, J. (2018). Changes in physiotherapy students' knowledge and perceptions of EBP from first year to graduation: a mixed methods study. *BMC Medical Education* 18 (1): 1–11.

21 Hughes, L.J., Mitchell, M.L., and Johnston, A.N.B. (2021). Moving forward: barriers and enablers to failure to fail – a mixed methods meta-integration, 104666. *Nurse Education Today* 98.

22 Fetters, M.D. and Freshwater, D. (2015). The 1 + 1 = 3 integration challenge. *Journal of Mixed Methods Research* 9 (2): 115–117.

23 Fetters, M.D., Curry, L.A., and Creswell, J.W. (2013). Achieving integration in mixed methods designs – principles and practices. *Health Services Research* 48 (6 Part 2): 2134–2156.

24 Åkerblad, L., Seppänen-Järvelä, R. and Haapakoski, K. (2021). Integrative Strategies in Mixed Methods Research. *J Mix Methods Res* 15(2):152–170.

25 Bazeley, P. (2012). Integrative analysis strategies for mixed data sources. *The American Behavioral Scientist* 56 (6): 814–828.

26 Campbell, R., Quilty, B., and Dieppe, P. (2003). Discrepancies between patients' assessments of outcome: qualitative study nested within a randomised controlled trial. *BMJ* 326: 252–253.

27 O'Cathain, A. (2015). Assessing the quality of mixed methods research: toward a comprehensive framework. In: *SAGE Handbook of Mixed Methods in Social & Behavioral Research* (ed. A. Tashakkori and C. Teddlie), 531–556. Thousand Oaks: SAGE Publications.

28 Ellaway, R. (2020). Mixed methods, crimes, and misdemeanours. *Advances in Health Sciences Education* 25 (4): 777–779.

29 Pluye, P., Gagnon, M.P., Griffiths, F., and Johnson-Lafleur, J. (2009). A scoring system for appraising mixed methods research, and concomitantly appraising qualitative, quantitative and mixed methods primary studies in mixed studies reviews. *International Journal of Nursing Studies* 46 (4): 529–546.

30 Lavelle, E., Vuk, J., and Barber, C. (2013). Twelve tips for getting started using mixed methods in medical education research. *Medical Teacher* 35 (4): 272–276.

12 Action research: improving clinical education programmes

Janet Lefroy and Emma Collins

Learning objectives

By the end of this chapter, you should be able to:
- Appreciate the nature of action research and identify its place in clinical education research.
- Formulate research questions about important topics to be answered by action research.
- Identify whom to involve in your action research.
- Conduct rigorous action research.

Introduction

Action research, as the name suggests, is both action and research. It involves critical analysis of problems (research) and testing out new solutions (action). In this chapter, we present the principles underlying action research and how it has been applied to education for curriculum development, institutional change, and the personal development of educators. We describe the steps involved in two forms of action research as they apply to the clinical educator and provide case studies of our own experiences of these: *Practical* action research (Janet's case study, Box 12.1) and critical (*practitioner*) action research (Emma's case study, Box 12.2).

The principles of action research were first outlined by Kurt Lewin (1890–1947), a social psychologist interested in improving social organisation of groups [1]. His underlying principle of action research was that groups collectively address and support social change together. Lewin's model is often presented as a cycle of *plan, act, observe and reflect*. Other action research models are often based on Lewin's concepts, for example, Carr and Kemmis's model (Figure 12.1) [2].

One important feature of action research is its participatory nature, involving individuals within institutions or societies in solving practical problems and contributing to knowledge in a participatory process [3]. Another key feature is change. Action research by practitioners aims to change one or more of three elements: the practitioners' practices, their understanding of their practice, or the conditions in which they practise [4]. The concepts of critical reflection and self-reflection are at the heart of action research [5].

Types of action research

There are many different types of action research [6]. Carr and Kemmis [2, 4] distinguish three broad approaches:
1. Technical action research (positivist, a social experiment changing practice and aiming for measurable improved outcomes).
2. Practical action research (interpretive, reflecting on and understanding what we do and incorporating and generating theory in useful solutions).
3. Critical action research (emancipating us from the conditions that constrain what we do, espousing conditions that enhance what we do and thus transforming practice).

Practitioner action research is a form of critical action research that aims to help other people and therefore has values and virtue at its core [7]. Practitioner action research concerns learning, knowledge creation, is educational, collaborative, critical and risky, and is always political according to McNiff [5].

While recognised schools of action research differ in the degree to which they are influenced by critical theory (that critical reflection upon the social and cultural assumptions underlying practice is how

---

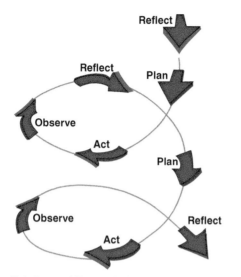

Figure 12.1 Carr and Kemmis's (1986) action research model. *Source*: [2] / Taylor & Francis.

changes in attitude can occur), they all have the following features in common: [3]

- Concerned with social practice.
- Aimed towards improvement.
- A cyclical process of incremental change and evaluation.
- Pursued by systematic enquiry.
- A reflective process.
- Participatory (although some accept action research as individual problem-solving and reflection).
- Determined by the practitioners.

Action research has been important to developments in healthcare, but has also been useful to the education sector, higher education, and clinical education as described in the next section.

In this chapter, we focus on *practical* action research and *practitioner* action research (a form of critical action research) as these are the most relevant for clinical education. For further information on other types of action research, see the further reading.

Action research by educators

Practical action research in education has allowed teachers to take ownership of research and to facilitate change in curricula and classroom teaching: the 'teacher as researcher' contributing to theory and increasing the generalisability of their action research findings as applied to curriculum development and institutional change [8–10]. One of the attractions of action research to the educational community is the shift in focus from 'outsider'

research to collaborative research [10] which chimes with the shift to regarding higher education students as adult learners actively involved as co-researchers and co-creators of knowledge. Teachers in higher education are therefore encouraged to regard students as rightful collaborators in action research for curriculum development or institutional change. Teachers and researchers do, however, need to be careful not to overload their learners with research activities when most will already be on full-time programmes of study.

Action research has been used in clinical education to bring about required curriculum changes and to ensure thoughtful innovation of learning and teaching methods. Action research can also be used to develop evaluation procedures and transform our ideas about institutional structures and culture [11–16].

Practitioner action research is another form of action research widely adopted by educators [17]. Personal professional development is core to the 'teacher as researcher' concept, answering the question 'How do I improve my professional practice?'. Although scholarship for personal professional development can be an individual activity for a teacher, when done in collaboration with others who act as critical friends, this is practitioner action research, critically examining what we are doing, why and what the effects have been [10, 18, 19]. These reflections can also promote a scholarly approach to developing our individual and collective teacher beliefs.

In the next section, we will outline the steps involved in each of these two types of action research. We have annotated the steps as they map onto the Reflect–Plan–Act–Observe–Reflect stages in the action research cycle (Figure 12.1). We then offer two case studies (Boxes 12.1 and 12.2) as illustrative examples of these two forms of action research.

Practical action research

Practical action research entails eight steps.

Step 1 (observe and reflect): Turning your problem to be solved into research questions

It is only worth putting effort into setting up an action research team and project if you need to make substantial change and it is not immediately apparent what the changes should be. You may have identified the need for change because of problems that arose in teaching sessions, or from student evaluations of learning, or in poor assessment outcomes. You can turn these into initial broad research questions by comparing the actual outcomes with intended learning outcomes and asking yourself what strategies might achieve the desired outcomes. You should then write an initial statement containing all this information and circulate it amongst key personnel in your organisation (e.g. programme leaders, teaching teams, and curriculum committee) seeking permission to innovate and to potential stakeholders to see whether they would be willing to get involved.

Step 2 (reflect): recruiting stakeholders

Your action research will benefit from involving individuals who have a stake in the programme you wish to change (see Chapter 5). In the clinical education context, this is likely to include teachers and students, but it could also include an educational psychologist if you are needing to change teaching methodology, a social scientist, and patient representatives if patient behaviour or care is part of the topic. We recommend keeping the number of stakeholders to a realistic team size (four to eight), as this makes stakeholder discussions more practicable and manageable.

Step 3 (reflect): critical and self-critical reflection on current state

Involve stakeholders in preliminary discussions of the problem(s) you have identified with your current curriculum, culminating in a draft research proposal. This will include modification of your initial statement, e.g. articulating a set of guiding objectives, making assumptions explicit. It will also include a review of the research literature to find how comparable curricula have covered similar objectives and what problems they have encountered.

Step 4 (plan): planning change

While you want your stakeholders to contribute their innovative 'grass roots' ideas, you should try to align them with theory, evidence from the literature, and the best practice from comparable programmes. When planning change, it is essential that your action research team maintains alignment between intended learning outcomes, teaching methods and content, and assessment strategies and items.

Your team's plans should include how the next stage of the action research cycle will be conducted so that the most useful observational data can be collected by rigorous methodologies. Plans may also include faculty development strategies and monitoring of the wider impacts of change on other areas of the curriculum. At this step, it is important to ensure ethical approvals are in place for the research.

Step 5 (act and observe): implementing and monitoring change using rigorous research methodologies

As the change is rolled out, your team should collect data to monitor outcomes and enable immediate small improvements to be made in repeat iterations. It is also important to step back and evaluate rigorously to discover whether the intended learning outcomes are now being achieved, and what other consequences there might be. Types of monitoring data may include assessment of knowledge and skills, student satisfaction scores, tutor monitoring of student engagement and behaviour, and student and tutor views.

Your action research team should carefully consider which research methods to use in your action research. There are likely to be few clinical education outcome measures amenable to meaningful statistical comparison. Assessment outcomes comparing different cohorts pre- and post-changes will be affected by factors other than the changes made, and measures of student likes or dislikes for an educational intervention and self-evaluation of learning may be biased by factors other than the quality of the learning experience. A convincing level of proof can, however, be reached from a body of evidence and mixed methods may be used to achieve this (see Chapter 11). The evidence you gain from qualitative research about the impact of change will be richer than quantitative measures alone.

Triangulation of methods and sources is normal procedure in action research, not only to enhance credibility but also to give a better depth of understanding by providing different types of information and information from different perspectives [8, 16].

You might find it possible to run a pseudo-experiment with a cross-over design involving student cohorts in qualitative or quantitative comparison trials of the old curriculum versus the new intervention where students can effectively act as their own controls. For example, when one cohort is taught one module using the 'new' methods and another module using the 'old' methods, while a comparison cohort is taught the first module with the 'old' and the second with the 'new' methods. You can then make comparisons within cohorts for their feedback on the two methods and also between cohorts for any outcome data.

There are no set approaches to analysis in action research. Use has been made of phenomenology, thematic analysis, grounded theory, and activity theory among others.

Realist evaluation (see Chapter 10) is another possible approach to data collection and analysis in action research [20]. Realist evaluation has an explanatory focus and involves participants in answering the question 'what works for whom in what circumstances and why?' [21]. If your team wants to incorporate realist principles into action research, you will aim to answer realist research questions – not just 'has it worked?' – but 'for whom has it worked and not worked?' 'In what circumstances does it work and not work?' and for both, 'why?'

Step 6 (reflect): critical and self-critical evaluation to answer the research questions

In order to bring a wide perspective to analysis, involve your stakeholder group in the process as much as possible. Action research often takes the position that we create meaning by interacting with the realities around us. As explained in Chapter 3, the constructivist approach does not aim to establish causality in the same terms that positivist research may, nor does it seek the generation of generalisable laws. The implications of this are that the findings of action research will not be universal. Although they arise from real-life experiences and not from experimental conditions, and therefore have validity for the people studied, recommendations to others can only be tentative and must be adapted to the context and circumstances of the reader.

If you decide to bring a realist approach to action research, you acknowledge that groups within a student cohort may react differently from each other in the same conditions. If the influence of context is discussed, this may enable a more nuanced curricular approach and interventions to be better adapted for use in other settings.

Step 7 (plan): cycle 2 planning

Your successful innovations can be retained, but those which did not work as expected will need to be problematised again and entered into another cycle of action research.

Step 8 (help others to reflect and act): disseminating your research findings

The findings developed by your action research team should be reported locally within the teaching team and to your organisation's curriculum committee (or equivalent). Your student body might also value hearing the report.

Such a report can be useful to larger audiences such as through a publication or a conference presentation. The advantages might include assisting individuals who find themselves in a similar predicament in resolving similar issues, as well as advancing educational theory and comprehension. The dissemination of action research innovations can also encourage similar self-critical reflection in other educators (see Chapter 28).

BOX 12.1   Case study of using practical action research in clinical education

Janet led three sequential practical action research projects as part of a PhD by published works.

The first project developed an undergraduate medicine consultation skills curriculum. The action research team had various members at different stages, as stakeholders found time to participate, but always had representation from teachers and students. Four meetings were required to complete the design part of the action research cycle. The first design group agreed a timeline for the design phase, the production of materials, the recruiting and training of tutors, seeking ethical approval and the implementation, and monitoring and evaluation of the first year of the consultation curriculum.

Reflecting

The overarching research question was 'How can the existing communication skills curriculum be optimised, in the light of experience here and elsewhere, and in congruence with the rest of the curriculum?'

The team conducted a review of current consultation skills teaching in the clinical education literature and visited two other medical schools to inform an initial critical review of the previous communication skills curriculum. Reflecting on their findings, the group highlighted the following problems for action:

- The Calgary Cambridge guide to the medical interview [22] incorporates the patient's perspective in a helpful way. However, there was a risk of mismatch between the framework 'exploring the presenting complaint' and students' experiences of meeting patients with chronic conditions (who were not presenting a complaint to be diagnosed).
- Simulated patient consultations were felt by student team members to be more useful than role-play with peers, but the group setting in skills classes induced high-performance anxiety.
- The need for integration of the consultation skills curriculum with the programme of placements for experiential learning was raised at the first design meeting and became an important feature of the design of year 1.

Planning

The team planned innovations for the first year of the new curriculum:

- A new first session about active listening and how to give and receive feedback.
- Students interviewing simulated patients in pairs.
- Simulated patient's emotional level to be chosen by students in one session.
- Tutor continuity.
- Placement providers were asked to provide opportunities for the skills learned in classes to be practised.

They also drafted a strategy document for the rest of the five-year curriculum with consultation skills milestones at the end of each of the five years. This had to be ratified by the wider school curriculum development meetings, and the draft was modified by these meetings. The team might therefore be seen as an extra layer in an already complex process of curriculum design and certainly did not have sole authorship of the consultation skills curriculum. What the action research process added was the in-depth examination of the previous curriculum. The student member of the group was a rich source of insights and would not have been involved if Janet did not deliberately invite stakeholders.

Acting and observing

The innovations they made to the consultation skills curriculum all needed to be evaluated. As the first iteration rolled out, they collected monitoring data from student evaluation forms and tutor debriefings. They triangulated these with focus group discussions with students.

Reflecting and reporting

The team reported what they learned from the student evaluations, tutor debriefings, and focus group discussions about the consultation skills curriculum internally and at national education conferences. They also produced three journal publications which enabled wider dissemination of some of their key findings [23–25].

They then undertook two more action research projects identifying the key consultation competencies required by students and feedback that can support consultation skill development [26–30].

Practitioner action research

Practitioner action research is action research for professional development, not just for an individual but also the community involved [7]. It consists of five key steps.

Step 1: reflect

You decide to critique your teaching with a view to improving educational outcomes. Examining your teaching will help you understand the situation more fully. This new understanding will help you to evaluate your teaching and make any changes that are necessary. Do not do this alone. You should find critical friends and check your perception of what is happening against their perceptions. One way would be for them to observe your teaching as part of a peer observation of teaching scheme.

Step 2: plan

You make changes to your teaching in light of the perceptions of your critical friends. You agree with them what changes to make. Your joint agreement about perceptions and changes helps you all to understand the situation better.

Step 3: act

You implement the changes, continuing to learn from colleagues, and they learn from you. They decide to try things out for themselves.

Step 4: observe

Your colleagues invite you in turn to become their critical friend and to help them evaluate their teaching. You observe them and provide feedback on their teaching.

Step 5: reflect

Collectively you have become a community of enquirers. You have changed your social situation, and this is bound to have consequences for your school as this is one form of organisational change. This can feel threatening to the leadership of the school unless they realise and welcome its beneficial potential for the institution its staff and learners. If managers encourage this form of collective enquiry and get involved in learning with the people they support, the individual learning becomes organisational learning. Your individual 'I-enquiry' has turned into a collective 'we-enquiry'.

BOX 12.2   Case study of using practitioner action research in clinical education

Emma conducted practitioner action research as part of a MA in Higher Education module. She followed the five steps of reflect, plan, act, observe, and reflect.

Reflecting

She gathered some initial anecdotal evidence suggesting that a personal and professional e-portfolio, which focused upon graduate attributes and was available to BSc preregistration nursing students was not fully integrated within the nursing curriculum. Both students and their personal tutors who were responsible for signing off the e-portfolio were unclear of its concept and purpose. The signing-off process of the e-portfolio occurred in year 3 of the nursing programme that Emma was responsible for leading and managing.

Planning

Identifying this practical workplace problem, Emma's action research project aim was to evaluate whether better information for personal tutors about the e-portfolio would promote its integration within the nursing programme. She chose practitioner action research as there was a practical workplace problem, a change in practice was required, and it was participant focused [17]. She started with a literature review, identifying gaps in the literature in relation to tutor perspectives of the advantages and challenges of e-portfolios. This informed her planning of a project exploring personal tutors' feedback on the e-portfolio and developing personal tutor guidance.

She only involved personal tutors in her stakeholder group due to the limited timescale of six months for the project, acknowledging that students could also be useful stakeholders and could be part of another action research project cycle.

She developed draft personal tutor guidance which was then reviewed by the personal tutors in the project to ascertain their opinions and thoughts about its use, demonstrating the value of collaboration within action research [18, 19].

She planned to keep a reflective diary and conclude each stage of the project with a reflective account to enhance the critical nature of the research [18]. The planning stage also involved getting ethical approval for the project's data collection.

Acting and observing

The action research project had two complete cycles involving different data collection methods in each cycle:

Cycle 1: She monitored use of the e-portfolio and made field notes from a personal tutor e-portfolio training session. These included general observation notes from the training session and a summary of the questions and general discussion generated.

Cycle 2: She held a focus group with personal tutors which discussed two topics – the cycle 1 data (a form of data triangulation) and the proposed personal tutor e-portfolio guidance. She transcribed the focus group, which was a personal research development point and also promoted researcher immersion in the data. She analysed the data by coding and then grouping codes into themes (see Chapter 19). She used an open coding system, counting up keywords and phrases used during the two cycles and then identified themes from this.

The focus group agreed that the proposed personal tutor guidance about the e-portfolio would be valuable and might help to integrate its use. Personal tutors also suggested some amendments to the guidance document.

The lack of understanding about the e-portfolio among the tutors was a larger problem than she had anticipated. This led her to the conclusion that the personal tutor information alone would not completely address this lack of awareness and understanding. Other measures were required. It was evident that she would need a school implementation strategy for the e-portfolio and to develop a formal training package for staff.

Reflecting

Her reflection on the project helped her identify limitations. It was a small-scale project and took place within one school of the University. Not all the original study objectives were achieved during the two cycles. However, the remaining study objective which was to disseminate the personal tutor information was addressed in a subsequent cycle. Although this delay meant the project was not complete after cycle two, in fact it proved advantageous for the project because it enabled the personal tutors to engage, suggest and comment on draft personal tutor information prior to producing a final version for their use. Her reflection from this was that flexibility is required in action research, and plans may need to be changed to complete as many cycles of action research as needed.

Summary

Action research aims to solve practical problems (to improve/change a social practice).

The process should involve those who are most concerned (participatory) in a journey – often a cycle of planning, acting, observing (data collection), and reflection. If sufficiently systematic and self-critical, this can also contribute to generation of knowledge of use to others.

Action research suits teachers wishing to improve their personal teaching practices and/or their institution's curriculum [3, 31–33]. Teachers can reflect self-critically, using existing knowledge from the literature. The reflect–plan–act–observe cycle helps to develop logically [33, 34]. Action research teams should involve key stakeholders such as students and patients as well as interested members of faculty. Curricula are always changing, faculty engagement in the observation and reflection processes can be good for team engagement and development; and if you do find something works well, the findings should be disseminated to help colleagues facing similar difficulties [3].

Our two case studies have demonstrated how action research can be used to improve curricula within clinical education for both students and educators. The case studies also highlight the various approaches of action research and the different methods of data collection and analysis.

Top tips

- Involve stakeholders in all stages of the project. Action research should be participatory.
- Make changes based on inquiry. Action research should be aiming for improvement.
- Consider triangulation to get a more thorough view of what is really happening.
- Be prepared to adapt and change focus. Action research is a journey – cyclical and ongoing. You may need to undertake additional cycles.

Common pitfalls

- Omitting the two key elements of action research which make success more likely – participation and critical reflection. Ensure to include these in your curriculum development projects.
- Lacking a clear focus. This may cause you to lose your way. If other problems are identified, the project may become too big.
- Not involving those who will be affected by your curriculum change. This can lead to resistance and unintended consequences.

Ethical issues

- If you do not get ethical approval before you start rolling out your innovation, you will not be able to publish the results of your evaluations in any peer-reviewed journal. That is a waste of good new knowledge which might benefit a wider audience than your local school.
- If planning an intervention/control study or a cross-over study, your ethics panel will want to be sure that students are not disadvantaged by being in one or other group, or by declining to participate in any research you are doing.
- It is worth considering whether there may be any unintended consequences of your changes. Ethics committees like to see that you have weighed up potential benefits and risks.
- Action research is an iterative approach. You may need to return to the ethics panel chair with a request to modify your application partway through the project.

Further reading

Coghlan, D. and Brydon-Miller, M. (ed.) (2014). *The SAGE Encyclopedia of Action Research*. London: SAGE Publications.

Hammond, M. (2013). The contribution of pragmatism to understanding educational action research: value and consequences. *Educational Action Research* 21 (4): 603–618.

Johannesson, P. (2020). Development of professional learning communities through action research: understanding professional learning in practice. *Educational Action Research* 30 (3): 411–426.

Kemmis, S. and McTaggart, R. (1992). *The Action Research Planner*, 3e. Geelong: Deakin University Press.

McKernan, J. (1996). *Curriculum Action Research: A Handbook of Methods and Resources for the Reflective Practitioner*, 2e. London: Kogan Page.

References

1 Lewin, K. (1948). *Resolving Social Conflicts*. New York, NY: Harper.

2 Carr, W. and Kemmis, S. (1986). *Becoming Critical: Knowing Through Action Research*. Lewes: Falmer.

3 Kember, D. (2000). *Action Learning, Action Research: Improving the Quality of Teaching and Learning*. London: Kogan Page.

4 Kemmis, S. (2009). Action research as a practice-based practice. *Educational Action Research* 17 (3): 463–474.

5 McNiff, J. (2010). *Action Research for Professional Development*. Dorset: September Books.

6 Jefferson, R.N. (2014). Action research: theory and applications. *New Review of Academic Librarianship* 20 (2): 91–116.

7 McNiff J. (2012). Action research for professional development: concise advice for new action researchers. http://www.jeanmcniff.com/ar-booklet.asp (accessed 3 May 2023).

8 Stenhouse, L. (1975). *An Introduction to Curriculum Research and Development*. London: Heinemann.

9 Cain, T. (2011). Teachers' classroom-based action research. *International Journal of Research and Method in Education* 34 (1): 3–16.

10 Simmons, M., McDermott, M., Eaton, S.E. et al. (2021). Reflection as pedagogy in action research. *Educational Action Research* 29 (2): 245–258.

11 Grant, A. and Robling, M. (2006). Introducing undergraduate medical teaching into general practice: an action research study. *Medical Teacher* 28 (7): e192–e197.

12 Ryan, C.L. and McAllister, M.M. (2020). Professional development in clinical teaching: an action research study. *Nurse Education Today* 1: 85.

13 Magee, D., Bramble, M., and Stanley, D. (2020). Expanding an action research framework for an evidence based mentoring program in nursing: an exploration of cooperative inquiry. *Educational Action Research* 28 (4): 597–608.

14 Coetzee, M., Britton, M., and Clow, S.E. (2005). Finding the voice of clinical experience: participatory action research with registered nurses in developing a child critical care nursing curriculum. *Intensive and Critical Care Nursing* 21 (2): 110–118.

15 Lee-Hsieh, J., Kuo, C.L., Turton, M.A. et al. (2007). Action research on the development of a caring curriculum in Taiwan: part II. *Journal of Nursing Education* 46 (12): 553–561.

16 van Schalkwyk, S.C., Couper, I.D., Blitz, J., and de Villiers, M.R. (2020). A framework for distributed health professions training: using participatory action research to build consensus. *BMC Medical Education* 20 (154): 1–10.

17 Kara, H. (2017). *Research and Evaluation for Busy Students and Practitioners*, 2e. Bristol: Policy Press.

18 McNiff, J. and Whitehead, J. (2010). *You and Your Action Research Project*. Oxon: Routledge.

19 Denscombe, M. (2010). *The Good Research Guide for Small-Scale Social Research Projects*. Maidenhead: McGraw Hill.

20 Westhorp, G., Stevens, K., and Rogers, P.J. (2016). Using realist action research for service redesign. *Evaluation* 22 (3): 361–379.

21 Wong, G., Greenhalgh, T., Westhorp, G., and Pawson, R. (2012). Realist methods in medical education research: what are they and what can they contribute? *Medical Education* 46 (1): 89–96.

22 Kurtz, S., Silverman, J., Benson, J., and Draper, J. (2003). Marrying content and process in clinical method teaching: enhancing the Calgary-Cambridge guides. *Academic Medicine* 78 (8): 802–809.

23 Lefroy, J., Brosnan, C., and Creavin, S. (2011). Some like it hot: medical student views on choosing the emotional level of a simulation. *Medical Education* 45 (4): 354–361.

24 Yardley, S., Irvine, A.W., and Lefroy, J. (2013). Minding the gap between communication skills simulation and authentic experience. *Medical Education* 47 (5): 495–510.

25 Yardley, S., Hookey, C., and Lefroy, J. (2013). Designing whole-task learning opportunities for integrated end-of-life care: a practitioner-derived enquiry. *Education for Primary Care* 24 (6): 436–443.

26 Lefroy, J., Gay, S.P., Gibson, S. et al. (2011). Development and face validation of an instrument to assess and improve clinical consultation skills. *International Journal of Clinical Skills* 5 (2): 115–125.

27 Lefroy, J., Thomas, A., Harrison, C. et al. (2014). Development and face validation of strategies for improving consultation skills. *Advances in Health Sciences Education* 19 (5): 661–685.

28 Lefroy, J., Roberts, N., Molyneux, A. et al. (2017). Utility of an app-based system to improve feedback following workplace-based assessment. *International Journal of Medical Education* 8: 207–216.

29 Lefroy, J., Hawarden, A., Gay, S.P., and McKinley, R. (2017). Positive impacts of written feedback: does formal workplace based assessment add value to informal feedback? *MedEdPublish* 6 (1): paper no. 27.

30 Lefroy, J., Hawarden, A., Gay, S.P. et al. (2015). Grades in formative workplace-based assessment: a study of what works for whom and why. *Medical Education* 49: 307–320.

31 Genn, J.M. (2001). AMEE medical education guide no. 23 (part 1): curriculum, environment, climate, quality and change in medical education – a unifying perspective. *Medical Teacher* 23 (4): 337–344.

32 Stringer, E. (2008). *Action Research in Education*, 2e. Upper Saddle River, NJ: Pearson Education Inc.

33 Norton, L. (2009). *Action Research in Teaching and Learning*. Oxford: Routledge.

34 McKernan, J. (1996). *Curriculum Action Research: A Handbook of Methods and Resources for the Reflective Practitioner*, 2e. London: Kogan Page.

13 Online data collection: emerging possibilities

Dominique Harz and Kristina Dzara

Learning objectives

By the end of this chapter, you should be able to:
- Identify and define online data sources for clinical education research projects.
- Design clinical education research projects using online data.

- Define and appraise differences between observational and interactive online data.
- Plan data collection and analysis using online data.
- Reflect on the strengths, limitations, and ethical issues of online data collection.

Introduction

The rapid internet expansion has enabled users to develop and interact with content and shifted the concept of the 'world wide web' to a new and collaborative 'read write web' or 'Web 2.0,' with emphasis on user-generated content, interactivity, and interoperability [1]. This paradigm change has provided clinical educators with the opportunity to rethink teaching methods and channels. Moreover, online platforms have given access to a wide range of information, broadening the possibilities of research and programme evaluation in clinical education. In this chapter, we define and use the term online platform as 'an internet-based virtual space, where applications, software, websites, and systems enable the delivery of information, services, and/or interaction between users, while also collecting and using data about these processes' [2]. Furthermore, we can also think of online platforms as a valuable resource to help us to identify topics, connect with collaborators, design and implement technology-based interventions, and obtain data [1, 3]. This chapter will focus on the latter and describe how online platforms can provide access to online data for research. When we refer to online data we mean 'all types of information that originate from online platforms, including but not limited to text, audio, video, images, and website traffic, usage, or engagement metrics' [1, 4, 5].

The use of online data for the development of clinical education practice has grown, as evidenced by multiple systematic and scoping reviews. For example, Curran et al. [6] reviewed the use of digital, social, and mobile technologies in clinical education and noted increasing positive commentary on their potential benefits and opportunities for enhancing teaching and learning. Guckian et al. [7] synthesised evidence related to social media (SoMe) interventions in undergraduate medical education, noting that use was associated with objective knowledge improvements and self-reported clinical and professional performance. Chan et al. [8] aggregated and reported on trends in the use of SoMe in knowledge translation and education for physicians and trainees, observing a steady increase in the literature, most commonly related to practice improvement, descriptions of technology, and evidence-based practice. These reviews point to an increased use and study of these technologies, but limited evidence of efficacy and few long-term outcomes reported in the current literature [6–8]. They also reveal a rise in online data generation and use, which has the potential to unearth new sources of data ripe for exploration. We encourage you to explore this new space and consider whether you can use online data within your research.

Throughout this chapter, we offer guidance for using online data as part of clinical education research. We start by providing specific considerations when designing a project that uses online data as an information source and describing their benefits and limitations. Then, we briefly describe the main sources of online data and the different

---

Starting Research in Clinical Education, First Edition. Edited by Eliot L. Rees, Alison Ledger, and Kim A. Walker.
© 2024 The Association for the Study of Medical Education (ASME). Published 2024 by John Wiley & Sons Ltd.
Companion website: www.wiley.com/go/clinicaleducation

types of online data available. Next, we present considerations for how to collect and analyse these types of data and interpret findings. To conclude, we discuss some specific ethical considerations associated with the use of online data.

Study considerations

When collecting online data, the same steps apply as when using traditional data. First you must identify a problem and review the existing literature to determine the problem's relevance and how further research can advance knowledge on the topic. Next, you should develop a clear question and devise a research plan, ensuring coherence between your research question, paradigm, and methodology as explained in Chapter 3. You should avoid improvising and making rushed decisions, which can negatively impact project quality.

When using online data within your research, it is important to justify the need for online data rather than traditional data and demonstrate how online data collection aligns with the research question. You may choose to use online data as the primary data source for a study, or as a complement to support traditional data sources to provide triangulation. An additional consideration relates to critically understanding the characteristics of online data and its implications for clinical education research. The decision to utilise online data to answer a research question should be undertaken after considering the benefits and disadvantages as compared to traditional data sources.

The first logical reason for choosing to use online data is when the main subjects of study are online platforms. In this case, the focus of analysis is likely to include online data. For example, Tackett et al. [9] described the reach of, and user preferences for, medical education videos on YouTube, which they assessed using online data. In this case, YouTube analytics data were collected, such as watch time and number of views. However, it is important to recognise that not all studies about online platforms collect online data. For example, Messman et al. [10] compared the effects of a podcast and a supplementary blog versus a podcast only, on emergency medicine junior doctors' learning. The authors implemented a randomised control trial in which participants completed knowledge application and acquisition tests. While the data in their study related to the efficacy of delivering content via online platforms, the data collected and used within the study were traditional.

Additional arguments that favour the use of online data are associated with recruitment (see Chapter 6) and data access. The magnitude and reach of online platforms offer researchers access to data from a potentially large and diverse participant population [5]. For example, for studies involving sensitive topics or personal opinions, online platforms can facilitate data gathering from individuals who would otherwise be difficult to reach [1]. Anonymous online platforms can foster high levels of self-disclosure and may be less affected by social desirability bias [5]. For example, Castro and Andrews [11] found that anonymous nursing blog posts provided valuable and longitudinal insights into how nurses felt about their work.

Another advantage of online data collection includes potentially rapid, sometimes even immediate, data collection. This, combined with the potential to reach a large number of participants, can translate into a great amount of quickly generated data, sometimes at a low cost, which can potentially diminish study duration and accelerate time to publication [3, 4]. Further cost savings can be made by eliminating travel, mailing, and other recruitment costs [1]. An additional benefit is that participants can choose when and where to participate, which can positively impact recruitment. Recruitment can also be enhanced if snowball sampling aligns with the research methodology. It is fairly easy for participants to reach out to their friends or acquaintances and recruit them online, leading to potentially fast growth in the number of participants and possibly a self-sustaining project, for example, where data collection autonomously continues over time [1, 12].

Potential disadvantages of using online data are related to concerns about generalisability of data derived from online platforms. Data obtained from the internet is potentially not representative, as access to the internet is not universal [13]. This was a common argument when internet use was skewed towards computer-literate, Caucasian males from higher socio-economic backgrounds [14]. However, internet use has widely expanded, is more diverse, and includes users from throughout the globe, which could result in minority or underrepresented groups now being included [12, 14].

Some additional concerns are related to reduced levels of researcher control in the online environment, which could negatively impact validity and reliability. There may be technological challenges, such as hardware configurations or network performance, which can impact how the participant experiences an online study intervention or participates in an online interview or focus group. You may have little control over where participants engage in the study, for example, in a crowded coffee shop, under the influence of alcohol or drugs, while multitasking, or with other personal or family demands, which may limit ability to focus on the study. While unlikely, some participants may try to cheat or sabotage data collection [14]. Despite these concerns, there is robust evidence that studies involving online platforms can gather valid and reliable online data, comparable to data obtained with traditional offline methods [13].

Lastly, depending on the online platform and data type, there may be some technologically related disadvantages. You may encounter unexpected problems deploying the study due to software or hardware failures [13]. Thus, your research team should have the technical expertise needed to execute and support the study. Fortunately, there are a range of software packages that can aid you in collecting online data [13]. We also suggest contacting the information technology (IT) team at your institution to determine what help they may be able to supply.

Due to the few drawbacks and numerous advantages that online platforms and data gathering might provide, there is a risk that you may be tempted to implement a rapid but methodologically flawed study. Instead, we recommend developing a well-considered research plan to ensure credible results. It is better to take time to plan in the initial project phase than to experience major or even devastating flaws in the implementation or analysis stages [5].

Types of online platforms

There are multiple different types of online platforms, ranging from websites to international companies. You should be aware of the characteristics and nuances of specific platforms. They can be classified based on the specific purposes they seek to serve. Common types are

- Social media (SoMe) networks (e.g. Twitter, Facebook, LinkedIn, Mastodon, and Instagram).
- Media sharing platforms (e.g. YouTube, Spotify, Apple podcasts, and Vimeo).
- Educational platforms (e.g. edX, Coursera, Khan Academy, and Udacity).
- Online learning platforms (e.g. Moodle, Blackboard, and Canvas).
- Blogging platforms (e.g. http://WordPress.com, Tumblr, and Weebly).
- Search engines (e.g. Google and Yahoo).
- Marketplaces (e.g. Amazon, eBay, and Booking.com).

- App stores (e.g. Google Play and Apple App Store).
- Service platforms (e.g. Uber, Lyft, and Airbnb).
- Organisational websites (e.g. for medical schools, hospitals, or advocacy organisations).

These different types of online platforms can host and share information in multiple formats: numeric, graphical, textual, audio, video, and usage or engagement metrics. Furthermore, they can also support interaction and socialisation between users. SoMe, for example, offers information in the form of user interaction by accessing online profiles ('friending', 'following'), supporting ideas or statements ('liking'), or opposing them ('disliking') [15]. Patro et al. [16] leveraged this information in their five-year retrospective cohort study to determine the relationships between programme reputation, SoMe activity, and popularity of otolaryngology residency programmes. For this, they aligned United States News and World Report rankings, with online data in the form of Doximity residency reputation scores, and SoMe use and growth metrics. The authors concluded that higher ranked programmes showed a more active presence on SoMe, had more followers, and started using SoMe earlier [16].

Types of online data

Online data can be classified into two categories based on your degree of involvement as the researcher in the data origination and collection: observational and interactive data.

Observational data

Observational data, or nonobtrusive data, is publicly available online information and requires no interaction between you and your study participants [6]. Hence, you play no role in the data generation and data collection takes place in a more naturalistic space. Usually, research that uses this type of data is retrospective; however, if data generation and collection are completed over time, observational data can also be used in cross-sectional or prospective studies.

Observational data can be obtained from a multitude of platforms, including but not limited to emails, webpages, blogs, SoMe, and podcasts. Thus, they can have different formats, such as text comments, audio-visual content, or scores [1, 6]. In some cases, these studies can be completely descriptive, for example, by presenting the number of specific residency programmes represented on unique SoMe platforms over time.

One advantage of observational data is they are usually publicly available, which makes the data collection process very time- and cost-effective [15]. Additionally, because the researcher's role is limited to nonobtrusive observation, social desirability bias may be reduced [17]. Furthermore, since data are usually generated in real-time, observational data have the advantage over surveys of reducing recall bias [4]. The key distinction here is that the researcher does not interact or engage with participants nor intervene in the development of the data.

Observational data usually focuses on two broad areas of information: human behaviour and static information. Regarding human behaviour, online data can provide valuable information to explore practices and interactions happening online. This can be achieved with real-time or archived data, found on discussion threads, via Altmetric scores, SoMe metrics, or other engagement metrics such as website traffic, session length, page views, and exit rate [18]. Altmetric scores (short for alternative metrics) are used to assess the attention given to a scholarly publication, beyond its citation in other scholarly articles. Their calculation is based on a variety of online outputs: number of downloads, shares, likes, among others [19]. SoMe metrics are measurements that indicate SoMe use, reception, and impact [20]. Examples of these are likes, comments, shares, clicks, impressions, and reach. Maggio et al. [21] examined Altmetric attention scores, associated outlets including Mendeley, Twitter, and Facebook, and top article characteristics from 6265 health professions education articles in 13 journals. They pointed to increased Altmetric attention, specifically for those articles topically related to SoMe or social networking [21]. Here, the authors used online data to assess online behaviours, without participant interaction, since the data were publicly available.

The second focus in observational data collection is appraising static online information, such as published documents and media related to people, institutions, or groups [17, 18]. Here, you intend to answer a research question with existing observational data. Maldonado et al. [22] sought to determine whether SoMe and digital scholarship were considered in promotion and tenure guidelines at medical schools in the United States. They acquired all guidelines publicly available online from medical schools, and then searched these to determine the absence or presence of relevant keywords, and subsequently reported SoMe and digital scholarship inclusive language identified through their work. Another example is Massanelli et al. [23] who utilised Google Analytics to measure website performance before and after implementation of a new department of surgery website, concluding a more modern website improves user engagement.

Interactive data

Interactive data, or obtrusive data, refer to online information collected when the researcher is involved in the data generation and/or actively interacts with the study participants [1]. This definition is broad and could include more traditional methods such as an online survey or virtual interview. Interactive online data are generally used in cross-sectional or prospective studies since the data are generated in real time.

These types of online data often include researcher and participant interactions in the form of written content, such as posted comments; or engagement in the form of hits or likes. For example, Chung et al. [24] acted as facilitators at an asynchronous, online journal club discussion of a published manuscript, hosted by the *Journal of Graduate Medical Education* and the *Academic Life in Emergency Medicine* blog, to explore the topic of resident wellness through their SoMe accounts. Multiple data sources including blog comments, tweets using the dedicated hashtag, and the transcript of a video panel discussion were brought together, thematically analysed, and aligned with web analytics to ultimately identify domains of discussion, gaps in the literature, and demonstrate reach.

More recently, Hall et al. [25] described how they gathered and analysed data from a monthly Twitter chat where scholars addressed topics relevant to medical and health professions education, guided by a moderator who tweeted guiding questions and served as a content expert [25]. The authors generated a qualitative dataset from the chat transcript obtained from Symplur (a healthcare SoMe analytics company that serves as a register and archive of healthcare hashtags and provides a large databank of Twitter conversations around healthcare). Aligned with descriptive data from Symplur and Twitter, they noted three key concepts that indicated the need for a professional learning network during the early COVID-19 pandemic, demonstrating the value of SoMe in supporting health professions educators during a global crisis.

The specific advantages of interactive online data include the ability to design a study involving participant interaction, which could include rigorous experimental designs. Thus, research questions and the focus of analysis can be more fully aligned because you can design the study in advance, engage with participants, and encourage robust data collection. This approach potentially requires more time and effort on your part because studies using interactive data are generally more complex and may involve more sophisticated methods of implementation [5]. Yet, data derived from these types of studies could lead to more meaningful and impactful results.

Data collection

Online data can be collected in a range of ways, depending on the research paradigm (see Chapter 3). Other factors to consider include the type, format, content, and magnitude of the online dataset, as well as the kind of online platform used to find and extract the data. Consequently, you must plan early and define a data collection strategy considering these factors. You must also take into account the technical skills and costs needed to gather online data. Scholars should search for guidelines, such as the Development of Reporting Guidelines for Social Media Research (RESOME), which is currently under development [26]. Additionally, we recommend you pilot data collection processes to avoid setbacks. Another important consideration is determining whether data collected from different platforms are comparable, as different platforms offer diverse engagement metrics [1].

Data extraction from webpages or blog discussion threads is often straightforward. Data can be collected by hand, through simple copying and pasting data into a document, spreadsheet, or database. Some software also enable you to extract information from web pages. For example, the qualitative data analysis software NVivo (QSR International Pty Ltd.) offers a browser extension that allows you to capture content from web pages, online PDFs, Twitter, and Facebook posts, for coding and analysis.

In the case of other online platforms and depending on how the data are organised, you may have the option to download multiple content or variables at once, for example, from Google Analytics [23, 27], Altmetric Explorer [21], or a social reference manager such as Mendeley [28]. You could then organise these data and perhaps even triangulate them with additional data to create a more robust dataset for analysis.

However, depending on the project aim, type of online data, and the dataset size, the extraction of online information can be sometimes more challenging and require special knowledge and technological skills [18]. If you need to collect data in the form of online metrics or are working with 'big

data', you may require the use of more sophisticated methods [5] (see Chapter 23). For example, application programming interfaces (APIs) are software intermediaries that allow interoperability among different computer systems. Some are freely available but offer restricted access to data; others offer broader access to data but are associated with fees, often costly [5, 15]. One example of the former is Twitter, which has two public APIs: streaming and representational state transfer (REST). The streaming API allows access to near real-time Twitter data, while the REST API enables the retrieval of historical data from the previous seven to nine days [29, 30]. Depending on the research question and robustness of the data, REST API may be sufficient for a broad research question. Nonetheless, it is not likely to be sufficient for a direct question related to a unique or underused hashtag [4, 5].

Data quality and integrity

As with traditional data, you must ensure that online data are reliable and valid. Moreover, with these types of data, you must consider some special quality and integrity features.

An important concern is related to the representativeness of the internet user population, which subsequently affects generalisability [1, 5]. Thus, you should decide whether generalisability is an important consideration in your study. If so, take special care when defining the population and sample (when relevant) during project planning and reflect on how representativeness and generalisability can define, impact, or limit your results.

We recommend being cautious regarding the authenticity of online comments, webpages, and/ or accounts. This is particularly important when social networks are the data sources, as individuals sometimes build fake accounts, thus rendering demographic information unreliable [1]. However, fake profiles are sometimes easy to detect, since real users connect with friends and collect likes over a long time period. In contrast, fake profiles usually add friends and likes in one single activity burst [12].

One last consideration regarding data quality and integrity relates to the potential for people to behave differently in an online environment compared to real life. This can especially occur when participants engage in SoMe platforms, when comments may not represent their opinion, nor be valid nor reliable [1]. If in doubt, consult with your supervisor or colleagues to determine whether data appear consistent and trustworthy and consider collecting additional information to corroborate initial findings. Furthermore, you should also be transparent with readers about any concerns and record this as a potential limitation of your study.

Data analysis

As online platforms can support the hosting and sharing of different data formats (text, image, audio, and video) and content (interactions, reflections, and static information), you can analyse data in a myriad of ways [1]. You must consider your paradigm, type of data, and whether your analysis will involve a quantitative, qualitative, or a mixed methods approach. You should define this when planning your project to ensure alignment between components of the research design (see Chapter 3).

Data analysis itself does not necessarily vary compared to traditional data analysis approaches. As an example, Yilmaz et al. [27] utilised student registration forms, interaction metrics, course feedback, and free-text responses collected via Google Analytics and Moodle to evaluate the effectiveness of a Massive Online Open Course (MOOC) in teaching medical students about COVID-19. The online data were analysed using descriptive statistics for the quantitative data and thematic analysis for the qualitative data.

However, there are some additional and lesser-known analysis methods that are worth highlighting. For example, sentiment analysis is a method of analysis that aims to identify, extract, and explore individuals' subjective and private experiences, such as emotions, opinions, attitudes, or judgement [5, 31, 32]. This type of analysis is usually textual, but some recent studies have also utilised audio and video [32]. The methodology has evolved and can include machine learning approaches, with lexicon-based, keyword-based, or concept-based foci [32]. Guha and Pande [33] explored well-being and mental health among PhD students by analysing the content of 1994 randomly selected tweets. The analysis involved a sentiment analysis to determine positive or negative qualities of the tweets. The authors determined that sentiments were 43% positive, 28% neutral, 19% negative, and 10% undetermined. They concluded that most tweets express positive sentiment, and that negative tweets highlight mental health concerns, problems with academic culture, or COVID-19 pandemic challenges.

Link analysis is another interesting method, focusing on the existence of interconnections between online data. Here, you analyse the links that connect websites to understand the networks that are formed or exist between webpages, groups, or individuals [5]. Fernandez-Luque et al. [34] designed and used a metric to determine the quality of blog posts and video content, which they then related to trustworthiness in an online health community, using link analysis.

Finally, data mining is growing in importance and can often include online data analysis. Data mining is the analysis of observational data sets – usually large-scale – that aim to find meaningful patterns between variables and present the data in novel ways to make them easier to understand and hence more useful [35]. Data mining approaches vary depending on analysis objectives: 'cluster analysis' aims to find the natural grouping of data records, 'anomaly and outlier detection' looks for unusual records, and 'association rule mining' searches for dependencies between data [35].

Ethical considerations

As with traditional data, all studies using online data should be reviewed by an appropriate research ethics committee prior to study initiation, including any data collection. You should never attempt to self-determine whether data can or cannot be used for research purposes. Hence, it is important to assess the nature of the data and determine the most relevant research ethics committee pathway for submission. In some cases, studies involving online data could be deemed 'not human subjects research', because there is indeed no interaction between researcher and participant [36]. However, you should expect to submit a complete research ethics committee proposal, with the understanding there is variation by board, and studies using online data might be deemed exempt, expected, or may even require a full research ethics committee review. We recommend you consult with your local research ethics committee to ensure you comply with all local, national, and international standards [37].

Unfortunately, there are no specific and clear guidelines about research stemming from online platforms or the use of online data in clinical education. Nevertheless, there are some existing guidelines about ethics in internet-mediated research that may be helpful [38, 39]. The section below details special ethical considerations when using online data in clinical education research.

First, there may be difficulties defining the benefits and harms associated with using online platforms and subsequently online data, both for participants and researchers. As with all studies, you have the responsibility to ensure that participants are not harmed [5]. However, this can be more difficult in the online environment, in part because there are fewer studies that report problems we can learn from, and also because it can be hard to determine participant reactions to the research and their risk of harm [5]. To address this, you must establish good rapport during live data collection. For example, with online group discussions, you must establish ground rules for respectful interaction among participants and ensure all participants know they can withdraw from the study at any time [5], which is not dissimilar from research using traditional forms of data (see Chapter 7). Additionally, as a researcher, you may experience distress due to exposure to sensitive and/or distressing information, including disclosures about grief, self-harm, or bullying, sometimes from anonymous sources. You must anticipate whether these risks could be encountered and design a strategy to avoid personal, ethical, or legal consequences [5].

The second ethical challenge concerns how participants consent to study inclusion. In an online environment, it can be difficult to assess the participant's ability to give informed consent, or if they belong to a 'vulnerable group'. Furthermore, once the participant consents, it also can be challenging to determine if they fully understand their rights, responsibilities, and opportunity for discussion [5]. Thus, it is fundamental that you establish an open communication process with participants [18]. We recommend providing an online platform that includes information regarding the project and the participant's rights and responsibilities. That information should be succinct and easy to read to encourage understanding. You can also include checkboxes for participants to fill out to confirm they comprehended key consent points. Vary whether a 'yes' or 'no' response is required to detect if they are reading content carefully or mindlessly checking boxes [18]. An additional alternative could be using offline methods for the informed consent process to support reliability and rigour [18].

Further difficulties around consent specifically relate to the use of online observational data. In this case, information can be collected from public platforms without informing the participant or requesting their consent. As participants post information knowing that it will be publicly available, a research ethics committee may decide that consent is implied, especially for low-risk studies [40]. Nevertheless, determining the degree of online data privacy can sometimes be difficult in the virtual setting. Although at first glance we may assume that all online content is public, it is not always the case [1]. Data can have different degrees of privacy, ranging

from being completely public and visible to all internet users and search engines, to completely private where only some selected users (usually followers or friends) have access [1]. Additionally, user-selected privacy settings vary. Thus, information privacy is related to the unique features of the digital space. Users' perceptions and expectations of the shared information should also be considered. In this regard, it can be helpful to appraise the sensitivity of the information posted online and the context of the platform used [18]. If the content of a post is rather personal or the topic is sensitive, and posted in a personal blog, for example, it may be wise to assume that the user who posted the information is not aware that the data are publicly accessible. We recommend that you always check with your research ethics committee to determine whether an informed consent process is needed.

A final consideration relates to confidentiality when reporting results. You should ensure that participants cannot be identified directly or indirectly, especially in qualitative designs. This can be difficult when using online data, where with a simple reverse search the participants might potentially be identified [18]. Qualitative studies using verbatim quotes, for example, can mitigate participant identification by overlapping information from different platforms and aggregating and combining data as part of triangulation and aggregation for reporting [5]. An additional strategy to avoid participant identification could be paraphrasing the quotes ensuring that the original meaning and the richness of the data are maintained [16].

Summary

Evolution in online platforms has provided researchers with novel and unique types of data. These new forms of data can be used in clinical education research as a primary outcome measure or aligned with traditional data. In both cases, online data can offer new perspectives and may result in more comprehensive knowledge development. As with traditional data, you must design studies using online data responsibly and with intent, to ensure outcomes are meaningful.

We acknowledge that the information and recommendations outlined in this chapter may become outdated because of the rapid and dynamic platform development and replacement. However, the core ideas and guidelines presented will remain applicable and set a foundation for you to continue expanding the breadth and depth of research using online data.

Top tips

- Have a clear rationale for the use of online data in your research.
- Develop a clear question, devise a plan, and ensure alignment between project elements, the same as when using traditional data.
- Consult with your local research ethics committee to ensure appropriate ethical standards in advance of any data collection.

Common pitfalls

- Making rushed decisions about study design and data collection, which can negatively impact project quality. Take time to plan your study.
- Starting data collection and analysis before piloting your approach. Ensure your plan is feasible and your findings will be sufficient to answer your research question(s).
- Overstating your results. Report findings that are in alignment with your project scope and context.

Ethical issues

- Weigh potential benefits and harms associated with your project, for both you and your participants.
- Assess participants' ability to grant informed consent and be clear about their rights and responsibilities.
- Consider the degree to which participants are identifiable. Refrain from reporting identifiable information from or about participants.

References

1 Lafferty, N.T. and Manca, A. (2015). Perspectives on social media in and as research: a synthetic review. *International Review of Psychiatry* 27 (2): 85–96.

2 OECD (2019). *Introduction to Online Platforms and Their Role in the Digital Transformation*. Paris: OECD Publishing.

3 Quinton, S. (2013). The digital era requires new knowledge to develop relevant CRM strategy: a cry for adopting social media research methods to elicit this new knowledge. *Journal of Strategic Marketing* 21 (5): 402–412.

4 Mccormick, T.H., Lee, H., Cesare, N. et al. (2017). Using Twitter for demographic and social science research: tools for data collection and processing. *Sociological Methods & Research* 46 (3): 390–421.

5 Fielding, N., Lee, R.M., and Blank, G. (2017). *The SAGE Handbook of Online Research Methods*, 2e. SAGE Publications.

6 Curran, V., Matthews, L., Fleet, L. et al. (2017). A review of digital, social, and mobile technologies in health professional education. *Journal of Continuing Education in the Health Professions* 37 (3): 195–206.

7 Guckian, J., Utukuri, M., Asif, A. et al. (2021). Social media in undergraduate medical education: a systematic review. *Medical Education* 55 (11): 1227–1241.

8 Chan, T.M., Dzara, K., Dimeo, S.P. et al. (2020). Social media in knowledge translation and education for physicians and trainees: a scoping review. *Perspectives on Medical Education* 9 (1): 20–30.

9 Tackett, S., Slinn, K., Marshall, T. et al. (2018). Medical education videos for the world: an analysis of viewing patterns for a YouTube channel. *Academic Medicine* 93 (8): 1150–1156.

10 Messman, A.M., Ehrman, R.R., and Gruppen, L.D. (2021). LIMEs and LEMONs: critically examining the effect of a blog post on junior faculty learners. *AEM Education and Training* 5 (3): e10553.

11 Castro, A. and Andrews, G. (2018). Nursing lives in the blogosphere: a thematic analysis of anonymous online nursing narratives. *Journal of Advanced Nursing* 74 (2): 329–338.

12 Kosinski, M., Matz, S.C., Gosling, S.D. et al. (2015). Facebook as a research tool for the social sciences: opportunities, challenges, ethical considerations, and practical guidelines. *American Psychologist* 70 (6): 543.

13 Hewson, C. and Laurent, D. (2008). Research design and tools for internet research. In: *The SAGE Handbook of Online Research Methods* (ed. N. Fielding, R.M. Lee, and G. Blank), 58–78. SAGE Publications, Ltd.

14 Hewson, C. (2008). Internet-mediated research as an emergent method and its potential role in facilitating mixed methods research. In: *Handbook of Emergent Methods* (ed. S.N. Hesse-Biber and P. Leavy), 543–570. New York, NY: Guilford Press.

15 Sinnenberg, L., Buttenheim, A.M., Padrez, K. et al. (2017). Twitter as a tool for health research: a systematic review. *American Journal of Public Health* 107 (1): e1–e8.

16 Patro, A., Carr, S., Stevens, M.N. et al. (2021). Otolaryngology residency program rankings and social media usage: a longitudinal analysis. *The Laryngoscope* 131 (11): 2455–2460.

17 Connelly, L.M. (2017). Unobtrusive measures. *Medsurg Nursing* 26 (1): 59.

18 Hewson, C., Vogel, C., and Laurent, D. (2016). Internet mediated research: state of the art. In: *Internet Research Methods*, 2e, 33–70. SAGE Publications.

19 Robinson, D.B., Powell, A.G., Waterman, J. et al. (2021). Predictive value of Altmetric score on citation rates and bibliometric impact. *BJS Open* 5 (1): zraa039.

20 Wouters, P., Zahedi, Z., and Costas, R. (2019). Social media metrics for new research evaluation. In: *Springer Handbook of Science and Technology Indicators* (ed. W. Glänzel, H.F. Moed, U. Schmoch, and M. Thelwall), 687–713. Springer.

21 Maggio, L.A., Meyer, H.S., and Artino, A.R. (2017). Beyond citation rates: a real-time impact analysis of health professions education research using altmetrics. *Academic Medicine* 92 (10): 1449–1455.

22 Maldonado, G., Smart, J., Wiechmann, W. et al. (2022). Frequency of social media and digital scholarship keywords in US medical schools' promotion and tenure guidelines. *Academic Medicine* 97 (1): 105–110.

23 Massanelli, J., Sexton, K.W., Lesher, C.T. et al. (2021). Integration of web analytics into graduate medical education: usability study. *JMIR Formative Research* 5 (12): e29748.

24 Chung, A., Battaglioli, N., Lin, M., and Sherbino, J. (2018). JGME-ALiEM hot topics in medical education: an analysis of a virtual discussion on resident well-being. *Journal of Graduate Medical Education* 10 (1): 36–42.

25 Hall, E., Kreuter, J.D., Sörö, T. et al. (2021). Harnessing the power of social media to support a professional learning network during the COVID-19 pandemic. *Journal of Continuing Education in the Health Professions* 41 (1): 10–12.

26 Kaushal A, Bravo C, Duffy SW, Lewins D, et al. Developing reporting guidelines for social media research (RESOME) by using a modified Delphi method: protocol for guideline development. JMIR Research Protocols 2022 11 5:e31739.

27 Yilmaz, Y., Sarikaya, O., Senol, Y. et al. (2021). RE-AIMing COVID-19 online learning for medical students: a massive open online course evaluation. *BMC Medical Education* 21 (1): 1–14.

28 Sugimoto, C.R., Work, S., Larivière, V., and Haustein, S. (2017). Scholarly use of social media and altmetrics: a review of the literature. *Journal of the Association for Information Science and Technology* 68 (9): 2037–2062.

29 Kumar, S., Liu, H., and Morstatter, F. (2014). *Twitter Data Analytics*. New York, NY: Springer.

30 Suh, S.C. and Anthony, T. (2018). *Big Data and Visual Analytics*. Springer International Publishing.

31 Mäntylä, M.V., Graziotin, D., and Kuutila, M. (2018). The evolution of sentiment analysis – a review of research topics, venues, and top cited papers. *Computer Science Review* 27: 16–32.

32 Qazi, A., Raj, R.G., Hardaker, G., and Standing, C. (2017). A systematic literature review on opinion types and sentiment analysis techniques: tasks and challenges. *Internet Research* 27 (3): 608–630.

33 Guha, P. and Pande, D. (2021). A sentiment analysis of the PhD experience evidenced on Twitter. *International Journal of Doctoral Studies* 16: 513.

34 Fernandez-Luque, L., Karlsen, R., and Melton, G.B. (2012). HealthTrust: a social network approach for retrieving online health videos. *Journal of Medical Internet Research* 14 (1): e1985.

35 Elatia, S., Ipperciel, D., and Zaiane, O.R. (2016). *Data Mining and Learning Analytics: Applications in Educational Research*, 1e. Hoboken, NJ: Wiley.

36 Moreno, M.A., Goniu, N., Moreno, P.S., and Diekema, D. (2013). Ethics of social media research: common concerns and practical considerations. *Cyberpsychology, Behavior, and Social Networking* 16 (9): 708–713.

37 Johansson, A.C., Durning, S.J., Gruppen, L.D. et al. (2011). Perspective: medical education research and the institutional review board: reexamining the process. *Academic Medicine* 86 (7): 809–817.

38 Franzke, A.S., Bechmann, A., Zimmer, M. et al. (2019). *Internet Research: Ethical Guidelines 3.0 Association of Internet Researchers*. Ethics Working Committee of AOIR. https://aoir.org/ethics/.

39 The British Psychological Society (2021). Ethics guidelines for internet-mediated research. https://www.bps.org.uk/guideline/ethics-guidelines-internet-mediated-research.

40 Hammer, M.J. (2017). Ethical considerations when using social media for research. *Oncology Nursing Forum* 44 (4): 410–412.

PART III

Qualitative research

Alison Ledger

Many new clinical education researchers are not only changing disciplines, but also undertaking qualitative research for the first time. This is because qualitative methods are especially fruitful in understanding the complex interactions and relationships that unfold in clinical education. Instead of measuring the performance or opinions of large populations, qualitative methods allow us to explore the varied experiences and perspectives of a small group of people in rich detail. They advance understanding of practice in specific contexts and communities and often reveal something about the language and cultures at play. When detailed insights from qualitative studies are shared, educators can consider whether research findings and recommendations are relevant to their particular setting and use this knowledge to inform their practice.

This part will introduce you to common qualitative research methods and inspire you to consider creative methods of data collection and analysis. It starts with the fundamentals of qualitative data collection. Chapter 14 defines research interviews and focus groups, when to choose them, and how to interact with participants to gather rich detail about their experiences. Chapter 15 extends this by promoting the use of drawing, photographs, or videos to develop deeper insights. In Chapter 16, ethnography is introduced as a means of surfacing taken for granted aspects of clinical and educational practice. This chapter highlights the different roles a qualitative researcher can occupy and the importance of considering your role in co-constructing meaning. The power of stories as research data, in analysis, or in dissemination is then conveyed in Chapter 17 on narrative methods. This chapter begins to address common questions about the nature of knowledge

in qualitative research, which you will no doubt encounter as you continue your research journey.

The part then moves on to qualitative analysis. We decided to focus on the family of thematic analysis approaches because they are frequently adopted by new researchers, yet often misunderstood. Chapter 18 clarifies essential differences between three types of thematic analysis approaches, once again stressing the value of understanding your research paradigm and undertaking qualitative research in an informed way. The journey to becoming a knowing qualitative researcher is not always easy. Chapter 19 supports you in this journey, by making common struggles explicit and offering strategies for navigating periods of uncertainty during the analysis phase.

What all these chapters share is a call to fully embrace the subjectivity afforded by qualitative research methods. This subjectivity may feel strange and unsettling at first, particularly if you have been taught good research is 'objective', 'unbiased', and 'generalisable'. The authors acknowledge these feelings yet encourage you to consider different markers of quality. As you read, note how the chapters promote rich contextual detail, authenticity, and reflexivity during the qualitative research process. Reflect on the ways you may take an active role in research decision-making, interacting with participants, and interpreting qualitative data, and consider how your position can indeed be a strength.

This part should be considered as a starting point. In qualitative research, it is likely you will change course at some point along the way. However, it is this freedom that makes qualitative research so rich and exciting. Trust in the process, seek every opportunity to discuss your thinking with supervisors and peers, and have faith that things will become clearer as you progress. Relish the chance to be creative!

Starting Research in Clinical Education, First Edition. Edited by Eliot L. Rees, Alison Ledger, and Kim A. Walker.
© 2024 The Association for the Study of Medical Education (ASME). Published 2024 by John Wiley & Sons Ltd.
Companion website: www.wiley.com/go/clinicaleducation

14 Interviews and focus groups: guided conversations

Lucy Wallis, Becky Petley, and Rachel Locke

Learning objectives

By the end of this chapter, you should be able to:
- Make informed choices between interviews and focus groups and their various types.
- Develop an interview or focus group topic guide.

- Conduct research using interviews or focus groups.
- Reflect on your role as a researcher within interviews or focus groups.

Introduction

This chapter explores interviews and focus groups and their role in clinical education research. The chapter begins by defining interviews and focus groups and outlining when to use each method. Initial considerations are then discussed, including intended beneficiaries of the research and specific sampling issues. Following this, the different types and forms of interviews and focus groups are described, along with practical guidance on how to use these methods. This includes designing an interview guide, conducting, recording, and transcribing, and reflections on researcher positionality and ensuring rigour. We then provide an example of using interviews in clinical education research and detail the process of undertaking an interview study.

What are research interviews and focus groups?

A research interview is a guided conversation between a researcher and participant. A researcher asks questions in order to explore and collect in-depth information on an individual's perceptions, opinions, feelings, and/or experiences about a particular topic [1]. An example of this data collection technique within clinical education is conducting interviews with patients to understand their experience of being cared for by students.

A focus group is a discussion between a group of participants guided by a facilitator. The facilitator

may or may not be the main researcher. Focus groups are used to obtain multiple views about a topic of interest, using the dynamics of the group to stimulate a deep exploration and jointly constructed understanding of a phenomenon [2]. Examples within clinical education include focus groups with students to explore how they collectively feel about financial pressures during their training. Relative strengths of interviews and focus groups are presented in Table 14.1.

Focus group or interview?

Interviews and focus groups are both key research methods for gaining in-depth insights into experiences and meanings of a particular phenomenon. However, it is important to know which method to choose when conducting clinical education research. For this, the aim of the research and the methodology must be considered (see Chapter 3). Focus groups are useful for learning a group perspective on a subject, observing the way particular groups converse and interact, as well as generating a broad understanding. Participants in a group discussion can receive support from each other, and this may contribute to them feeling emboldened to contribute to the discussion. In contrast, an interview works best for learning about an individual's perspective or experience of a phenomenon [3]. Interviews enable an in-depth exploration into an individual's feelings on a topic, where the researcher can explore a response in detail without affecting a group dynamic. With the emphasis of focus groups on group discussion, an interview is

---

Starting Research in Clinical Education, First Edition. Edited by Eliot L. Rees, Alison Ledger, and Kim A. Walker.
© 2024 The Association for the Study of Medical Education (ASME). Published 2024 by John Wiley & Sons Ltd.
Companion website: www.wiley.com/go/clinicaleducation

Table 14.1 Strengths and considerations when using interviews and focus groups

Method	Strengths	Considerations
Interviews	Useful method to discuss a sensitive topic Flexibility: you can modify your line of enquiry and follow up on interesting responses	Can be time consuming to arrange, conduct, and transcribe the interviews Your assumptions are difficult to rule out, and it is important for you to reflect Structured interviews are easier to replicate and analyse, but semi-structured and unstructured interviews allow greater flexibility
Focus groups	Cost and time efficient: can include variety within a population, from a number of people in one sitting Participants can elaborate but also disagree with other viewpoints You can capture participants' reactions to comments and views made in the group	Sensitive topics may be inappropriate for group discussions A risk that individual differences/opinions are not voiced owing to the group setting and peer pressure Participants' contributions may not be equal: individuals may dominate the discussion or not contribute

more appropriate for sensitive or highly personal topics that a participant may be unwilling to talk about in front of peers [4].

The resources and time you have for data collection need to be considered before choosing the research method. For example, focus groups allow for discovering variety within a population and a range of opinions in a short time. In contrast, if a researcher has a longer time frame for their data collection and analysis of individual experiences, conducting multiple interviews over a longer time period may be better. It is also important to consider your participants when deciding which method to choose. For example, the practicality of organising a focus group with six ward managers may mean that individual interviews are a more feasible option. Additionally, if it is imperative that you obtain a detailed perspective of every participant in your sample, interviews would allow for this as group dynamics of a focus group may be difficult to predict.

Sampling in interview and focus group data collection

Sampling is covered in Chapter 6; however, specific sampling considerations for interviews and focus groups are discussed here. It is worth considering whether you want a homogenous (similar) or heterogeneous (varied) sample. Do you wish to recruit individuals from a specific demographic group, for example South Asian nurses, or nurses from all levels of seniority, any geographical area and any age group (see Wozniak [5]). You will need to make this decision in relation to the aim of your research, but if doing focus groups, this decision may impact the group dynamics. When conducting focus groups, factors such as the hierarchy of the group composition need to be considered. Participants may be less open to sharing their true opinions if supervisors, colleagues, or supervisees are also in the group [6] and therefore homogenous groups may be more effective. Conversely, heterogenous groups may be more useful in stimulating discussion through a variety of perspectives with differing opinions [6]. Homogenous or heterogenous group composition also extends to professions. For example, is it beneficial to hold focus groups with members of a single profession, or a range of different professions? Familiarity is also a consideration. The dynamics of a focus group are affected if there are a few participants who know each other within a group of strangers [7]. However, when conducting focus groups with young people, we find it is beneficial to have familiarity between participants to ensure confidence to share as well as challenge each other's opinions.

The extent of homogeneity or heterogeneity in a focus group will also affect the number of focus groups required. For example, when the population of interest is largely homogenous with a straightforward research question, fewer focus groups will be required. In contrast, a more complex research question and a more heterogenous population of interest will require more focus groups. Focus groups usually comprise six to ten participants [6], although we have found they work most effectively with six participants. Online focus groups (which will be explored later) are more successful with smaller numbers: Lobe [8] suggests three to five participants online. This relates to smaller groups allowing 'courteous turn taking' which becomes more challenging online with larger numbers [9]. Hennink et al. [10] suggest deciding how many focus groups to conduct should be based on factors such as the purpose of your study, group composition, and whether you aim to reach data or thematic saturation (the point in data collection when issues begin to be repeated and 'further data collection is redundant', see Chapter 6).

These factors are also important to consider with an interview sample. Hanson et al. [11] suggest 10–20 interviews as an estimated range of participants, but state that determining sample size should be based on whether the researcher decides they have collected sufficient data to develop meaningful findings. As with focus group research, you do not necessarily know how many interviews you will need in advance of starting data collection. The ideal number of interviews is debated, along with whether it is possible or desirable to achieve saturation (for more on this topic, see [12, 13]). For your first clinical education project, your best guide may be the number of interviews it is possible for you to conduct within your time and resource constraints and we recommend seeking advice from supervisors, collaborators, or peers who have undertaken the same course of study.

Choosing specific interview or focus group methods

Online versus face-to-face interviews and focus groups

During the COVID-19 pandemic, the need to continue research projects meant the growth of remotely conducted research methods [14]. Interviews and focus groups can now take place through a range of means: face-to-face, on the phone, through online video calling software such as Zoom, Microsoft Teams, or Skype [15], via email [16], through Mobile Instant Messaging Interviews [14] including WhatsApp [17], or online word processors such as Google Docs [18]. The researcher needs to consider their sample, time and cost restraints, the aim of their research, the topic and their chosen analysis tool in deciding which means of data collection is most appropriate.

A key advantage of undertaking online interviews or focus groups is the broader range of participants which can be reached. Online interviews or focus groups allow the possibility of collecting data in an evening or weekend; this flexibility is especially useful when recruiting healthcare professionals who may not have time for research participation during work time. Conducting interviews or focus groups online removes the need for travel, which can reduce costs for you, participants, and the environment. Video calls enable you to see the participants (where cameras are on), pick up on non-verbal communication (such as facial expressions

and body language), and build rapport which may be lacking in phone or email interviews. However, depending on the topic, you may decide that a phone or email interview would be more appropriate than a video or face-to-face interview. Online approaches are not a direct replacement for face-to-face approaches and different researcher skills are needed [19]. For example, you may need to make decisions around connectivity issues and participants' background distractions which threaten participant privacy [9].

Face-to-face methods of data collection still hold a number of benefits. Online methods may limit relationship building between participants and between you and your participant(s) [19]. For example, before an in-person focus group begins there is likely to be small talk between participants which can help create an atmosphere of ease. This element may be missing in the online format where participants are unable to have private conversations. It is also important to consider the needs of your participants when choosing the means of delivery, for example, considering their extent of technological knowledge and internet access.

Different types and formats of interview

Interviews can be conducted with individuals (the most common method), pairs, or in groups. A group interview is different from a focus group. In a focus group, the researcher encourages participants to interact with each other. In a group interview, the researcher interacts with each participant in the group but only occasionally asks for the level of group consensus [20]. Various types of interviews are explained in Table 14.2, with clinical education examples cited.

Interviews also vary in their degree of structure; they can be unstructured, semi-structured, or structured. Semi-structured interviews are increasingly prevalent in clinical education research [3], as they allow similar topics to be discussed across interviews, whilst leaving room for flexibility in the order and phrasing of questions [23]. Study objectives, and the planned method of analysis, will determine the extent of structure in the interview [6]. Table 14.3 explores these different forms of interview. Unstructured interviews may be used, for example if the interviewer is an occupational therapist interviewing other occupational therapists to gain an exploratory account about the experience of their first clinical placement. An example of using semi-structured interviews may be if a researcher is exploring the experience of panel members (with different professional backgrounds and seniority) of an ARCP (Annual Review of Competence Progression).

Table 14.2 Different types of interviews

Type of interview	Description
Traditional seated one-on-one interview [21]	You ask an interviewee questions from an interview guide
Narrative interview [22]	You help an interviewee tell their story
Vignettes [4, 20]	You provide hypothetical scenarios for interviewees to read or watch and then respond to
Walking interview [23]	You and the interviewee walk through landscapes, or structured walks designed to gather responses and reflections from specific places
'In situ' interview [24, 25]	You follow your interviewee in their daily routine and ask questions (this could also happen virtually) For example, interviewing doctors 'in situ' to allow for discussion about and observation of strategies to work around dyslexia in real time in clinical practice [24]
Interview to the double [26, 27]	You ask the interviewee to pretend that you (the interviewer) are to act as their body double the next day at work. The interviewee is asked what you need to know to be able to replace them the next day at work. This is a way of uncovering workplace learning or practice

Though uncommon in clinical education research, structured interviews could be used if it is important that all participants answer the same questions, or to speed up analysis.

How to conduct interviews and focus groups

Developing and piloting a topic guide

Regardless of format, an important early step is developing a topic guide, a list of topics, questions, themes, or areas to be covered in the interview. For a focus group, the topic guide establishes the agenda and provides direction for the group discussion [7]. You should balance its use with supporting the conversation to flow naturally and promoting interaction between participants [30, 31].

Questions for the topic guide will develop from your literature review and research questions. Questions should not be a verbal version of a questionnaire [7]. A good question should prompt considerable interaction among the participants in a focus group and detailed reflection from an interviewee. Questions should be open-ended and the wording should encourage the participant(s) to talk freely and at length. However, it is also important to consider prompts in the event a participant provides short answers or an answer they think the

Table 14.3 The different formats of interviews

Format of interview	Interview guide	Analysis	Further comments
Structured	A set of questions in a strict order and posed in the same wording to all participants	This format makes coding and analysis most straightforward [28], owing to the same set of questions for each interview	The format may be constraining for interviewees and tends to be less common owing to the exploratory nature of qualitative research [6]
Semi-structured	A flexible interview guide with some predetermined questions, but you are not limited to the guide as you are in structured interviews	The flexibility means data analysis requires greater interpretation than for structured interviews	You can change the question order and wording, ask follow-up questions and omit questions. This format involves more shared control between you and the interviewee
Unstructured	Unstructured interviews are informal and involve open conversations with one or two predetermined questions	Analysing this format of interview is the most challenging, owing to the time-consuming process of assessing and coding data which has not come from a standard set of interview questions as in more structured interviews [29]	What is discussed at the interview is led by the interviewee. You can follow up on points raised by the interviewee, but have less control over the direction of discussion than in the other two interview types

Table 14.4 Examples of open and closed wording of questions

Open question	Closed (leading) question
Tell me your experience of undertaking the independent and supplementary prescribing short course?	Do you think that the independent and supplementary prescribing short course benefited your prescribing practice?
When did you first start thinking about a career in healthcare?	Did you start to consider a career in healthcare in primary school?

interviewer wants to hear, rather than their own perspective. When designing a topic guide, it is important to remember that you need to collect rich quotes to later present in your findings. It is also critical that the question wording gives no clues to the researcher's own opinion on the topic (see Table 14.4).

Questions should be in a logical order, but a guide is only a guide. Topics will be determined by the direction of the discussion. You should begin with easy non-threatening questions which enable the participant(s) to become comfortable talking. Following this, the bulk of the interview/focus group involves asking the key questions and covering the main purpose of the data collection. A couple of straightforward questions should be asked to close the interview but also to allow the interviewee to feel encouraged from their contributions.

It is challenging to judge the number of questions needed. For focus groups, different groups will spend varying lengths discussing their opinions on a topic. Similarly, for interviews, interviewees will vary in the extent to which they answer different questions depending on their experiences, their investment in the topic, and their degree of openness. It is good practice to have more questions than needed, but you also need to be prepared to identify the key questions if time is running out (see example interview guides on the companion website). A common pitfall for new researchers is planning too many questions in the time available. Participants need enough time to elaborate on their answers without feeling hurried and you should not feel you have to rush to fit in all your questions. Piloting will help with this, as you need to develop skills and judgement to make the data collection process a success.

Piloting a topic guide is an essential task, especially for new researchers. It can be useful to pilot your topic guide with someone who is likely to have knowledge of the topic, but who you will not recruit for your study. In addition, it is useful to obtain feedback on your interview/focus group guide from your supervisor, or to be interviewed with your questions to explore your own perspective on the research topic. Piloting and obtaining feedback allow for determining question clarity, to see if a question is understood in the intended way, if certain words need defining, the kind of response a question may elicit and may give an indication of the number of questions needed. Guides can then be modified. Piloting will also allow you to gain practice and develop your skills in steering a discussion, making a note of a follow-up question whilst listening to participants, and becoming comfortable with embracing silences rather than filling them unnecessarily.

Recording the interviews or focus groups

When conducting a focus group or interview, a key consideration is how data will be recorded. Audio or video recording assists you in the collection, analysis, and interpretation of the data by ensuring the participants' words are captured accurately, reduces the amount of notes you are required to take, and allows you to focus on listening to the participant(s). When taking a digital recording, you should ensure the equipment is in position and working prior to the start of the interview and that participants give informed consent for its use (see Chapter 7). Additionally, it is essential to ensure that the interview or focus group cannot be overheard and that there is no background noise that may interfere with the sound quality of the recording. Following the interview or focus group, it is essential you store the recording safely, abiding by local and national guidelines. Transcription can then be used to turn the audio into a written format.

Conducting the interview or focus group

When the participant(s) have arrived and are ready for the data collection you can proceed through a number of steps.

Getting Started

- Introduce yourself and the topic (including the purpose of the research).
- Thank the participant(s) for their time.
- Ensure the participant(s) have read the information sheet and signed a consent form.
- Remind the participant(s) that the interview/focus group is being recorded (if applicable) and about anonymity and confidentiality.
- For a focus group, set up some ground rules, such as ensuring what is said remains confidential within the group or respecting each other's contributions regardless of seniority or profession.
- Ask if there are any questions.
- Define key concepts in order to prevent ambiguity during and after the interview/focus group.
- Clarify timings for the interview/focus group, i.e. how long the session will take.

Promoting participation

- Use positive body language, such as appropriate eye contact, and repeat what a participant has said to show that you understand and value a participant's contributions [32]. If using video-based software, observe yourself to ensure you are showing active listening (but do not get too distracted by analysing your own performance).
- Manage the group dynamic, for example by supporting all participants to contribute to the discussion [33]. If it appears that one participant is dominating, phrases such as 'what do others think of what "participant x" has just said?' provide a way to open the conversation up to all members whilst ensuring the 'dominator' feels their contributions are acknowledged and valued [34].
- Develop awareness of when to bring closure to a particular discussion that is no longer contributing new points or is leading to inappropriate conflict in a focus group. This could be achieved by summarising the discussion and posing the next question.
- If the topic is particularly sensitive, look out for a participant becoming distressed by the conversation. For focus groups, it may be beneficial to have an additional facilitator present to help with this and the logistics [35].
- If a question leads to a brief answer, prepare prompts, probes, or related/follow-up questions to encourage participants to expand on their answer. Ask for an example from their own experience to illustrate their answer.
- Seek clarification for an answer or reflect back an understanding, asking 'have I understood correctly?' Gaining clarification during data collection can ensure the participants' views are accurately recorded and assist with subsequent data analysis.

Ending the interview or focus group

- Summarise key points to ensure the participant(s) feel(s) they have been listened to.
- If the topic is sensitive, conduct a debrief that allows the participant(s) to reflect on the discussion and where to seek support if required [36].
- Ask for any final contributions or if there are any questions.
- Thank the participant(s) for their time again and remind them of anonymity and confidentiality.
- Upload the recording to a secure location and if necessary, write up any notes (for example about the interview/focus group context or dynamics).
- Reflect on the topic guide and adapt it for future focus groups/interviews if necessary, for example changing the structure, wording of questions, or adding additional questions.

Transcribing the focus group or interviews

When preparing for interviews and focus groups, you also need to consider how you are going to transcribe the data. For example, you may focus only on the words spoken by a participant, or you may also include comments on their tone and pauses [37]. To decide, it may be helpful to consider what you feel the transcript represents, for example is it a direct representation of reality or a construction of the environment in which the data was gathered? (see Chapter 3). Though some researchers employ someone else to undertake transcription, there are benefits to transcribing your own interviews or focus groups. While video meeting platforms often offer an automated transcript of the recording, these usually need to be tidied up for accuracy. When transcribing yourself, you can ensure the transcription is accurate and begin immersing yourself in the data and start the process of analysis while listening back to the recordings. The analysis and write up of data are covered in subsequent chapters (see Chapters 18, 19, 26 and 27).

Researcher reflexivity and positionality

When conducting interviews and focus groups, you should be reflexive. Reflexivity involves a specific type of critical thinking whereby you identify how your values, beliefs, identity, experiences, and reasoning shape the research you are conducting [38, 39]. Reflexivity is traditionally associated with qualitative methods; however, all forms of research involve decisions and interpretations by the researcher and therefore these are also important considerations when using quantitative methods [40, 41]. If undertaking interviews or focus groups from a post-positivist orientation (see Chapter 3), the aim is to limit the impact of the researchers' subjectivity on the research process, thereby reducing bias (unintended errors that influence the research outcomes) [42]. For example, multiple researchers may analyse the data to confirm the accuracy of the findings. For those using interviews or focus groups from a constructivist stance, the aim is not to eliminate your impact on the research, but to create an explicit awareness of your influence to help readers interpret and apply the findings [43]. This awareness supports understanding of how the findings and conclusions were constructed through the researcher's active engagement with the research process.

A key part of reflexivity is identifying your positionality: your worldview and position in relation to the subject being studied, the participants, and the research context and process [38] (see Chapter 4). An example of this is when you are an insider and share certain characteristics with the participants, such as a social group, or when you are an outsider and do not have characteristics in common with the participants. An example to illustrate the importance of reflexivity when conducting interviews and focus groups is a nurse who has a clinical academic role and whose work is split between the university and practice setting. If the nurse were to interview other nurses as part of their research, they could be considered an insider due to their shared role within nursing. However, the researcher's role in academia may also lead to the clinically based nurses perceiving them as an outsider. By reflecting on their positionality, the researcher would be able to consider how they influence their research. For example, considering how their insider role within nursing creates the advantage of a shared language with the participants, but may also lead to them making inaccurate assumptions about the participants' knowledge of nursing. A way to promote reflexivity is to keep a journal that can be used to document and audit your reflections on how your position is influencing the research process [44]. You can also discuss your reflections with outside individuals to consider alternative interpretations of what was said. When writing up an interview or focus group study, it is recommended that you report how reflexivity was incorporated, for example by stating that a reflexive journal was kept.

How to ensure rigour in focus groups/interviews

As you plan and undertake interviews or focus groups, you need to maximise the rigour and trustworthiness of your research process [45, 46]. In addition to engaging with the method and data reflexively, you will also need to meet other criteria of quality research. If working from a post-positivist stance, you would increase rigour by focusing on the criteria of reliability and validity, for example through multiple researchers analysing one interview transcript and evaluating the degree of inter-rater reliability, i.e. whether all researchers agreed [47]. If working from a constructivist paradigm, you would seek to increase trustworthiness through criteria such as credibility and dependability [48], for example by having a prolonged engagement with the research participants (see Chapter 3). Whichever criteria you use to determine the rigour and/or trustworthiness of your research, this should be transparently reported within your write up.

An illustrative case study in Box 14.1 provides an example of the process.

Box 14.1   A case study

In 2019, Lucy led a study to evaluate the assessment of trainee advanced clinical practitioners (ACPs) in a county in England [21]. In the United Kingdom, ACPs are healthcare professionals who are educated at master's level and have advanced skills allowing them to work in an expanded role. Exploring attitudes of educators or learners [11] and programme evaluation are both recognised as areas best explored through qualitative study design. The study comprised case studies of different health sectors where ACPs were employed (e.g. primary care, secondary care), with interviews as the main data collection technique. Interviews were chosen over focus groups, to account for the diverse sample and limit the influence of differences in roles or levels of seniority on the data collection process, whilst obtaining detailed perceptions of the individual training experience and assessment.

An initial scoping study reviewed the literature, consulted national organisations, and helped to identify key local stakeholders. These included training leads, supervisors, and lay representatives (referred to collectively as assessors) and also trainees. Phone interviews reduced the travel required and allowed Lucy to arrange interviews at short notice in a consistent way. However, phone interviews presented challenges, for example through limiting non-verbal communication. This reduced Lucy's capacity to build rapport and support the participants in feeling comfortable enough to be honest about their thoughts. In order to account for this challenge, Lucy employed active listening, for example by summarising an answer or asking follow-up questions. She used a semi-structured interview guide in all interviews to provide some structure whilst allowing the questions to be adapted according to the different roles/sectors of the assessors and trainees.

Interviews took place with 11 trainees and six assessors over a three-month period. Organising the interviews required Lucy to be persistent and flexible enough to conduct interviews at short notice. Each interview lasted approximately 50 minutes. This led to a total of 300 minutes of assessor interviews and 510 minutes of trainee interview recordings. The sheer volume of recording and subsequent data highlights a key challenge with interview research, which needs to be factored in when designing and costing a study. Where often a researcher needs to transcribe their own recordings, in this case a professional transcriber was used because of the volume of data collected and the funding available for this service. Lucy and the research team coded the

Box 14.1   (continued)

interview data and developed themes. Using multiple coders provided a way to achieve agreement on the analysis and limited the impact of the subjectivity of the interviewer, thus increasing the rigour of the research within this post-positivist study. Based on the findings, the importance of triangulating the research through interviewing a number of different stakeholders was evident, as the assessors and the trainees had varying views on the effectiveness of the assessment process. Only interviewing the assessors or the trainees would have given only one perspective and resulted in different findings to the ones which were reported.

Summary

This chapter has outlined the purpose of interviews and focus groups in research, highlighting strengths and considerations when using these methods and providing guidance on when each should be used. It has also described the skills required to use these methods and given advice on how to create a topic guide. Furthermore, this chapter has supported you to reflect on your role as a researcher in relation to interviews and focus groups. Whilst there is some transferability between clinical skills such as medical history taking and undertaking interviews or focus groups, there are also significant differences. Therefore, if you choose to use these methods to conduct clinical education research, it is important you practise applying the principles presented in this chapter. With experience, you will grow in confidence and ability as an interviewer or focus group facilitator.

Top tips

- Make an informed choice as to whether an interview or a focus group is most appropriate for meeting your research aim. Weigh up the relative strengths and considerations.
- Select an appropriate sample for your research aim, time, and resources.
- Develop and pilot a topic guide, to practise, gain feedback, and refine your questions.
- Employ active listening throughout your interviews or focus groups.
- Reflect on the interview or focus group process, including your involvement in the data collection and analysis.

Common pitfalls

- Planning too many questions. Factor in time for the participant to think and elaborate on their answers.
- Insufficient probing or clarification. Ask follow-up questions to gather detail and ensure there are the quotes to support your findings.
- Expressing judgement or testing the knowledge of the participant(s). Instead, remain focused on accessing the participants' perception of a topic, not yours.
- Interviewing efficiently as if taking a clinical history. Allow time and space for rich stories, specific examples, and reflections.
- Ending the interview too soon. Often participants relax and offer new insights towards the end.

Ethical issues

- Interviews and focus groups vary in the degree to which confidentiality can be assured. Explain to focus group participants that you cannot promise confidentiality on behalf of other participants, but request that responses are not shared outside the group.
- Safety of participants must be ensured. Whether online or face-to-face, undertake interviews or focus groups in safe, private spaces where participants feel comfortable to share their experiences or views.
- Power imbalances may exist. Carefully consider focus group allocation and take extra steps to build rapport when hierarchies are at play.

References

1 Kvale, S. (1996). *InterViews: An Introduction to Qualitative Research Interviewing*. Thousand Oaks, CA: SAGE Publications.
2 Salmons, J. (2017). Janet Salmons defines focus groups. In: *SAGE Research Methods Video*. SAGE Publications. https://methods.sagepub.com/video/janet-salmons-defines-focus-groups.
3 McGrath, C., Palmgren, P.J., and Liljedahl, M. (2019). Twelve tips for conducting qualitative research interviews. *Medical Teacher* 41 (9): 1002–1006.
4 Cristancho, S.M., Goldszmidt, M., Lingard, L., and Watling, C. (2018). Qualitative research essentials for medical education. *Singapore Medical Journal* 59 (12): 622–627.

5 Wozniak, W. (2014). Homogeneity of focus groups as a pathway to successful research findings? Methodological notes from the fieldwork. *Przegląd Socjologii Jakościowe* 1: 6–22.

6 Ramani, S. and Mann, K. (2016). Introducing medical educators to qualitative study design: twelve tips from inception to completion. *Medical Teacher* 38: 456–463.

7 Stewart, D.W., Shamdasani, P.M., and Rook, D.W. (2007). *Focus Groups*. Thousand Oaks, CA: SAGE Publications.

8 Lobe, B. (2017). Best practices for synchronous online focus groups. In: *A New Era in Focus Group Research: Challenges, Innovation and Practice* (ed. R.S. Barbour and D.L. Morgan), 227–250. Palgrave Macmillan.

9 Daniels, N., Gillen, P., Casson, K., and Wilson, I. (2019). STEER: factors to consider when designing online focus groups using audiovisual technology in health research. *International Journal of Qualitative Methods* 18: 1–11.

10 Hennink, M.M., Kaiser, B.N., and Weber, M.B. (2019). What influences saturation? Estimating sample sizes in focus group research. *Qualitative Health Research* 18: 1–11.

11 Hanson, J.L., Balmer, D.F., and Giardino, A.P. (2011). Qualitative research methods for medical educators. *Academic Pediatrics* 11 (5): 375–386.

12 Braun, V. and Clarke, V. (2021). To saturate or not to saturate? Questioning data saturation as a useful concept for thematic analysis and sample-size rationales. *Qualitative Research in Sport, Exercise and Health* 13 (2): 201–216.

13 Varpio, L., Ajjawi, R., Monrouxe, L.V. et al. (2017). Shedding the cobra effect: problematising thematic emergence, triangulation, saturation and member checking. *Medical Education* 51 (1): 40–50.

14 Kaufmann, K., Peil, C., and Bork-Hüffer, T. (2021). Producing in situ data from a distance with mobile instant messaging interviews (MIMIs): examples from the COVID-19 pandemic. *International Journal of Qualitative Methods* 20: 1–14.

15 Lo Iacono, V., Symonds, P., and Brown, D.H.K. (2016). Skype as a tool for qualitative research interviews. *Sociological Research Online* 21 (2): 103–117.

16 Fritz, R.L. and Vandermause, R. (2018). Data collection via in-depth email interviewing: lessons from the field. *Qualitative Health Research* 28 (10): 1640–1649.

17 Gibson, K. (2022). Bridging the digital divide: reflections on using WhatsApp instant messenger interviews in youth research. *Qualitative Research in Psychology* 19 (3): 611–631.

18 Opara, V., Spangsdorf, S., and Ryan, M.K. (2021). Reflecting on the use of Google Docs for online interviews: innovation in qualitative data collection. *Qualitative Research* 1–18.

19 Davies, L., LeClair, K., Bagley, P. et al. (2020). Face-to-face compared with online collected accounts of health and illness experiences: a scoping review. *Qualitative Health Research* 30 (13): 2092–2102.

20 Bernabeo, E.C., Holmboe, E.S., Ross, K. et al. (2013). The utility of vignettes to stimulate reflection on professionalism: theory and practice. *Advances in Health Sciences Education: Theory and Practice* 18: 463–484.

21 Wallis, L., Locke, R., Sutherland, C., and Harden, B. (2022). Assessment of advanced clinical practitioners: a short report. *Journal of Interprofessional Care* 36 (6): 946–950.

22 de la Croix, A., Barrett, A., and Stenfors, T. (2018). How to do research interviews in different ways. *The Clinical Teacher* 15: 451–456.

23 Evans, J. and Jones, P. (2011). The walking interview: methodology, mobility and place. *Applied Geography* 31 (2): 849–858.

24 Locke, R., Alexander, G., Mann, R. et al. (2017). Doctors with dyslexia: strategies and support. *The Clinical Teacher* 14 (5): 38–53.

25 White, J. (2007). Supporting nursing students with dyslexia in clinical practice. *Nursing Standard* 21: 35–42.

26 Sheridan, L., Price, O., Sheridan, L.. et al. (2018). Interview to the double: a methodological tool for practice-based research. https://ro.uow.edu.au/uowbooks/26/ (accessed 8 May 2023).

27 Bekti, R. (2022). Exploration of medical professionalism across postgraduate medical education in Indonesia. https://etheses.whiterose.ac.uk/31862/ (accessed 8 May 2023).

28 Doody, O. and Noonan, M. (2013). Preparing and conducting interviews to collect data. *Nurse Researcher* 20 (5): 28–32.

29 Zhang, Y. and Wildemuth, B.M. (2009). *Unstructured Interviews: Applications of Social Research Methods to Questions in Information and Library Science*, 222–231. Libraries Unlimited.

30 O'Nyumba, T., Wilson, K., Derrick, C., and Mukherjee, N. (2018). The use of focus group discussion methodology: insights from two decades of application in conservation. *Qualitative Methods for Eliciting Judgements for Decision Making* 9 (1): 20–32.

31 Morgan, L. (1997). *Focus Groups as Qualitative Research*, 2e. London: SAGE Publications.

32 Rogers, C.R. and Farson, R.E. (1987). Active listening. In: *Communication in Business Today* (ed. R.G. Newman, M.A. Danziger, and M. Cohen). Washington, DC: Health and Company.

33 Luke, M. and Goodrich, K.M. (2019). Focus group research: an intentional strategy for applied group research? *The Journal for Specialists in Group Work* 44 (2): 77–81.

34 Liamputtong, P. (2011). *Focus Group Methodology: Principles and Practice*. London: SAGE Publications.

35 Krueger, R. (2002). *Designing and Conducting Focus Group Interviews*. Minnesota: University of Minnesota.

36 Sim, J. and Waterfield, J. (2019). Focus group methodology: some ethical challenges. *Quality and Quantity* 53: 3003–3022.

37 Willig, C. (2008). *Introducing Qualitative Research in Psychology*, 2e. Maidenhead: Open University Press.

38 Holmes, A.G.D. (2020). Researcher positionality – a consideration of its influence and place in qualitative research – a new researcher guide. *Shanlax International Journal of Education* 8 (4): 1–10.

39 Råheim, M., Magnussen, L.H., Sekse, R.J. et al. (2016). Researcher-researched relationship in qualitative research: shifts in positions and researcher vulnerability. *International Journal of Qualitative Studies on Health and Well-being* 11 (1): 30996.

40 Lakew, Y. (2017). Statistical tales: bringing in reflexivity to make sense of quantitative data. In: *Present Scenarios of Media Production and Engagement* (ed. S. Tosoni, N. Carpentier, M.F. Murru, et al.), 225–238. Lumière.

41 Sikes, P. (2004). *Methodology, Procedures and Ethical Concerns. Doing Educational Research: A Guide for First Time Researchers*. London: SAGE Publications.

42 Pannucci, C.J. and Wilkins, E.G. (2010). Identifying and avoiding bias in research. *Plastic and Reconstructive Surgery* 126 (2): 619–625.

43 Florczak, K.L. (2021). Reflexivity: should it be mandated for qualitative reporting? *Nursing Science Quarterly* 34 (4): 352–355.

44 Nowell, L.S., Norris, J.M., White, D.E., and Moules, N.J. (2017). Thematic analysis: striving to meet the trustworthiness criteria. *International Journal of Qualitative Methods* 16: 1–13.

45 Morse, J.M., Barrett, M., Mayan, M. et al. (2002). Verification strategies for establishing reliability and validity in qualitative research. *International Journal of Qualitative Methods* 1 (2): 13–22.

46 Heale, R. and Twycross, A. (2015). Validity and reliability in quantitative studies. *Evidence-Based Nursing* 18: 66–67.

47 O'Connor, C. and Joffe, H. (2020). Intercoder reliability in qualitative research: debates and practical guidelines. *International Journal of Qualitative Methods* 19: 1–13.

48 Lincoln, Y. and Guba, E.G. (1985). *Naturalistic Inquiry*. Newbury Park, CA: SAGE Publications.

15 Visual elicitation: techniques for digging deeper in qualitative interviews

Gerard J. Gormley, Sayra Cristancho, and Katherine Crook

Learning objectives

By the end of this chapter, you should be able to:
- Recognise how visual elicitation techniques can enrich data derived from qualitative research interviews.

- Describe the principles and practicalities of using various visual elicitation interview techniques.
- Consider whether visual elicitation techniques may be useful in your own clinical education research project.

Introduction

Interviews are a commonly used method of data collection in qualitative research (see Chapter 14). They enable researchers to gain data about participants' experiences and provide textual material for analysis. Whilst the traditional qualitative research interview will serve most individuals starting out in qualitative research, there are times it can fall short of providing rich and nuanced insights into participants' experiences. This is no truer than in the field of clinical education research. Clinical education and practice are often complex and mediated by a bewilderment of factors. Moreover, participants' experiences are personal, multi-layered, and at times difficult to access and articulate. How often have we heard the phrase 'It's just hard to put into words. . .!' Given the inherent complexities of clinical education, it is right that we represent our participants, and their experiences, well in our research. At the point of obtaining interview data, we must strive to provide a sufficient and in-depth representation about participants' experiences. This provides a meaningful foundation for analysis. Qualitative research interviews are much more than a series of linear questions and responses. From a constructivist position, qualitative research interviews are a dynamic process in which data is co-constructed between interviewer and interviewee. Interview elicitation techniques, including visual elicitation, offer ways of enhancing the quality and richness of data created through this process.

Drawing from disciplines such as anthropology and social sciences, interview elicitation techniques are gaining popularity in clinical education research. They represent a group of methods you can utilise to augment the traditional qualitative research interview. There is a wide array of elicitation techniques, from *guided walks* [1] (where a participant and interviewer walk in a place of interest while conducting a qualitative interview to gain insights of self and place) to *artefact elicitation* [2] (where a participant brings a previously created physical artefact to act as a prompt in an interview). Such visual stimuli then form an anchor through which interviewer and interviewee find common ground to co-explore the various angles of a story during the interview.

There are several visual elicitation techniques you can choose from. In this chapter, we introduce three visual elicitation techniques, which may be used to dig deeper in clinical education research interviews: rich pictures, photo-elicitation, and point of view elicitation. Rich pictures are hand-drawn representations of a particular experience by a research participant. In photo-elicitation, photographs created by the researcher or participant are used within an interview to encourage discussion and elicit rich data. Finally, point-of-view elicitation involves video footage, captured from a research participant's point of view, to enrich data obtained during an interview.

Starting Research in Clinical Education, First Edition. Edited by Eliot L. Rees, Alison Ledger, and Kim A. Walker.
© 2024 The Association for the Study of Medical Education (ASME). Published 2024 by John Wiley & Sons Ltd.
Companion website: www.wiley.com/go/clinicaleducation

Some of the advantages of visual elicitation techniques include

- Opening up other communication channels to convey and elaborate on experiences that are difficult to access and articulate by words alone (i.e. visualising what you cannot verbalise).
- Enhancing the relational dimensions of interviews by promoting rapport and reducing power gradients.
- Promoting the interviewer's and interviewee's ability to be present, focused, and able to dwell on a subject matter.
- Stimulating deeper reflection on an area of interest.
- Enhancing the interviewer's ability to empathise with interviewees' experiences, concepts and ideas.
- Supporting exploration of a sensitive subject matter.
- Producing powerful, expressive artefacts which can be analysed and/or included when communicating and disseminating your research findings.

In addition to enhancing the traditional interview, visual elicitation techniques can also provide a powerful means of communicating and disseminating your research findings. For example, incorporating elicitation photographs or pictures into publications and presentations (see Chapters 27 and 28). Moreover, the visual elicitation materials can also be used as data in their own right for analysis [3–5].

In the remainder of this chapter, we aim to further introduce and illustrate the basis of visual interview elicitation techniques and how they can enhance the richness, trustworthiness, and quality of your interview data. We hope you are inspired to try visual elicitation techniques and experience that they are worth the additional effort in implementation.

Rich pictures

A rich picture is a pictorial hand-drawn representation of a particular experience. It is both a tool and a form of expression for unpacking and articulating complex, problematic, or significant aspects of an experience [6]. Rich pictures are very specific to the people who draw them. Therefore, the goal is not to depict an objective documentation of all features of a situation; rather, to gain insights of how research participants view and understand an experience, particularly around its unspoken/hidden aspects [7]. It can include the participant's perspective on what happened, who was involved, how people felt, how people acted, how people behaved, and what external pressures were present [8].

In clinical education research, rich pictures have been paramount in exploring how medical educators experience governance in curriculum change processes [9], what patients with terminal illnesses are willing to share about their experiences for educational purposes [10], how surgeons make sense of and resolve complex operations [11], and how trainees navigate moral dilemmas and emotional responses during complex clinical situations [12]. Using rich pictures, researchers can probe, not only for the physical/technical aspects but also for the conceptual and emotional components of the participant's story. Figure 15.1 shows an example of how a rich picture can help elucidate the various components of a complex surgical operation from the perspective of the surgeon.

Knowing when to use rich pictures in your qualitative research study can be challenging. If you follow a constructivist perspective, you will believe that rich pictures, as a type of visual method, are socially constructed, and their meaning depends on both the creator and the viewer [14]. As such, rich pictures are a powerful conduit for understanding. Therefore, they are particularly useful for questioning deeply held assumptions, for discovering overlooked connections, traps, possibilities, and contradictions of an experience, and for stimulating perspective taking when exploring participants' experiences of working, learning, or receiving care in complex and dynamic environments. Based on these premises, rich pictures are best utilised to explore topics that are emotionally, politically, or socially charged that make them difficult to access or articulate, for example, the struggles that residents go through while learning to navigate difficult conversations with parents in the neonatal intensive care unit [15].

Key considerations when using rich pictures

As drawings activate different parts of the brain from words, the conversations that unfold around a rich picture can generate multiple perspectives and interpretations because of the ability to both *hear* about and *see* how those perspectives are depicted. Visual metaphors add a complementary language to words that help people articulate their insights. This is particularly critical in research with vulnerable populations or individuals with communication barriers. Rich pictures can also be used in combination with other elicitation methods to add richness to the data [16]. However, despite these qualities, drawing rich pictures can be intimidating to many participants. Participants may feel they lack the necessary artistic skills and without

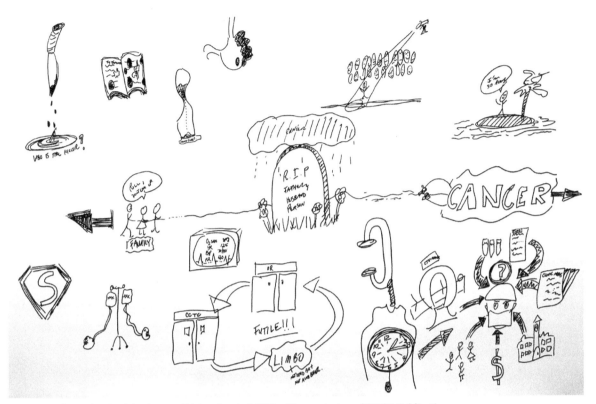

Figure 15.1 Example of a rich picture. Cristancho et al. [13] with permission of SAGE Publications.

proper guidance from the part of the researcher, the sole idea of drawing may deter many from participating. Ethical concerns about confidentiality, consent, and authorship also impose challenges. As the meaning intended by the participant may be misinterpreted when a rich picture is published, you need to exercise careful attention in describing the context. Therefore, clear discussions with participants about how the drawings may be disseminated, and for what audience, should be judiciously conducted [17].

How to use rich pictures

During data collection, research participants are usually asked to recall a memorable situation related to the specific research question and to draw everything they deem important. It is common practice to include a pre-drawing conversation with participants about the context of their personal or professional experience. The purpose of this pre-drawing conversation is twofold: (i) to inspire participants' thinking and (ii) to examine how the verbal accounts of participants influence what they draw and what they share about their experiences. After this set up is complete, participants are shown and walked through an example

of a rich picture from a previously published paper or textbook to ease any concerns about the need for artistic skills. The rich picture activity is followed by a semi-structured interview where participants elaborate on the story behind it and answer specific probes from the researcher [7]. Depending on the research question, data analysis may focus on the content of the interviews, or on a combination of both the rich picture and interview data [7]. For interview text, thematic analysis, content analysis, grounded theory, and various forms of discourse analyses may be appropriate. When analysing visual and interview data in combination, iconographic analysis [8] can be used.

Photo-elicitation

Photo-elicitation is the use of photographs within an interview, often at the start, to encourage discussion and elicit rich data [18]. The interview can incorporate a single image or multiple images, which can be created by the researcher or the participant [19]. If researcher-generated, the photograph is taken or gathered by the researcher based on their understanding of the research topic, its aims, and the research questions. If participant-generated, volunteers are asked to take a photograph or multiple images related to the research topic in response to a question or prompt. Images produced by participants can be diverse and unique to each individual; for example, participants from a recent physiotherapy study produced photographs ranging from drawings to a photograph of a work desk to convey what 'psychology' meant to them in

physiotherapy practice (see Figure 15.2). The image can also be incorporated into the analysis alongside the interview transcription.

There are numerous benefits of using this method. Asking a participant to take a photograph can encourage reflection on the research topic prior to the interview. Photo-elicitation can also increase engagement during the interview, as the participant has invested time and effort to take their

(a)

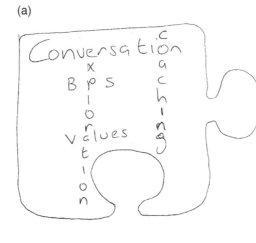
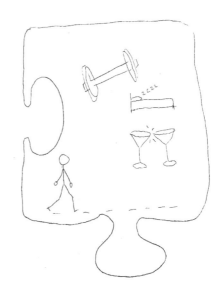

(b)

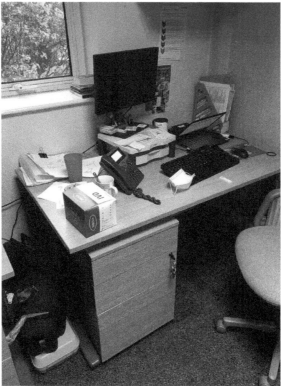

Figure 15.2 (a, b) Images produced by participants in a photo-elicitation study. *Source*: Katherine Crook.

photograph. It may also place the participants in a position of power [20], as experts on the topic through their photographs. Thus, using photo-elicitation can amplify the collaborative nature of knowledge production [18] and help you to build rapport with participants [21]. Other, more pragmatic benefits of using photo-elicitation include aiding memory and reducing tiredness during potentially longer interviews [22]. These advantages can be particularly beneficial if undertaking research remotely with minimal or no face-to-face contact with participants.

Key considerations when using photo-elicitation

Flexibility is one of photo-elicitation's greatest strengths and is demonstrated by its variety of applications. Photographs can be used at different stages of a project, including data collection and data analysis [18]. Analysis of the image can be undertaken in isolation or combined with other data such as interview transcriptions, using a suitable method of co-analysis. Additionally, photo-elicitation can be valuable for dissemination activities [20], enabling evocative dissemination methods such as an art exhibition or a video compilation.

Photo-elicitation can also be useful when studying sensitive topics. For example, Edmondson et al. [23] aimed to explore the use of a non-verbal and non-written method with participants discussing why they self-harm. Photo-elicitation may also be beneficial with participants who are considered vulnerable due to age, health condition, or social, economic, and educational status. For example, Platzer et al. [24] utilised researcher-generated photo-elicitation with older individuals of low socioeconomic status to explore their perceptions of health. In this instance, a visual rather than written method helped the researchers to navigate challenges related to variable cognitive capacities and literacy. These examples demonstrate how this method may be particularly useful if you are working on healthcare or community-based projects and working with adults, children, or older individuals. On a practical level, photo-elicitation can be completed face to face, or undertaken remotely. Photographs can be taken digitally, emailed before an interview, and/or shared via an online meeting platform, meaning you can recruit interviewees nationally or internationally.

How to use photo-elicitation

Once participants have been recruited, attention turns to the device for taking photographs. This may be a disposable camera provided by the research team, or the participant's own camera such as a mobile phone or tablet. If it is the latter, it is important to ensure that everyone has access to a similar device which they are familiar with to ensure equity. Instructions to take photographs can then be presented; this can be in the form of a prompt or question, and sufficient time should be provided to ensure that everyone understands the task. Instructions should include what to do with the photograph(s) once the task is completed, for example requesting that participants send their photograph(s) to the research team prior to the forthcoming interview. If multiple photographs have been taken, participants may be asked to choose a sample which best represents their response to the prompt. Once received, and prior to the interview, you should familiarise yourself with the photograph(s) and begin to generate potential questions. Recording initial impressions of the photograph(s) at this time will help to develop the interview and encourage in-depth discussion.

Point of view video elicitation

Point of view video elicitation is a technique that has been used for many decades in disciplines such as the humanities and anthropology. In essence, participants video record, usually from a first-person perspective, an activity of interest they are engaged with. The activity could be in a naturalistic setting such as a clinical environment, or a more constructed setting such as a simulation laboratory. Point of view video footage can be captured by a number of methods, including wearing a body-camera or video glasses. The footage captured provides a representation of what the participant was actually seeing as the activity unfolded, i.e. a *trace* of their engagement with the activity and environment. Following the activity, this footage can then act as a stimulus during a qualitative interview, allowing you to observe the participant's point of view and listen to them talk aloud their lived experiences. By so doing, you can develop a greater connection and empathise with their experiences.

Moreover, video elicitation can promote verbalisation of aspects of experiences that might not normally be accessed in traditional interviews, particularly bodily practices and tacit knowledge [25]. An important advantage of this approach is that participants rely less on memory, recall, and distortions of post hoc rationalisation. For example, Behrens et al. [26] employed point of view elicitation to explore the complex emotions that were experienced by medical students in a simulation activity. Investigators attached video glasses to capture video footage of medical students as they engaged in a complex simulation. Following the simulation, participants were interviewed using their point of view video footage. The footage provided a powerful stimulus for medical students to reflect on their experiences and express emotions they often found challenging to articulate. For example, one of the outcomes was medical students shared a desire to externally conceal any signs of their intense emotions, in case this was interpreted as a sign of weakness and a threat to their professional identity.

Key considerations when using point of view video elicitation

There are a wide variety of instances in which point of view video elicitation is well suited. However, it particularly lends itself to in-person activities that naturally unfold as the individual engages in that activity. For example, placing a video device on a patient to capture their healthcare experiences or placing video glasses on a student as they take part in a simulation-based learning activity. Compared to video footage from a static camera, point of view video footage provides a closer representation of the individual's experiences, capturing a trace of their experiences as the activity unfolds. It also removes the possibility that a separate videographer influences the activity under investigation.

How to use point of view video elicitation

On the companion website, we have provided a step-by-step guide on using point of view video elicitation in qualitative interviews. Preparation is key to this process. It is important you obtain a suitable portable video camera with audio recording facilities (e.g. video glasses). A trial run of using such equipment is always advised, ensuring you have adequate data storage space. Prior to video recording a participant's point of view, we would advise time for the participant to become accustomed to wearing the portable video camera. When the participant is ready to take part in the activity under investigation, make sure to switch on the portable video camera. Once the activity is concluded, switch the video camera off and immediately transfer the video footage data to a computer for viewing. The most common approach to using point of view video footage in interviews is for both interviewer and interviewee to observe the footage together, with the interviewee talking aloud about their experiences. Either individual can pause the video at any stage, at a point of interest, even rewinding the video to review again. At these points, interviewers are encouraged to use probing questions to gain a deeper understanding of interviewees' experiences. For example, 'I'm really intrigued to know what you were experiencing at this moment. Can you elaborate on this for me? I'm curious to know what happened here and why you did this?' Following the interview, it is important you ensure participants remain content and comfortable with the process. Finally, make sure to comply with your research governance policies by securely saving and/or erasing the video footage.

Summary

We hope this chapter has piqued your interest into some of the visual-based interview elicitation techniques available in qualitative research. Whilst such elicitation techniques require some additional effort to integrate into your interviews, they have the potential to augment and enrich the data you obtain. Moreover, the visual creations can also be used as data in their own right and be a powerful vehicle to communicate your research findings. We encourage you to reflect on your research question and if suitable for visual elicitation, have a go at these methods. In the process, make sure to do justice to those generous individuals who offer their experiences and images in your interviews.

Top tips

- Pilot your methods. Ask a colleague to draw a rich picture for you, try out your photo-elicitation prompt, or test the equipment to record participants' points of view. Piloting will help you to understand potential concerns of interviewees and develop strategies for promoting participation and producing rich data.

- Create a habit of writing reflective memos as a strategy to regularly question your own assumptions about the phenomenon of study and the visuals produced.

- Expect the unexpected. Even with the most carefully honed prompt, your participants may produce visuals you would never have imagined. Embrace any surprises that arise.

Common pitfalls

- Not putting sufficient time and thought into preparing your instructions for participants. Aim to strike a balance between promoting confidence and allowing room for creativity and personal interpretation.
- Neglecting to consider the participant's physical and psychological comfort when using point of view equipment. Allow time for the participant to wear the device prior to recording and reassure them about the security of any footage obtained, to enhance trust.
- Missing opportunities for rich discussion. Familiarise yourself with your participants' rich pictures/photographs/video footage and ask curious questions. Often what might seem mundane on first observation, could actually be quite important in helping you to address your research question.

Ethical issues

- Conversations about ethics may need to be revisited throughout the study, as new concerns about participant confidentiality may arise.
- Visual elicitation can offer a range of new dissemination possibilities. When designing your study, think about how you may present participants' visuals and ask for their consent before disseminating them.
- When using photo-elicitation, make sure participants are aware of the need to gain consent if they are taking photographs of people or a specific location. To mitigate risks of identification, you can ask participants to avoid taking photographs of recognisable locations or people's faces.
- When possible, ask for feedback from participants and colleagues while drafting your manuscript or preparing a presentation to ensure key ethical concerns are addressed.

Further reading

Cristancho, S., LaDonna, K., and Field, E. (2022). Visual methods in health professions research: purpose, challenges and opportunities. In: *Researching Medical Education*, 2e (ed. J. Cleland and S.J. Durning), 139–152. Wiley.

Gormley, G.J. and Fenwick, T. (2016). Learning to manage complexity through simulation: students' challenges and possible strategies. *Perspectives on Medical Education* 5: 138–146.

Lauck, S.B., Oliffe, J.L., Stephenson, A., and Adhami, N. (2021). Can you picture it? Photo elicitation in qualitative cardiovascular health research. *European Journal of Cardiovascular Nursing* 20 (8): 797–802.

Molinaro, M.L., Cheng, A., Cristancho, S., and LaDonna, K. (2021). Drawing on experience: exploring the pedagogical possibilities of using rich pictures in health professions education. *Advances in Health Sciences Education* 26 (5): 1519–1535.

Skinner, J. and Gormley, G.J. (2016). Point of view filming and the elicitation interview. *Perspectives on Medical Education* 5: 235–239.

References

1 Clark, A. and Emmel, N. (2010). Using walking interviews. *Realities* 13: 1–6.

2 Abildgaard, M.S. (2018). My whole life in telephones: material artifacts as interview elicitation devices. *International Journal of Qualitative Methods* 17. https://journals.sagepub.com/doi/pdf/10.1177/1609406918797795.

3 Bell, S., Berg, T., and Morse, S. (2019). Towards an understanding of rich picture interpretation. *Systemic Practice and Action Research* 32: 601–614.

4 Padgett, D.K., Smith, B.T., Derejko, K.-S. et al. (2013). A picture is worth. . .? Photo elicitation interviewing with formerly homeless adults. *Qualitative Health Research* 23 (11): 1435–1444.

5 Booton, C.M. (2018). Using rich pictures to verify, contradict, or enhance verbal data. *The Qualitative Report* 23 (11): 2835–2849.

6 Guillemin, M. (2004). Understanding illness: using drawings as a research method. *Qualitative Health Research* 14 (2): 272–289.

7 Cristancho, S.M. and Helmich, E. (2019). Rich pictures: a companion method for qualitative research in medical education. *Medical Education* 53 (9): 916–924.

8 Bell, S., Berg, T., and Morse, S. (2016). *Rich Pictures: Encouraging Resilient Communities*. Routledge.

9 Velthuis, F., Dekker, H., Coppoolse, R. et al. (2021). Educators' experiences with governance in curriculum change processes; a qualitative study using rich pictures. *Advances in Health Sciences Education* 26 (3): 1027–1043.

10 Bood, Z.M., Scherer-Rath, M., Sprangers, M.A. et al. (2019). Living with advanced cancer: rich pictures as a means for health care providers to explore the experiences of advanced cancer patients. *Cancer Medicine* 8 (11): 4957–4966.

11 Cristancho, S.M., Bidinosti, S.J., Lingard, L.A. et al. (2014). What's behind the scenes? Exploring the unspoken dimensions of complex and challenging surgical situations. *Academic Medicine* 89 (11): 1540.

12 Ribeiro, D.L., Costa, M., Helmich, E. et al. (2021). 'I found myself a despicable being!': medical students face disturbing moral dilemmas. *Medical Education* 55 (7): 857–871.

13 Cristancho, S., Bidinosti, S., Lingard, L. et al. (2015). Seeing in different ways: introducing "rich pictures" in the study of expert judgment. *Qualitative Health Research* 25 (5): 713–725.

14 Crotty, M. (2020). *The Foundations of Social Research: Meaning and Perspective in the Research Process*. Routledge.

15 Cheng, A., LaDonna, K., Cristancho, S., and Ng, S. (2017). Navigating difficult conversations: the role of self-monitoring and reflection-in-action. *Medical Education* 51 (12): 1220–1231.

16 Hartel, J., Noone, R., Oh, C. et al. (2018). The iSquare protocol: combining research, art, and pedagogy through the draw-and-write technique. *Qualitative Research* 18 (4): 433–450.

17 Cox, S., Drew, S., Guillemin, M. et al. (2014). *Guidelines for Ethical Visual Research Methods*. Visual Research Collaboratory. https://socialequity.unimelb.edu.au/__data/assets/pdf_file/0006/1981392/Ethical-Visual-Research-Methods-WEB.pdf.

18 Glaw, X., Inder, K., Kable, A., and Hazelton, M. (2017). Visual methodologies in qualitative research: autophotography and photo elicitation applied to mental health research. *International Journal of Qualitative Methods* 16 (1): 1–8.

19 Bignante, E. (2010). The use of photo-elicitation in field research. *EchoGéo* 11. https://doi.org/10.4000/echogeo.11622

20 Bates, E.A., McCann, J.J., Kaye, L.K., and Taylor, J.C. (2017). "Beyond words": a researcher's guide to using photo elicitation in psychology. *Qualitative Research in Psychology* 14 (4): 459–481.

21 Meo, A.I. (2010). Picturing students' habitus: the advantages and limitations of photo-elicitation interviewing in a qualitative study in the city of Buenos Aires. *International Journal of Qualitative Methods* 9 (2): 149–171.

22 Collier, J. Jr. (1957). Photography in anthropology: a report on two experiments. *American Anthropologist* 59 (5): 843–859.

23 Edmondson, A.J., Brennan, C., and House, A.O. (2018). Using photo-elicitation to understand reasons for repeated self-harm: a qualitative study. *BMC Psychiatry* 18: 98.

24 Platzer, F., Steverink, N., Haan, M. et al. (2021). The bigger picture: research strategy for a photo-elicitation study investigating positive health perceptions of older adults with low socioeconomic status. *International Journal of Qualitative Methods* 20. https://journals.sagepub.com/doi/full/10.1177/16094069211040950.

25 Skinner, J. (2012). Four part introduction to the interview: introducing the interview; society, sociology and the interview; anthropology and the interview. In: *The Interview: An Ethnographic Approach* (ed. J. Skinner), 1–49. Oxford: Berg Publications.

26 Behrens, C.C., Driessen, E.W., Dolmans, D.H., and Gormley, G.J. (2021). 'A roller coaster of emotions': a phenomenological study on medical students lived experiences of emotions in complex simulation. *Advances in Simulation* 6 (1): 24.

16 Ethnography: sense and sensibilities in conducting fieldwork

Lisa Dikomitis and Brianne Wenning

Learning objectives

By the end of this chapter, you should be able to:
- Recognise key features, principles, and applications of ethnographic research.
- Plan your first ethnographic study.
- Prepare for challenges associated with conducting participant observation.
- Recognise the ethical dilemmas in doing ethnographic fieldwork.

Introduction

An ethnography is a descriptive, detailed, written account of a particular culture, group, or community, situated in a specific context, time, and place. By *culture*, we refer to a range of characteristics that can indicate belonging, such as religion, politics, history, language, and various practices, including clinical and educational practices. It is important to note that culture is dynamic and members of one culture are likely to be members of many other cultures too. A community can include those living in a particular geographical area, attending a particular clinical practice, working in a specific healthcare setting, belonging to a specific group of health professionals, or attending the same university. In ethnography, the researcher observes and interacts with a community, revealing unexpected or hidden aspects of the community members' day-to-day life.

This chapter introduces ethnography, including its history and contributions, different types of ethnographic fieldwork, and the practicalities of participant observation. We provide an example from clinical education to support you in considering whether ethnography may be appropriate for your own research topic and question. Throughout, we stress the importance of ongoing reflexivity and ethical considerations when working as an ethnographer.

History and value of ethnography

The origins of ethnography lie in the nineteenth century. It has been historically associated with anthropology, and, later in the twentieth century, with qualitative sociology. Since the early twentieth century, ethnographers carried out fieldwork, commonly in a society very different from their own, usually in a community geographically located far away from the ethnographer's own community.

Ethnography means, in its most literal translation, 'writing people'. Indeed, both 'writing' and 'people' are central to ethnographic practice. Ethnography can be both a noun and a verb. The noun refers to the holistic description of a group, a community, or a culture. This can take different formats: a book-length monograph, an academic journal article, an audio-visual documentary, or a podcast, to name some examples. The verb denotes the 'doing' of ethnographic fieldwork, and this traditionally involved long-term immersion in the community under study.

Ethnography is still the methodological hallmark and characteristic feature of anthropology as a discipline, but, in recent decades, ethnographic fieldwork has become common in different social science disciplines, such as marketing, journalism, higher education, health research, and clinical education. It is also increasingly undertaken outside academia,

Starting Research in Clinical Education, First Edition. Edited by Eliot L. Rees, Alison Ledger, and Kim A. Walker.
© 2024 The Association for the Study of Medical Education (ASME). Published 2024 by John Wiley & Sons Ltd.
Companion website: www.wiley.com/go/clinicaleducation

in civil society, non-governmental organisations, and the private sector [1, 2].

Why do ethnographic fieldwork?

The basis of ethnographic fieldwork is direct and sustained contact with people as they go about their daily lives. Because of the ethnographer's level of familiarity with people and their lives – or key aspects of it such as professional activities or educational practices – ethnographic fieldwork produces rich, detailed accounts of experience (see Box 16.1). It offers a perspective that many other methods simply cannot provide.

Ethnography is particularly well-suited to exploring the mundane – the ordinary, seemingly unimportant everyday occurrences – that structures people's (working) lives, education, training, and professional engagements. There is, for instance, a long tradition of conducting ethnographic fieldwork in clinical settings [4]. It can often be difficult for study participants to answer questions about their clinical education work when directly asked. The behaviour of most people is so embedded in their day-to-day experience that they lack active awareness of and reflection on it [5]. Because of this, it can be difficult for people to describe their experiences during conventional interviews or focus groups. Ethnographic fieldwork, therefore, is incredibly useful at exploring these phenomena in depth in a way that other methods cannot.

BOX 16.1   Example of ethnographic writing

The first time I interviewed Andrena was in the main lobby of a large urban hospital. A cavernous space. Strangely dark, even formidable. Later, I could see that the gloom had its comforts. A good place for quietly crying, or for staring into nothing. High ceilings, clusters of permanently fixed plastic chairs lined up in rows of three or four, or set together in L shapes. Chairs as neutral as could be, in tones of beige and practical brown, placed neatly on the wall-to-wall grey carpet. Some leafy potted plants (plastic too, but the realistic kind) helped divide the room into smaller waiting areas. The lobby always felt empty, odd for a hospital full of children. At one end, almost unnoticeable, was the receptionist's desk – not the busy centre of this clinical space, as one might expect, but far away, giving the impression of a waiting room with nothing to wait for.

Source: Mattingly [3] / The Regents of the University of California.

Ethnographies of clinical education

There is a long tradition of ethnographic research focusing on clinical education studying medical students. Classic examples include *The Student-Physician* [6] and *Boys in White* [7], an ethnographic account of medical student culture when most medical students in the United States were predominantly male. Paul Atkinson [8] conducted long-term ethnographic fieldwork in clinical education and studied how medical work and medical knowledge are (re)produced. The late clinician-cum-anthropologist Simon Sinclair [9] carried out ethnographic fieldwork in a London medical school, which resulted in *Making Doctors: An Institutional Apprenticeship*. In *Bodies in Formation*, anthropologist Rachel Prentice [10] explored how trainees become physicians, through ethnographic observations in anatomy laboratories and operating rooms. Sophie Bolt [11] and Maria Olejaz [12] both studied body donation, the construction of body donor monuments and the handling of cadavers in dissection labs. Ethnography is now extending into clinical education globally and in a range of health professions. For example, Claire Wendland [13] wrote *A Heart for the Work: Journeys Through an African Medical School*, the first ethnography of medical training in the Global South, and Anna Ruddock [14] conducted ethnographic fieldwork in the All India Institute of Medical Sciences, an iconic institution of Indian healthcare.

Ethnographic fieldwork methods

Ethnography, as a methodological approach, is iterative-inductive, meaning it evolves throughout the duration of the study [15]. This type of research, where the researcher (ethnographer) is embedded in the everyday reality of a particular cultural context, is usually guided by serendipity rather than a hypothesis. This means that there is no magic formula for conducting fieldwork, instead the ethnographer adapts unilaterally to the context of the people they study. As Madden [16] puts it, 'Ethnographers study people in typical circumstances, where people interact with each other in routine or event ritualised ways, but in ways that are typical of that situation'. Ethnographic fieldwork can combine multiple data collection methods, including participant observation, interviews, focus groups, archival research, collecting audiovisual materials, and documents. Crucially, however, it always includes some type of participation in the everyday life of the social world under investigation [17]. The ethnographer collects data in situ, in the community's natural context. This allows them to develop an insider perspective, certainly in comparison to conducting a one-off interview.

Participant observation versus observation

In ethnographic fieldwork, participant observation is the most common data collection method. Here ethnographers typically live in, or as close to the field site as possible, and participate in daily communal life as well as observing interactions in the community. This can help bridge barriers and foster trust between researchers and community members [18], to listen to and engage in conversations to develop an understanding of the culture of the people being observed, within the context of that culture.

Ethnographic interviews are part and parcel of participant observation, occurring as a result of what is observed and happening spontaneously. They can appear more like a conversation, in contrast to the one-off semi-structured interviews conducted in other qualitative research projects (see Chapter 14). Ethnographic interviews allow you to gain a deeper understanding of several aspects of the daily life and interaction just observed or capture an individual's experience in the community [18]. They are often conducted with community members with whom you have already developed a deep rapport and established trust.

Observation (or 'non-participant observation') differs from participant observation. As the terms suggest, the difference lies in the researcher's level of engagement. In participant observation, you take an active role and engage directly with participants: doing what they do, asking questions, experiencing the situation first-hand. Participant observation provides you with an embodied, insider perspective. By contrast, in non-participant observation, you are a fly on the wall, so to speak, and are not directly involved with the activities taking place, nor engage actively with participants. In certain clinical contexts, it is not possible to participate in the community under study. For instance, Higginson et al. [19] conducted an ethnographic study on uncertainty in critical illness, based on non-participation observation in two intensive care units.

Ethnographic fieldwork may include both types of observation depending on the specific fieldwork context, and the balance of these may shift over time. For instance, it is common for ethnographers to first observe, getting to know a particular group and setting, before fully engaging [20]. Generally, however, some amount of participant observation is central to 'doing' ethnography.

Planning an ethnographic study

If you choose ethnography as your research methodology, it is important to think through the practical aspects. This section introduces key considerations.

Choosing from types of ethnography

Anthropologists usually conduct long-term ethnographic fieldwork in one, or multiple, field site(s) through in-depth and sustained immersion in specific settings. Outside of anthropology, however, the model has been adapted to reflect the realities and constraints of other disciplines. Shorter rounds of ethnographic fieldwork are now seen as an effective way of engaging with the community under study without the caveat of long-term fieldwork. An overview of the different types of ethnographies, along with a brief description of each, is provided in Table 16.1. Considerations on which type to choose include the amount of time spent in the field, the number of researchers involved, and the types of data collection methods used.

This overview is not exhaustive and while it does not include online ethnographic work like netnography or cyber ethnography which are conducted in virtual spaces [35–37], it represents the most used terms. It is important to be aware of the different forms ethnographies can take and to be cognisant of the different terms under which these are known. From this table, it is evident that these categories lack bounded distinctions and often overlap with one another on several key characteristics. Furthermore, the home discipline of the researcher(s) may also influence which type of ethnography is used. For instance, health researchers more often conduct variations of rapid or focused ethnographies, while those in organisational studies and education research may use a variation of case studies. Finally, and perhaps most important to note is that adopting a shorter variation of ethnography does not mean conducting a traditional ethnography in a shorter time frame. Rather, it often requires a narrower focus of inquiry and more background and preparatory research before commencing fieldwork.

Choosing a field site

It is important to select an appropriate field site in which to conduct your fieldwork. This will depend on the topic of inquiry and be influenced by the time available to complete research. As previously explained, conventional ethnographies require long-term fieldwork immersion. In this case, it may be appropriate to choose a larger field site, such as a city, healthcare region, or country, or it may

Table 16.1 Types of ethnographic research

Type	Key features
Rapid ethnography [21–23]	• Ethnographic research (participant observation, semi-structured interviews, and document analysis) carried out over a short or intensive period • Captures relevant social, cultural, and behavioural information • Data collected from multiple sources • More than one field researcher to save time
Focused ethnography [24, 25]	• Short-term, intense field visits • Data collection more focused on a specific area of inquiry • Centres around communicative activities • Often carried out by a lone researcher
Quick ethnography [26, 27]	• High-quality ethnographic research collected and analysed in a short period (usually less than 90 days) • Lone researcher collects the data
Short-term ethnography [28]	• Rich ethnographic research carried out in a short period of intensive fieldwork • Research methods are adapted • Outline of what constitutes the field explicitly marked • Data often collected by a lone researcher
Micro-ethnography [29–31]	• Largely used by linguists and those interested in social interactions • Studies microscopic everyday activities and interactions in a highly specific, 'micro' culture (i.e. individual classrooms) • Often uses audio-visual records, to focus on what people do in real time
Ethnography-informed case study [32, 33]	• Combines case studies with ethnography • Uses ethnographic methods to examine sociocultural phenomena • Generally takes place over a longer time scale, similar to traditional ethnographies
Mini-ethnographic case study [34]	• An ethnographic approach that is confined within a case study protocol • Bound in a particular time and place, making the duration shorter than a traditional ethnography • Designed for those with limited time and finances

be feasible to work across multiple clinical and healthcare sites. If working to a shorter time frame, however, it is better to narrow the geographical focus. For instance, the field site may be a particular hospital, community setting, university, or office.

Remember, field sites need to be suited to the research topic. Ensure that you plan accordingly and have obtained appropriate permissions to conduct the research, particularly if working with an organisation (see Chapter 7). Organisations can often act as gatekeepers to participants you wish to include in your study, and they can greatly facilitate or hinder the research process. This last point is particularly important when time is a constraint.

Setting realistic expectations is paramount in choosing a field site, as what you can achieve is closely linked with time available for research. It is not possible to conduct ethnographic research in only a few days. It may take time to identify suitable informants and building rapport with them is crucial. When choosing a field site, select a location where you can maximise your time interacting and experiencing the culture. As with other qualitative research approaches, it is best to start analysis before data collection is complete, to ensure an iterative process of collecting and analysing data.

Choosing participants and building rapport

A final key aspect in planning an ethnographic study lies in identifying participants and building rapport with them. In anthropology, participants are often referred to as informants or interlocuters. They are often selected based on their knowledge, experience, and skill set. Some study participants will become the ethnographer's key informants [15]. As an ethnographer, you build relationships with your key informants who will introduce you to others. Relationships with key informants become increasingly informal as the relationship strengthens and rapport is built.

Building rapport should be one of your first priorities. This is marked by confidence and trust – trust that what community members are saying is true, and trust that the researcher will do no harm to the study participants [38]. To build this rapport, it is important to focus on open communication. You should be honest with your informants about the purpose of your research. Researchers often openly share thoughts and interpretations of the research data with informants in order to gain their feedback and involve them in the process. The length of time it takes to build rapport is dependent on your research topic, your background and experience, and will vary from informant to informant. If you are known to the study participants, then a relationship may already be established. If you are an outsider entering into a community, it could take considerably more time and effort. Cultural customs, personal interaction styles or preferences, and language styles all influence rapport building [39]. However, it is critical to work at building rapport, as it is through relationships that one is able to collect rich ethnographic data.

Conducting ethnographic fieldwork

Recording fieldnotes

Fieldnotes are central to ethnographic fieldwork. These are often recorded in a field diary, a journal you keep in the field, which contains detailed descriptions of your conversations, impressions, and observations [40]. These descriptions will be used later to write the ethnography. A key point to consider is that detailed, vibrant fieldnotes provide a foundation for detailed, vibrant ethnographies [41].

Fieldnotes may be kept in a variety of formats, depending on the research setting. They can be in notebooks, on scraps of paper, typed on a computer, recorded as audio, or a mix of all of these. Fieldnotes serve as a way to capture initial reactions and to ensure that information is not lost or forgotten. Box 16.2 contains some strategies for recording fieldnotes.

Using audio/visual materials

Ethnographic researchers will often draw on other qualitative data collection methods. This triangulation provides a richer, more nuanced understanding of the social phenomena under investigation. Audio/visual materials may provide a rich source of information to understand the cultural setting. These can be music, film, radio, television, photography, art, etc. Visual ethnography is a branch of ethnography that focuses on images, primarily photographs or videos, and how they form an integral part of experience and knowing [42].

BOX 16.2   Strategies for recording ethnographic fieldnotes

- Make diagrams.
- Write while travelling to/from your field site.
- Note what you see/hear/smell/taste/touch/feel.
- Label everything, i.e. date, time, where, who, etc.
- Avoid being a 'strange' stranger. Be present with your informants rather than writing all of the time.
- Build in writing time whenever possible. Type up your thoughts so you can later search for key terms.

Collecting documents

Ethnographers often work with existing documents. These consist of data that already exist and were generated for another purpose. This data is referred to as secondary data and may consist of annual reports, committee reports, emails, letters, notes, postcards, books, journals, or newspapers. These types of data are useful for three main reasons. First, they are often readily available and contain large amounts of information; second, they are socially constructed, meaning they can reveal much about the context outside of the document; and third, researchers can establish comparisons across time and space or establish what is already 'known' [43]. It is important, however, to be aware that documents present merely a 'snapshot' of a particular context.

Analysing and writing up ethnographic research

Fieldnotes from participant observation and non-participant observation should be approached in a systematic way. Both written and typed notes should be appropriately analysed through coding the dataset, creating sub-themes which can then be grouped to create overarching themes. This can be done manually or with specialist software such as QSR NVivo [44]. Further detail on analytic methods can be found in Chapters 18 and 19.

The fieldwork that a researcher engages in is only validated through the reports that result from it [45]. Ethnographies represent interpretations of informants and their lives [46]. When writing an ethnography, it is common practice to write from your personal standpoint and use the first person 'I' throughout. Fook [47] explains that ethnographic writing requires 'an ability to locate yourself in the picture, to understand, and factor in, how what you see is influenced by your own way of seeing, and how your very presence and act of research influences the situation in which you are researching'.

It can also be helpful to think of your informants as characters: describe them in more than merely physical and emotional terms, instead focusing on their actions [41]. Situate these characters in a time and place. For ethnographic texts to draw in readers, it is important that they contain rich details about people, places, and events [41].

Writing well is a key component of this process. One way to write well is to read more, especially other ethnographies [48]. Ethnographers are writers, and the best way to cultivate a storytelling voice is to read examples of how others do it.

Special considerations

Reflexivity as an ethnographer

Reflexivity is crucial for conducting social research, particularly ethnography. Reflexivity refers to a researcher's self-conscious awareness of their position in the research process [49] (see Chapter 3). Your social class, ethnicity, gender, professional background, and educational attainment all influence how others perceive and interact with you as an ethnographer and vice versa. Awareness of your position is important, as it will shape the type of data collected, received, perceived, attended to during analysis, and ultimately written about in the ethnography.

A researcher has three main types of positions upon which they need to reflect [50]. The first of these are fixed positions and include many of the characteristics mentioned above. Your personal context – such as age, gender, class, nationality, education, and ethnicity – are things which do not and will not change during the research process. This does not mean, however, that they should be accepted without being questioned. A good ethnographer considers how these personal circumstances influence data collection.

The two other positions are subjective and textual positions [50]. Subjective positions include your life story and experiences, for example whether you grew up in a rural or urban setting. These experiences are likely to shape your interpretations. Textual positions refer to the use of language and how the voice you create in your writing reveals your level of reflexive practice. Reflexivity is an active, ongoing process that is embedded throughout the research process, from collecting and analysing data to disseminating your findings.

Ethics and informed consent

All projects require appropriate ethical considerations. This almost always includes applying for institutional ethics approval, from an academic and/or healthcare board. Protecting informants' confidentiality and privacy is paramount. Obtaining informed consent is central to this.

While ethical considerations were introduced in Chapter 7, it is important to consider the particularities surrounding ethics and informed consent in an ethnographic setting. Since you are immersed in a particular place and interact frequently with the same people, informed consent takes a different form than in other methodologies. It is simply not practical to seek formal consent before each interaction with

an informant. While it is important that informants fully understand your research and how you will collect data before you begin, specific codes of ethics have been established for ethnographers. The American Anthropological Association (AAA) Code of Ethics recognises a form of 'rolling consent'. Because informed consent can be a dynamic and continuous process, it should continue via dialogue and negotiation with informants [51, 52]. This means periodically reminding participants of the study and confirming they still consent to participate by interacting with you.

Consent obtained during observation will take different forms depending on where the observation takes place. If you are observing public settings, then it is not appropriate nor even feasible to ask consent of everyone involved beforehand. Observing public interactions and noting details in your fieldnotes can be an acceptable practice. If, however, you are observing a specific group of people in a particular setting (such as a hospital, classroom, or primary care practice) then you will need consent not only of the institution but of those who will be observed.

Participant burden

When conducting an ethnography in the form of participant observation, it is important to avoid burdening a participant excessively. It may be that participating in your research requires more time and effort than prospective informants are able to give. Some researchers, on the other hand, have found that participants welcomed the opportunity to be involved [53]. The presence of an ethnographer in a community can be both an asset and a burden for the research participants [54]. Because of this, you should be constantly assessing the potential burden of your presence and adhere to what has been coined the 'hierarchy of responsibility' in which the rights, safety, and comfort of research participants are paramount [54].

Challenges of ethnography

The main challenges in conducting ethnographic research stem from its advantages. The time required can be prohibitive for many. The subjective, reflexive nature of ethnography and lack of a testable hypothesis can also leave those new to the method quite uneasy or unsure of the process. Depending on the context, it may be difficult to gain consent from an organisation to conduct an ethnography (particularly in busy environments or if sensitive information is likely to be revealed) and building rapport may be tricky, especially if there exists a large difference in terms of culturally appropriate ways of interacting.

A major challenge comes from the data that is produced through this approach. While it contains detailed information about a particular setting, it cannot be definitively presented as representative [20]. It is entirely possible that findings may hold true in whole or part for other situations, but that is for others to determine conclusively [55].

A further area to consider stems from how familiar the researcher already is with their place of study and potential participants (Box 16.3). Whilst familiarity may facilitate rapport building and make it easier for you to navigate the field site, conducting fieldwork in a familiar environment also poses particular challenges. The setting and participants may be too 'close', leading you to miss or dismiss important observations. Furthermore, though it might make building rapport very easy, participants may see the researcher as embedded in that environment, making them reluctant to share certain information for fear of others finding out. Both of these situations – conducting ethnography in a familiar or unfamiliar environment – are completely valid ways of doing ethnographic research. However, depending on the context, it is important to think through the issues that might arise in either situation.

Summary

It is the immersion in a particular social group, engaging in social activities for the purpose of research, that defines ethnography [45]. It is a fluid, flexible, reflexive process which begins with a broad

---

BOX 16.3   An example of ethnographic research in clinical education

Lisa Dikomitis (co-author) conducted ethnographic research in a medical school in the United Kingdom. The research topic centred on how one of the core components of a medical school – behavioural and social science (BSS) content – was perceived and understood by undergraduate medical students. This research included aspects of a traditional ethnography combined with other qualitative research methods. She chose to conduct participant information in a place that was very familiar to her – the medical school where she was teaching – because she wanted to gain insights into how medical students engaged with BSS, a core component of the undergraduate medical curriculum.

She conducted long-term ethnographic fieldwork in the medical school over a two-year period [56]. Participant observation was undertaken in problem-based learning (PBL) sessions, during clinical and community placements, in a variety of lectures, and during assessments. As Dikomitis was embedded in the medical school herself as a lecturer, she also conducted participant observation in her own classroom. To gain an insider student perspective, however, she engaged with students outside of classroom settings as well. For example, she conducted fieldwork during office hours, at local conferences, at non-mandatory educational events, and during extracurricular activities the medical students organised, such as a debate evening and charity events. She connected with several key informants and built deeper relationships with them through email, text messages, and catch-up meetings. It was also important to capture views from students outside her own teaching sessions. Engaging with medical students in such activities allowed her to carefully consider her position as both an educator and an ethnographer. Dikomitis conducted ethnographic interviews and semi-structured interviews with medical students she was not teaching.

Participant observation formed the first part of data collection. This allowed Dikomitis to familiarise herself with the environment and to build relationships with informants. The insights gained from this cultural immersion and these conversations provided guidance and structure when introducing later methods, particularly focus group discussions and interview questions. This was possible because she began analysing her fieldnotes early on and began constructing early themes from the data.

To supplement her fieldnotes from participant observation, Dikomitis included additional methods to gain an even deeper perspective on student perceptions. For instance, she asked students on a specific module to complete critical incident questionnaires after each session. For another course, students wrote a reflective essay at the beginning and end of a short intensive module. Dikomitis also conducted 1 focus group and a total of 11 individual semi-structured interviews. These supplementary methods enabled comparison between the insights gained from different sources and helped Dikomitis to consolidate the story she wrote in her ethnographic article [57].

topic and guiding questions rather than with a concrete hypothesis to be tested [58]. The iterative nature of ethnography means that as data is collected and patterns constructed, the focus of the study adapts accordingly. As the researcher is the primary 'tool' of data collection, they must be reflexive on how their own positionality, including both fixed and subjective characteristics, may have influenced the research process.

Ethnography helps us answer 'how' questions by viewing phenomena through the lens of those living in particular cultures. In this way, we can see the knowledge and meaning blueprints that underpin social interactions in particular settings [55]. This research methodology has underpinned much research in health, education, and beyond. It can be adapted to suit a particular researcher's needs in terms of time, resources, and research interest and when done well, offers rich and nuanced accounts of taken for granted cultures and practices.

Top tips

- Choose a topic and field site based on the time you have available for research.
- Spend time building relationships with gatekeepers and informants.
- Record rich and thorough fieldnotes. These provide the foundation for rich and detailed ethnographies.
- Read ethnographies as examples to cultivate your own storytelling voice. It may help to think of your informants as characters.

Common pitfalls

- Getting confused by the various terminology used to describe different types of ethnography. Look to your own discipline for the terminology used most consistently.
- Attempting to undertake a traditional ethnography in a shorter time frame. If your time is tight, you will need to narrow your focus.
- Knowing the community you are studying too well. If you are already an insider, implement reflexive strategies to ensure you do not miss important observations about the culture.

Ethical issues

- It is not possible to record formal consent for every fieldwork encounter in advance. Instead, reinforce information about your study at key time points and continue to confirm participants' consent to participate.
- Different field sites have different informed consent requirements. You may not require permissions to observe in public settings, but always seek organisational and individual permissions when observing specific groups in healthcare and education settings.
- Monitor the burden of your ethnography on informants and revise your plans if their rights, safety, or comfort is compromised.

References

1 Pelto, P.J. (2013). *Applied Ethnography: Guidelines for Field Research*. Routledge.
2 Ladner, S. (2014). *Practical Ethnography: A Guide to Doing Ethnography in the Private Sector*. Routledge.
3 Mattingly, C. (2010). *The Paradox of Hope*. University of California Press.
4 Long, D., Hunter, C., and van der Geest, S. (2008). When the field is a ward or a clinic: hospital ethnography. *Anthropology & Medicine* 15 (2): 71–78.
5 Blommaert, J. and Jie, D. (2010). *Ethnographic Fieldwork: A Beginner's Guide*. Bristol: Multilingual Matters.
6 Merton, R.K., Reader, G., and Kendall, P.L. (1957). *The Student-Physician: Introductory Studies in the Sociology of Medical Education*. Harvard University Press.
7 Becker, H.S. (ed.) (1961). *Boys in White: Student Culture in Medical School*. Transaction Publishers.
8 Atkinson, P. (1997). *The Clinical Experience: The Construction and Reconstruction of Medical Reality*. Routledge.
9 Sinclair, S. (2020). *Making Doctors: An Institutional Apprenticeship*. Routledge.
10 Prentice, R. (2013). *Bodies in Formation: An Ethnography of Anatomy and Surgery Education*. Duke University Press.
11 Bolt, S. (2012). Dead bodies matter: gift giving and the unveiling of body donor monuments in the Netherlands. *Medical Anthropology Quarterly* 26 (4): 613–634.
12 Olejaz, M. (2017). When the dead teach: exploring the postvital life of cadavers in Danish dissection labs. *Medicine Anthropology Theory* 4 (4): 125–149.
13 Wendland, C.L. (2010). *A Heart for the Work: Journeys Through an African Medical School*. University of Chicago Press.

14 Ruddock, A. (2021). *Special Treatment: Student Doctors at the All India Institute of Medical Sciences*. Stanford University Press.

15 O'Reilly, K. (2009). *Key Concepts in Ethnography*, Sage Key Concepts. London: SAGE Publications.

16 Madden, R. (2010). *Being Ethnographic: A Guide to the Theory and Practice of Ethnography*. SAGE Publications.

17 Atkinson, P. (2015). *For Ethnography*. London: SAGE Publications.

18 Munz, E. (2017). Ethnographic interview. In: *The SAGE Encyclopedia of Communication Research Methods* (ed. M. Allen), 454–457. SAGE Publications.

19 Higginson, I.J., Rumble, C., Shipman, C. et al. (2015). The value of uncertainty in critical illness? An ethnographic study of patterns and conflicts in care and decision-making trajectories. *BMC Anesthesiology* 16 (1): 1–11.

20 Strudwick, R.M. (2021). *The Ethnographic Radiographer*. Singapore: Palgrave Macmillan.

21 Ackerman, S.L., Sarkar, U., Tieu, L. et al. (2017). Meaningful use in the safety net: a rapid ethnography of patient portal implementation at five community health centers in California. *Journal of the American Medical Informatics Association* 24: 903–912.

22 McElroy, T., Konde-Lule, J., Neema, S. et al. (2007). Understanding the barriers to clubfoot treatment adherence in Uganda: a rapid ethnographic study. *Disability and Rehabilitation* 29 (11–12): 845–855.

23 Vindrola-Padros, C. and Vindrola-Padros, B. (2018). Quick and dirty? A systematic review of the use of rapid ethnographies in healthcare organisation and delivery. *BMJ Quality & Safety* 27 (4): 321–330.

24 Knoblauch, H. (2005). Focused ethnography. *Forum Qualitative Social Research* 6: 3.

25 White, K.L. (2009). Meztizaje and remembering in Afro-Mexican communities of the Costa Chica: implications for archival education in Mexico. *Archival Science* 9: 43–55.

26 Mullaney, T., Pettersson, H., Nyholm, T., and Stolterman, E. (2012). Thinking beyond the cure: a case for human-centered design in cancer care. *International Journal of Design* 6 (3): 27–39.

27 Handwerker, P. (2001). *Quick Ethnography: A Guide to Rapid Multi-Method Research*. Lanham, MD: AltaMira Press.

28 Pink, S. and Morgan, J. (2013). Short-term ethnography: intense routes to knowing. *Symbolic Interaction* 36 (3): 351–361.

29 Leeds-Hurwitz, W. (2005). Ethnography. In: *Handbook of Language and Social Interaction* (ed. K.L. Fitch and R.E. Sanders), 327–353. Psychology Press.

30 Streeck, J. and Mehus, S. (2005). Microethnography: the study of practices. In: *Handbook of Language and Social Interaction* (ed. K.L. Fitch and R.E. Sanders), 381–404. Psychology Press.

31 Garcez, P.M. (2017). Microethnography in the classroom. In: *Research Methods in Language and Education* (ed. K.A. King, Y.-J. Lai, and S. May), 435–447. Cham, Switzerland: Springer International Publishing.

32 Rian, S.Ó. (2009). Extending the ethnographic case study. In: *The SAGE Handbook of Case-Based Methods* (ed. D. Byrne and C.C. Ragin), 289–306. Thousand Oaks, CA: SAGE Publications.

33 Schwandt, T.A. and Gates, E.F. (2018). Case study methodology. In: *The SAGE Handbook of Qualitative Research*, 5e (ed. N.K. Dezin and Y.S. Lincoln), 341–358. Thousand Oaks, CA: SAGE Publications.

34 Fusch, P.I., Fusch, G.E., and Ness, L.R. (2017). How to conduct a mini-ethnographic case study: a guide for novice researchers. *The Qualitative Report* 22 (3): 923–942.

35 Bowler, G.M. Jr. (2010). Netnography: a method specifically designed to study cultures and communities online. *The Qualitative Report* 15 (5): 1270–1275.

36 Hallett, R.E. and Barber, K. (2014). Ethnographic research in a cyber era. *Journal of Contemporary Ethnography* 43 (3): 306–330.

37 Kozinets, R. (2009). *Netnography: Doing Ethnographic Research Online*. SAGE Publications.

38 Glesne, C. (1989). Rapport and friendship in ethnographic research. *International Journal of Qualitative Studies in Education* 2 (1): 45–54.

39 Zaman, S. (2008). Native among the natives: physician anthropologist doing hospital ethnography at home. *Journal of Contemporary Ethnography* 37 (2): 135–154.

40 Picken, F.E. (2013). Ethnography. In: *Social Research Methods* (ed. M. Walter), 337–350. Australia: Oxford University Press.

41 Ghodsee, K. (2016). *From Notes to Narrative: Writing Ethnographies That Everyone Can Read*. University of Chicago Press.

42 Pink, S. (2020). *Doing Visual Ethnography*. SAGE Publications.

43 Macdonald, K. (2008). Using documents. In: *Researching Social Life* (ed. N. Gilbert). SAGE Publications.

44 QSR International Pty Ltd (2018). NVivo (version 12). https://www.qsrinternational.com/nvivo-qualitative-data-analysis-software/home (accessed 9 May 2023).

45 Wolcott, H.F. (2004). The ethnographic autobiography. *AutoBiography* 12 (2): 93–106.

46 Geertz, C. (1973). *The Interpretation of Cultures*. New York, NY: Basic Books.

47 Fook, J. (1999). Reflexivity as method, annual review of health. *Social Science* 9 (1): 11–20.

48 Behar, R. (2020). Read more, write less. In: *Writing Anthropology: Essays on Craft and Commitment* (ed. C. McGranahan), 47–53. Duke University Press.

49 Willis, K. (2013). Analysing qualitative data. In: *Social Research Methods* (ed. M. Walter), 315–336. Oxford: Oxford University Press.

50 Goodall, H.L. Jr. (2000). *Writing the New Ethnography*. AltaMira Press.

51 American Anthropological Association (2012). Principles of professional responsibility. http://ethics.americananthro. org/category/statement/ (accessed 9 May 2023).

52 American Anthropological Association (2009). Code of ethics. https://www.americananthro.org/Participate AndAdvocate/Content.aspx?ItemNumber=1656 (accessed 27 May 2023).

53 Iphofen, R. (2013). *Research Ethics in Ethnography/ Anthropology*. European Commission. https://ec. europa.eu/research/participants/data/ref/h2020/ other/hi/ethics-guide-ethnog-anthrop_en.pdf

54 Madden, R. (2017). *Being Ethnographic: A Guide to the Theory and Practice of Ethnography*. London: SAGE Publications.

55 Herbert, S. (2000). For ethnography. *Progress in Human Geography* 24 (4): 550–568.

56 Dikomitis, L., Wenning, B., Ghobrial, A., and Adams, K.M. (2022). Embedding behavioural and social sciences across the medical curriculum: (auto) ethnographic insights from medical schools in the United Kingdom. *Societies* 12 (4): 101.

57 Dikomitis, L. (2021). How medical students in the United Kingdom think: about anthropology, for example. In: *Anthropology in Medical Education* (ed. I. Martinez and D.W. Wiedman), 91–113. Cham: Springer.

58 O'Reilly, K. (2005). *Ethnographic Methods*. London: Routledge.

17 Narrative research: from the general to the particular

Kathleen E. Leedham-Green, Alexandra Wright, and Giskin Day

Learning objectives

By the end of this chapter, you should be able to:
- Explain what is meant by 'narrative' in clinical education research.
- Articulate philosophical and ethical arguments for and against using narratives as data.
- Compare different ways of gathering, curating, analysing, and presenting narratives.

- Describe core features of plot-based, linguistic, functional, and sociological narrative analysis.
- Reflect on how narratives have shaped your own educational practice and leverage their strengths to inform and transform the practice of others.

Introduction

This chapter introduces a family of methods with stories at their heart. Qualitative researchers often come across stories as this is the way people communicate, but sometimes the meaning and power of these stories are lost through reductive analytic processes. Narrative research is a means of exploring, interpreting, and/or presenting stories as a whole. Doing so can be a powerful way of achieving impact through clinical education research. This chapter explains what is meant by 'narrative', introduces the philosophical underpinnings of narrative research, and offers strategies for gathering, choosing, analysing, and presenting narratives. We begin with our own stories of becoming narrative researchers (Box 17.1).

What is a narrative and narrative research?

The term narrative can be used to denote a wide variety of linguistic expressions, from everyday conversations to full biographies of people's lives. Chase [2] defines a personal narrative as a distinct form of communication:

> . . .it is meaning making through the shaping of experience; a way of understanding one's own or others' actions; of organizing events, objects, feelings or thoughts in relation to each other; of connecting and seeing the consequences of actions, events, feelings, or thoughts over time (in the past, present, and/or future).

In everyday life, we all use stories to organise, make sense of, and evaluate our experiences; to express the person we want to be; to consider antecedents, modulating factors, and consequences; and to persuade, shock, or inspire others. Similarly, we can use stories in clinical education research to make sense of teacher, learner, and patient experiences, identities, and the events that led to a particular outcome, such as an adverse clinical event.

Narrative research is an umbrella term, encompassing both research that treats stories as data (e.g. diary entries), and research in which the analysis phase entails the creation of stories, perhaps recounting an event from multiple perspectives. There are also a wide range of analytic approaches and ways of presenting narratives, which depend on factors such as the type of data collected and the research question.

In this chapter, we use narrative to refer to any kind of story, small or big, and narrative research to refer to any research that collects narratives as data, or creates narratives from other forms of data (e.g. semi-structured interviews, published texts) during the analysis phase.

Starting Research in Clinical Education, First Edition. Edited by Eliot L. Rees, Alison Ledger, and Kim A. Walker.
© 2024 The Association for the Study of Medical Education (ASME). Published 2024 by John Wiley & Sons Ltd.
Companion website: www.wiley.com/go/clinicaleducation

BOX 17.1   Becoming a narrative researcher

Kathleen's story

I was a junior teaching fellow and had inherited an undergraduate course element called 'opportunistic health promotion in primary care'. This included an assignment inviting medical students to recount and reflect on a consultation they had either conducted or observed where obesity was discussed. Over the course of three years, I read more than a thousand of these accounts, and I received ethical approval to analyse them for research purposes. Some of the stories were so powerful, they transformed the way I taught my course. I could see what my students were doing with their learning. I could also see their unmet needs and vicariously how patients were responding. I read vivid accounts of confrontations, collaboration, consternation, and complexity, as well as truly transformative personalised care. I developed insights into my students' thinking through their reflections as well as the language they used. Initially, I published a thematic analysis of these accounts [1]. The themes were useful as an abstraction of the content but did not do justice to the richness and informational power of the underlying stories.

This led me to reflect on how and why I had developed my educational programme promoting patient-centred conversations about obesity. Looking back, none of the major changes had been driven by my thematic analysis of the general cohort. They were driven by my emotional and cognitive response to perhaps one or two stories that I had found particularly powerful out of the many I was reading. These stories had grasped me, and I could not put them down until I had done something about them. With this in mind, I decided to explore narrative research within clinical education, so that I could share and distil the essence of how I had constructed my teaching model.

Alex's story

I was introduced to the concept of narrative early in my intercalated BSc in medical humanities. I had always been interested in stories, but there was something about the unique nature of narratives that really intrigued me. My first experience of narrative research was a short assignment which I found engaging and frustrating in equal measure. The knowledge and experiences brewing from the narratives captured me, but I felt limited by the assignment's scope, word count, and short deadline.

For the project component of the course, I explored experiences of loss and grief during the COVID-19 pandemic. The volume and intensity of the topic were daunting. I was worried that an academic approach may not do justice to the humanity of people's experiences. Again, narratives offered me a way in. They were accessible, engaging, and full of the complexities and nuances I sought to explore. They were all unique, rich and detailed, and finally I could engage with narratives on their terms, as living entities with so many insights to offer, and to see what I could understand and voice through my research.

Alex's story continues throughout this chapter.

Philosophy of narrative research

Spector-Mersel [3] has argued that narrative research is not a methodology, but an entire research paradigm with its own beliefs about truth, knowledge, and values. Can stories ever be considered to be 'true'? Does it matter? What forms of useful knowledge do they bring? By paying attention to individual experiences, what values do we bring to our research?

Clinicians are often educated to understand reality and knowledge from a positivist stance, that is, good research can reveal objective 'truths' about real things. You too may have been taught to think of meta-analyses of randomised controlled trials as the highest form of evidence, where results are aggregated across huge cohorts to produce increasingly robust scientific knowledge. Individual or personal stories may have been dismissed as providing 'weak evidence'. However, stories can be clinically powerful because they are situated in specific populations and contexts. Rather than asking relatively shallow 'true or false' questions of thousands of participants, narrative research asks deeper contextualised questions to a smaller number of individuals, often collecting rich detail about situations in chronological order (see Figure 17.1). Analysis and presentation of these stories can promote understanding and challenge us to consider situations from a different perspective.

Why choose narrative research?

Narratives provide immense potential within clinical education research. They can be used to illuminate the clinical learning environment, evolving professional identities, patient perspectives, sociocultural contexts, interprofessional dynamics, how learning is enacted, and the hidden curriculum, to name just a few areas. Health professional students and workers often learn through narratives, exploring clinical cases in depth. Narratives emphasise the

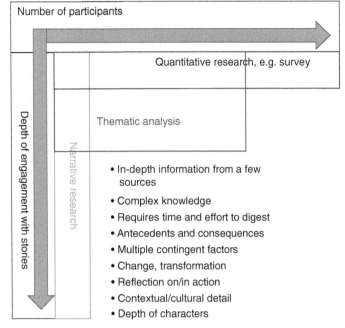

Figure 17.1 What is different about narrative research?

individual, make hidden experiences visible, and can be so powerful they transform perspectives and practices. They are one of the few types of data that include detailed characterisation, providing the reader with what is known as an insider 'emic' perspective on an event. We are invited to identify with the main protagonist, seeing the world through their eyes, and to evaluate occurrences as we would in everyday life. Narrative research can also provide outsiders with insights into hard to access contexts, including things that happen behind closed doors such as discrimination, abuse, grief, sexuality, and bullying. This emphasis on hidden stories aligns some narrative researchers with the values of critical theory and social reform: aiming to improve society by bringing to light suppressed stories and voices. Strengths of narrative research are summarised in Figure 17.2.

Countering critiques of narrative research

As you explore narrative data for the first time, you may be concerned whether stories are true or exaggerated: how can good research be based on subjective data? You may worry that they are muddied by the selective memory of the storyteller and the quality of their expressive skills. There is also the added layer of sense-making by the reader – you may be concerned that you or your audience will misinterpret meanings or project personal subtexts onto what is being described. Greenhalgh [4], one of the foremost proponents of narratives as a data source

in health services research, explained that narratives 'are not true in any simple sense'. Narratives do not offer a fixed truth. They change over time, with variations in memory, perspectives, and the context in which they are being told.

Questions of 'truth' can be countered with two arguments: first, Greenhalgh's concept of *verisimilitude*, where the story contains enough contextual detail and realistic human behaviour to simply resonate as true. Second, does it matter? If the story itself is the unit of study, and it is clearly not factual, that may be of interest. Stories can also contain emotional truths that resonate with our lived experience, despite having fictional characters and contexts. As a clinical education researcher, you may want to research subjectivity. How else could we study deeply personal phenomena such as cultural exclusion if not through narratives of lived experience? Any narrative is carefully crafted – we select what we tell based on the audience, the purpose of telling the story and what we consider is important to say. Narratives are told for a reason and one of your research objectives might be to explore the reasoning of the participant(s).

Doing narrative research

There are numerous possibilities when undertaking narrative research. You can collect data in narrative form, or you can create a narrative from the data

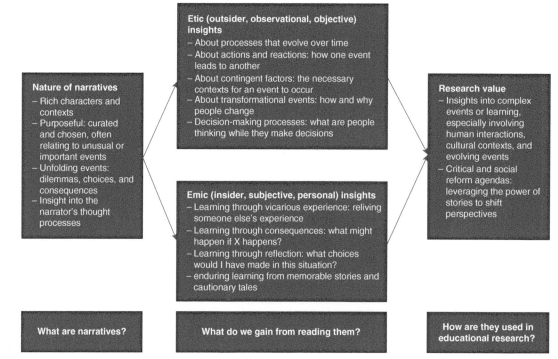

Nature of narratives
– Rich characters and contexts
– Purposeful: curated and chosen, often relating to unusual or important events
– Unfolding events: dilemmas, choices, and consequences
– Insight into the narrator's thought processes

Etic (outsider, observational, objective) insights
– About processes that evolve over time
– About actions and reactions: how one event leads to another
– About contingent factors: the necessary contexts for an event to occur
– About transformational events: how and why people change
– Decision-making processes: what are people thinking while they make decisions

Emic (insider, subjective, personal) insights
– Learning through vicarious experience: reliving someone else's experience
– Learning through consequences: what might happen if X happens?
– Learning through reflection: what choices would I have made in this situation?
– enduring learning from memorable stories and cautionary tales

Research value
– Insights into complex events or learning, especially involving human interactions, cultural contexts, and evolving events
– Critical and social reform agendas: leveraging the power of stories to shift perspectives

What are narratives?

What do we gain from reading them?

How are they used in educational research?

Figure 17.2 Strengths of narrative research.

collected [5]. Equally, there are a variety of options available when selecting an analytical approach and disseminating your findings. Different choices may lead to different ethical considerations. In Box 17.2, Alex explains how this can be a little overwhelming at first.

Though initially overwhelming, most narrative researchers come to value the flexibility of narrative research, delighting in its creativity. To help you in navigating decision-making, we have drawn on the work of McCance et al. [6] to outline five key steps in the narrative research process, which require careful thought (summarised in Figure 17.3).

Gathering narratives

Narratives can be gathered through an individual interview or recording, or pieced together through documentary evidence, such as diaries, blogs, letters, or written observations. When the aim is to collect data in narrative form, you are typically less directive than in other forms of qualitative research. You respect the narrator's own mode of storytelling

---

BOX 17.2   Alex's experiences of doing narrative research

The lack of strict rules in narrative research soon became my concern. Every stage of the process was wrought with questions of theory, methodology, and ethics. Finding the answers to these questions led me to spending hours in the library, making notes from Mishler's, Chase's, and Greenhalgh's works to name a few. The more I read, the less defined everything became, even the very definition of what constituted a narrative. I had no choice but to listen to my own instincts and thoughts, which terrified me. I had always been distanced from research in the past, observing and theorising from 'controlled' experiments. This was very different – I was forming my own questions and answers, purposefully selecting narratives, reading, and interpreting them through my own lens.

I found one of my biggest challenges was learning to trust the narratives and my interpretations. This was very different to having preformed hypotheses to accept or refute. Being a part of the research process was both uncomfortable and a comfort, as it meant that I could acknowledge my own humanity and use it judiciously to hear, learn from, and present insights into another's experience. It meant I could honestly reflect on that entire process, bringing more nuance, depth and, in my opinion, authenticity to the research. The rich, idiosyncratic, and multi-layered nature of these narratives was engaging and offered so much to work with. Their complexities offered deep, and often unexplored, insights and I felt privileged to work with them.

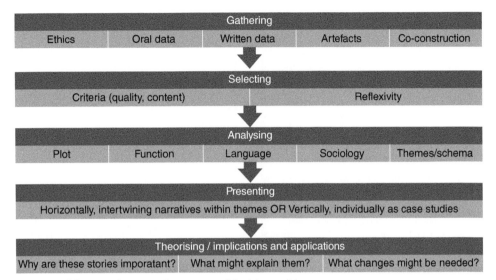

Figure 17.3 Summary of the narrative research process and decision-making.

about a topic and allow them to tell what matters to them on that particular day. For example, you may start with an open invitation to 'tell me the story of X' and allow the narrator to speak with minimal interruption. However, if your aim is to explore multiple interpretations of a specific event, or to co-construct a collaborative narrative, then you might take a more active clarifying and storifying role, adopting the role of a biographer or ethnographer. Regardless of the approach you choose, it is important to consider ethical issues such as ensuring participants cannot be identified and consent has been obtained (see Chapter 7). The risk of identification may be higher if complete narratives are gathered and presented, than when parts of individual stories are combined.

Selecting narratives

As a narrative researcher, you can choose how many stories you analyse and present. You may not present all the stories you have gathered in their entirety. If your focus is on a single person or event, the number of competing or complementary narratives you gather are likely to be relatively small and the selection process simple. If, however, you are adopting a more phenomenological approach, for example, exploring lived experiences of discrimination in surgical education, you might engage with dozens of narratives before you come across a story that serves as an exemplar or communicates a specific sub-phenomenon powerfully. To demonstrate academic rigour at the selection stage, you need to be transparent about your selection processes, engaging reflexively and either trying to mitigate any personal assumptions or agendas, or making

them explicit. Mitigating strategies might include demonstrating your chosen narratives are representative of the larger set, or inclusive of contrasting experiences or narrative styles. You may also attempt to score narratives against criteria. This is complex as some narrative-specific criteria such as rich contextual detail, vivid characterisation, a good 'plot', emotional authenticity, or verisimilitude too involve subjective judgement. We therefore suggest it may be more appropriate to engage in explicit reflection on your own subjectivities. This means the research is clearly situated as an interpretation through the researcher's lens, which should be regarded as a feature rather than a flaw of narrative research.

Analysing narratives

There are few clear accounts of how to systematically analyse narrative data, and there are multiple approaches which differ in their analytic focus. Your analysis can focus on the narrative content, form, or the social/performative function of the stories [7]. Hyvärinen presents a useful summation of trends in narrative analysis and adds auto-ethnography as an emergent form [8]. Questions to consider include to what extent your own subjectivity should be acknowledged as part of the analysis, whether to try to build a general understanding from the data, or to treat each narrative as a unique entity [9]. Mishler [10] proposed there are three main types of narrative analysis: plot-based, linguistic, and functional. While there is often overlap, these forms can serve as a useful starting point when beginning narrative analysis for their flexibility of approach. Other sociological analytic approaches, described

> **BOX 17.3 Alex's experiences of analysis**
>
> After immersing myself in literature of 'how to analyse a narrative', I was quite unsure of where I stood in the research process and, even, how to start. I tried focusing on each method in turn, but always ended up in a tangle as these raw experiences as told did not conform quite so diligently to theoretical models. So I chose to attend to another of Mishler's [10] suggestions: to treat these frameworks as a reference, perhaps a starting point, from which I could take any route which arose from the narratives. I returned to the narratives and began building my interpretation with each reading over several weeks, until the dots began to join together.

by Bury [11] and Plummer [12], may also be useful in studying the complexities of clinical education. Alex's experiences of the analysis phase are presented in Box 17.3 and offered as a worked example on the companion website.

Plot based

Plot-based analyses focus on ordering temporal data and can be useful for conducting retroductive explanatory analyses, for example, exploring what happened and why after a significant event where there were multiple contingent factors. Polkinghorne [5] described an approach in which a story is created from data by arranging the data chronologically and developing a plot. Details may be left out if they are not pertinent to the story or refute the plot. Clandinin and Connelly [13] also reported the constructing of narratives through observation, ethnographic fieldwork, mutual story-telling, and re-storying. A clinical education example might entail selecting parts of interviews and reordering them chronologically, to develop three contrasting stories of the journey through medical school – failing, just about managing, and flourishing.

Linguistic

Riessman's approach to narrative analysis [14] dissects a story 'as told', stanza by stanza, focussing on the way the story is told. This heavily linguistic form of analysis is concerned with the structure of the story, its metaphors, and forms of language. It treats the way the story is told as the unit of inquiry. Freeman [15] also emphasised linguistic interpretation, treating the text as the object of inquiry, exploring the use of language, cultural or social references, inferences and subjective meaning-making, thoughts, and acts. For example, a linguistic analysis of online

chronic pain diaries may explore patients' use of metaphors and what these metaphors may convey to nursing students about the phenomenon of chronic pain and palliation. Alternatively, close analysis of the language used by healthcare professionals when recounting their day-to-day work may give clues to the hidden curriculum or culture in a particular clinical setting.

Functional

As explained earlier, narratives are told for a purpose and an audience. They can be analysed functionally and also be used functionally. Charon [16] explored narratives as a form of healing for the writer and as a way of returning medicine to its humanistic roots. Greenhalgh and Hurwitz [17] have also explored narratives *as* medicine, but also *for* medicine: as tools for teaching and learning. For example, a functional analysis may explore the learning arising from stories about patient safety incidents for multiple parties, including patients, students, interprofessional teams, and institutions.

Sociological

Bury [11] concentrated more on the sociological reasons for why patients tell stories about their experiences, and what can be learnt about people and society from the stories they construct about health and healthcare. Plummer [12] invited us to consider multiple sociological dimensions:

1 The nature of the narrative: what impact does the narrator intend it to have, what points are they attempting to make?
2 The making of the narrative: in what context was the story elicited, and by whom and for what purpose? Are there any power imbalances or inducements to fictionalise the narrative?
3 The consuming of the narrative: who is the intended audience?
4 Narrative strategies: what strategies does the narrator use to coax or persuade?
5 Wider world: how does our sociocultural context and the narrator's position within it influence the story? Are there any unspoken meta-narratives that this story exists within, for example, geopolitical events?

On the companion website, we invite you to try your own sociological analysis of a text, exploring the ways a narrator has constructed their story of interactions and relationships with hospital staff.

Presenting narratives

Next, you need to consider how to present your findings. There is no prescriptive formula for doing this, and the form will depend on the scope and purpose of your research. Some authors adopt a thematic or horizontal approach, intertwining excerpts from each story within common themes. These themes are not groups of content codes, as in some forms of thematic analysis (see Chapter 18), but reflect the higher level meanings that can be constructed from whole narratives [18]. Others adopt a vertical approach where each story is presented as a case study, finishing with overall sense making across all narratives [19]. An increasingly common approach is to present *composite narratives*, combined stories which illustrate shared experiences rather than any one individual's story [20]. This minimises the risk that individuals will be identified, particularly when participants have shared personal stories related to sensitive topics. Composite narratives can also be shared in creative formats, such as comics, infographics, or videos.

Theorising from narrative data

If you have a strong background in post-positivist research, you may be wondering how conclusions can be drawn from the small, purposeful samples who participate in narrative research. The implications of narrative research need not be grand or generalisable, they can be micro-theories that explain local phenomena. Simons [21] argued that paradoxically, in the social sciences, in-depth case studies can be more informative than huge integrative studies that lose contextual and temporal detail. If a narrative is presented in sufficient detail, the reader can construct personally relevant conclusions, knowing their own context. You should also highlight any knowledge you deem to be transferrable and suggest implications and applications for others.

Quality criteria

There are few quality criteria specific to narrative research, however, generic criteria for qualitative studies apply such as trustworthiness, rigour, reflexivity, ethical approach, quality of writing, and relevance [22, 23]. Andrews [24] suggested additional narrative criteria. These include co-construction of meaning between narrator and researcher, attention to whose story is heard and whose might be untold, awareness of how findings are fluid and situated in a specific time and place, and awareness that stories are multi-layered with micro-stories situated within untold but implied overarching macro-stories. Some criteria may be specific to certain types of narrative research. For

example, checking details with participants (*member checking*) may be important if you are concerned about the 'accuracy' of individual accounts, but less relevant if you are clear that the stories created through the narrative research process are an interpretation (Boxes 17.4 and 17.5).

BOX 17.4   How Alex maintained quality

I continuously reflected and noted down any factors that could have skewed my lens (consciously or unconsciously). From my first reading and selection of the narratives, I felt a sense of duty to their authors. I had developed a set of criteria for selecting the narratives, but I still felt a sense of responsibility as I whittled down my choices. Each narrative portrayed authentic, valid, and often heart-wrenching experiences. That sense of duty weighed on me further as I began my analysis. Each narrator had given their permission for me to analyse their narrative, their recounted experience of loss, as part of my research. Just like having a conversation, I did not want to miss the point, misconstrue their writing, or portray any interpretation that could be untrue, unjust, or harmful to them or others. I found it helpful to keep a grounding – in the narratives, in my self-awareness, and in keeping a balance with the rest of my life. Check-ins with my supervisor and course team helped me to stay focused and keep perspective in my research. I analysed the narratives in discrete blocks of time over several weeks. Each time I returned there was more to find, the pages were soon worn with highlights and scribbles. This chance to step back gave opportunities to question and reflect on my interpretations, refining them into coherent and consistent insights grounded in the narratives.

BOX 17.5   Alex concludes her story

Within narrative research, there are infinite possibilities: infinite experiences, narrators, readers, contexts, and so on. Though at times frustrating, chaotic, and challenging, the learning and value I have found with this narrative lens is something I hope to hold onto and cultivate further in future learning, research, and practice. The diversity of experience is what makes this line of inquiry so exciting. It is an iterative process. I can keep attending to narratives; refining my listening ear, reflecting on my interpretations, and discerning new understandings through the most human modality of storytelling.

Summary

This chapter has explored a powerful but underutilised approach to clinical education research: narrative research. Narratives can be written, oral, or constructed from a range of artefacts and are shared for a reason. They can provide unique insights into a wide range of educational topics. They highlight the particular rather than the general, which is their strength. They can also be used to give voice to under-represented groups and reform practices through their lingering impact. Narratives take time to digest and are often presented in small numbers, so they must be chosen carefully and reflectively. They are powerful and memorable so they must also be chosen with ethical care and intent. They can be analysed for their plot, their language, their function, and socio-cultural context. They can be presented horizontally across narratives, picking out specific features or themes, or vertically down each individual narrative followed by an integrative analysis. When disseminated, narratives can foster new understandings and transform learning and practice in meaningful ways especially when using creative methods of dissemination.

Top tips

- There are multiple ways of doing narrative research. Make sure your methods match your purpose.
- Embrace subjectivity. You cannot take yourself out of narrative research. Bring yourself in – write in the first person and make your assumptions visible. Work with colleagues to co-construct meaning and reflect on your own assumptions.
- When gathering, selecting, and analysing narratives, focus on what is important to the narrator. The more meaningful the story, the more powerful the content.
- When presenting narratives, go for quality over quantity. Narratives take time to digest, and only a limited number can be absorbed by the reader within a single article. Do not be afraid to theorise from a single or small number of narratives.
- Enjoy the process: story telling can provide new insights for both the narrator and the researcher!

Common pitfalls

- Losing the power of narratives through overly reductive approaches. If coding narratives, be sure to attend to the sequence of events, characters, context, language, or storyteller's intent.
- Not explaining your methodology and design decisions sufficiently when presenting your research. Audiences may not be familiar with narrative research, so you need to articulate your research philosophy and justify your choices clearly.
- Lack of academic rigour. Address quality criteria at the research design phase and ensure your conclusions are logical based on the data that was analysed.

Ethical issues

- Revolutions have been started and governments, institutions, and politicians brought down by stories. Narratives are powerful, so should be chosen carefully, critically, reflectively, and ethically.
- Avoid using narratives for a purpose that the narrator had or would not reasonably consent to. When recruiting participants, explain how you intend to use the narratives and recontact participants if your plans change.
- Individual stories tend to be identifiable. Consider ways that you can share participants' stories without identifying them if they choose to be anonymous, such as crafting composite narratives.
- When reporting narrative research findings, be transparent about the context-specific nature of narratives and your role in creating and interpreting them. Findings should not be presented as a single, fixed truth.

References

1 Leedham-Green, K.E., Pound, R., and Wylie, A. (2016). Enabling tomorrow's doctors to address obesity in a GP consultation: an action research project. *Education for Primary Care* 27 (6): 455–461.

2 Chase, S.E. (2017). Narrative inquiry: toward theoretical and methodological maturity. In: *The SAGE Handbook of Qualitative Research*, 5e (ed. N.K. Denzin and Y.S. Lincoln), 546–560. SAGE Publications.

3 Spector-Mersel, G. (2010). Narrative research: time for a paradigm. *Narrative Inquiry* 20 (1): 20.

4 Greenhalgh, T. (2016). *Cultural Contexts of Health: The Use of Narrative Research in the Health Sector*. Copenhagen: WHO Regional Office for Europe.

5 Polkinghorne, D. (1995). Narrative configuration in qualitative analysis. *International Journal of Qualitative Studies in Education* 8 (1): 5–23.

6 McCance, T.V., McKenna, H.P., and Boore, J.R.P. (2001). Exploring caring using narrative methodology: an analysis of the approach. *Journal of Advanced Nursing* 33 (3): 350–356.

7 Elliot, J. (2005). Interpreting people's stories: narrative approaches to the analysis of qualitative data. In: *Using Narrative in Social Research*, 35–69. London: SAGE Publications.

8 Hyvärinen, M. (2016). Narrative and sociology. *Narrative Works* 6 (1): 38–62.

9 Andrews, M., Squire, C., and Tamboukou, M. (2013). *Doing Narrative Research*. Los Angeles: SAGE Publications.

10 Mishler, E.G. (1995). Models of narrative analysis: a typology. *Journal of Narrative and Life History* 5 (2): 87–123.

11 Bury, M. (2001). Illness narratives: fact or fiction? *Sociology of Health & Illness* 23 (3): 263–285.

12 Plummer, K. (1995). An invitation to a sociology of stories. In: *Studying Culture: An Introductory Reader* (ed. A. Gray and J. McGuigan), 333–345. London: Arnold.

13 Clandinin, D.J. and Connelly, F.M. (1999). *Narrative Inquiry: Experience and Story in Qualitative Research*. Wiley.

14 Riessman, C.K. (1993). *Narrative Analysis*. Newbury Park, CA; London: Sage Publications.

15 Freeman, M. (2015). Narrative hermeneutics. In: *The Wiley Handbook of Theoretical and Philosophical Psychology* (ed. J. Martin, J. Sugarman, and K.L. Slaney), 234–247. Wiley Blackwell.

16 Charon, R. (2001). Narrative medicine: form, function, and ethics. *Annals of Internal Medicine* 134 (1): 83–87.

17 Greenhalgh, T. and Hurwitz, B. (1998). *Narrative Based Medicine*. Wiley.

18 Price, S.L., McGillis Hall, L., Angus, J.E., and Peter, E. (2013). Choosing nursing as a career: a narrative analysis of millennial nurses' career choice of virtue. *Nursing Inquiry* 20 (4): 305–316.

19 Haydon, G. and Van Der Riet, P. (2014). A narrative inquiry: how do nurses respond to patients' use of humour? *Contemporary Nurse* 46 (2): 197–205.

20 McElhinney, Z. and Kennedy, C. (2022). Enhancing the collective, protecting the personal: the valuable role of composite narratives in medical education research. *Perspectives on Medical Education* 11: 220–227.

21 Simons, H. (1996). The paradox of case study. *Cambridge Journal of Education* 26 (2): 225–240.

22 Cohen, D.J. and Crabtree, B.F. (2008). Evaluative criteria for qualitative research in health care: controversies and recommendations. *The Annals of Family Medicine* 6 (4): 331.

23 Tracy, S.J. (2010). Qualitative quality: eight "big-tent" criteria for excellent qualitative research. *Qualitative Inquiry* 16 (10): 837–851.

24 Andrews, M. (2021). Quality indicators in narrative research. *Qualitative Research in Psychology* 18 (3): 353–368.

18 Approaches to thematic analysis: becoming a knowing researcher

Virginia Braun and Victoria Clarke

Learning objectives

By the end of this chapter, you should be able to:
- Appreciate that thematic analysis is a family of methods.
- Distinguish between codebook approaches and more organic, open, and reflexive approaches to coding data.
- Recognise the difference between topic summaries and shared meaning-based themes.
- Discuss the role of the researcher in thematic analysis, including the active role in reflexive thematic analysis.
- Reflect on and make appropriate conceptual, procedural, and language choices for different thematic analysis approaches.

Introduction

Thematic analysis is a common choice for analysing qualitative data, involving processes of coding and theme development to generate understanding around patterned meaning. It is typically understood as an analytic *method* (a theoretically flexible tool or technique for analysis), rather than an analytic methodology, such as discourse analysis, which comes with an inbuilt theoretical framework (see [1]). However, these apparently straightforward descriptions conceal complexity. Thematic analysis is not a method (singular) so much as a group of methods, which share some aspects, but can diverge significantly in procedure and philosophy. Certain iterations of thematic analysis are aligned with different research values or 'paradigms' (the belief systems that shape your research design decisions, see Chapter 3). Understanding these paradigmatic differences is crucial for making appropriate decisions in research using thematic analysis. This chapter aims to explain different approaches for clinical education researchers, who are likely to encounter very different examples and explanations of thematic analysis across disciplines and publications. This chapter offers a framework for understanding these differences so that you can make informed decisions in your own projects and achieve alignment between your stated paradigm and analytic methods. For further practical guidance, please see our book [1].

The spectrum of thematic analysis approaches

Thematic analysis approaches exist on a spectrum from the 'scientifically descriptive' to the 'artfully interpretive' [2], or positivist to non-positivist. The ways paradigms are referred to vary by discipline and geographic location [3, 4]. We have chosen to use broad terms in this chapter rather than the terms used in Chapter 3. Another useful way to map the thematic analysis spectrum is a small q-Big Q qualitative differentiation [5]. Big Q captures the use of qualitative data and analytic techniques within a qualitative paradigm or values framework; small q refers to a narrower orientation to qualitative research, focused on data and technique. There is no one set of values that all Big Q researchers agree on, but most would reject the possibility of objective knowledge, view qualitative research as inherently subjective, and meaning and truth as contextually situated, partial and multiple [6]. In small q, qualitative research tends to default to the disciplinary dominant values framework – usually some version of positivism (a conceptual framework that – depending on the version – values producing or striving to produce objective knowledge about an-assumed-to-be-independent-of-human-practices reality; it often now appears in a modified form referred to as post-positivism, see Chapter 3). Whether your qualitative approach is Big Q or small q, non-positivist or post-positivist, there is an

---

Starting Research in Clinical Education, First Edition. Edited by Eliot L. Rees, Alison Ledger, and Kim A. Walker.
© 2024 The Association for the Study of Medical Education (ASME). Published 2024 by John Wiley & Sons Ltd.
Companion website: www.wiley.com/go/clinicaleducation

aligned thematic analysis approach. This chapter gives you the tools to figure out which approaches do and do not fit with your research paradigm and values, and (thus) how to do conceptually coherent thematic analysis.

What do thematic analysis methods share? Typically, they encompass processes of coding and theme development, with the end result a set of themes capturing important meanings in the data. They allow you to engage more inductively or deductively with the data, basing your analytic interpretations very strongly in the data content (inductive) or in ideas somewhat external to the dataset, such as ideas developed through other scholarly engagement, or theoretical constructs (a more deductive approach). They also offer the possibility for you to explore and code meaning in more semantic (manifest, explicit) or more latent (hidden, implicit) ways (see [1]). Where thematic analysis methods diverge is in the conceptualisation of core constructs, and the process of coding and theme development – and the role of the researcher in this. Across different approaches, procedural differences reflect underlying research values, which legitimate their use. Understanding the differences in core concepts and procedures for different methods is essential to being a 'knowing' practitioner of thematic analysis. In this chapter, we illustrate our discussion of key differences in conceptualisation and procedure using an example study, introduced in Box 18.1 from one of our students. We chose this study as it has broad relevance to health research and education, highlighting the value of insights generated across disciplinary contexts – such as health psychology – where different research questions are likely being asked.

What is a theme and why does how we conceptualise themes matter?

Producing a set of themes is the purpose of thematic analysis, but what a theme is, is all too often implicit rather than explicit. This matters, as there are almost oppositional conceptualisations of 'a theme' in different methods, and failure to explicitly understand this can result in incoherent and poor-quality thematic analysis (see [8]). A common definition of a theme is a pattern of meaning identified or developed across a dataset. However, this definition obscures variation in what 'patterned meaning' is understood as, and in practices for 'identifying' such patterning. We highlight divergence by briefly describing three – not mutually exclusive – theme conceptualisations: (1) themes-as-topic summaries;

> **BOX 18.1   Experiences of diagnosis and self-treatment for people with pernicious anaemia**
>
> Conducted by Valentina Acquaviva, this study explored people's experiences of seeking a diagnosis of, and self-treating, pernicious anaemia. Pernicious anaemia is a chronic auto-immune disease that limits the body's capacity to absorb B12 from food and supplements. Symptoms overlap with those of other conditions, making diagnosis difficult. Within the UK National Health Service, treatment typically involves a B12 injection every two to three months. Anecdotally, some patients report requiring more frequent injections, but their doctors are often unsympathetic. Valentina's MSc Health Psychology project took a broadly experiential approach, aligning with much qualitative health psychology research that emphasises listening to the voices of patients and their illness and treatment experiences, and making empathetic interpretations of participants' sense-making (see [1]). Participants were recruited through the Pernicious Anaemia Society and advertising on social media. Because the participant group was geographically dispersed and likely to experience fatigue and other symptoms that could limit their capacity for more demanding data generation, Valentina opted for an online qualitative survey [7]. The survey was kept short (three substantive questions), and participants were asked to indicate their willingness to take part in further data collection; those participants were sent a follow-up survey with an additional three questions, developed following familiarisation with the initial survey data. Responses from the two surveys were treated as a single dataset and analysed using a reflexive version of thematic analysis.

(ii) themes as shared-meaning-based interpretative stories (see [1]); and (iii) themes as diamonds scattered in the sand.

What we call a topic summary theme is one centred on a particular topic or domain within the data. It often summarises what participants reported in relation to that topic, which might be closely aligned to a data generation question. For instance, participants in the pernicious anaemia study were asked a question about their experiences with General Practitioners (GPs) and other health professionals. A classic topic summary theme would be 'Experiences with GPs', with the theme overviewing the main points raised by participants describing their encounters, illustrated with data extracts.

BOX 18.2 Data extracts from the pernicious anaemia study that could illustrate 'negative experiences' or 'GPs are dismissive and obstructive'

I still continued to feel unwell even with thyroid treatment and went back to the GP who told me there was nothing serious wrong with me and sometimes we just have to put up with things.

My GP was, as so often is the case, totally useless – saying that 'it had been caught early because I only had mild macrocytosis' and dismissing the fact that I was experiencing some significant neurological issues as not being anything to do with B12.

My GP insisted I was depressed and became annoyed when I said I did not want to take antidepressants as I thought it was something else... This condition has significantly impacted on my life [...] This is not recognised or addressed by my GP. I have to manage it alone.

It might be divided into two subthemes – 'Positive experiences' and 'Negative experiences' (Box 18.2 provides some examples of the latter from the data). What unites material included in a topic summary theme (or subthemes) is the shared *topic*. Because of how they are conceptualised, such 'themes' can be developed early on in, or even *before*, the analysis process, making them more like analytic 'inputs' than 'outputs'.

A theme as a shared-meaning-based interpretative story captures something fundamentally different. A theme here conveys variation and nuance across the dataset related to, or united by, a central idea or concept. A shared meaning theme from the pernicious anaemia study was 'GPs are dismissive and obstructive', which captured the various ways GPs were experienced as dismissing participants' health concerns and obstructing their access to meaningful treatment (see Box 18.2). Echoing the use of 'postcode lottery' to depict regional disparities in healthcare, a theme which captured *unpredictability* around GP support was termed 'GP lottery'. This included that even good GPs could not be relied on (because they were a locum, they left the practice or retired), meaning participants who were currently supported by their GPs still experienced substantial anxiety about their treatment being withdrawn. The participant experience of GP care captured in these themes overlaps with the topic summaries just noted, but here we home in on a central aspect of interaction/experience, which illuminates something crucial for understanding

the particulars of the experience of pernicious anaemia-related care. Within our approach to thematic analysis, which we now term reflexive thematic analysis [9], the researcher tells an interpretative story about what this meaning helps us understand about our topic, rather than offering a descriptive account of data content [2], differentiated into positive and negative experiences. In contrast to topic summaries, shared-meaning-based themes cannot be developed early on in the analytic process because they require sustained analytic engagement to understand which patterns may be significant and offer useful insights (see [10, 11]). Developing this type of theme requires you to really get to know your dataset and to spend time noting and reflecting on different facets of meaning contained therein. Such themes are often quite different from what might have been imagined at the start of the process.

Our third conceptualisation orients to a different-but-related issue: are themes real, or are they produced (which isn't the same as made up!)? We have called the (implicit) conceptualisation of themes as *real* as a 'diamonds scattered in the sand' [12] approach. Here, themes are treated as real in the sense that they pre-exist analysis, they can be 'extracted from' data, and your role is to 'discover', 'identify', or 'find' these themes in the data. This understanding of themes often intersects with themes-as-topic summaries. It does not align with reflexive thematic analysis, as it evokes the researcher as (ideally) neutral conduit from data to results. Furthermore, it obscures how important being an active, reflexive researcher, who understands that you produce the analysis through your engagement with the data, is for reflexive thematic analysis (this active role is captured by the shorthand phrase: 'themes do not emerge'). The themes as diamonds conceptualisation does appear in research exploring meaning-based themes, but it is not well aligned with Big Q qualitative research values (see [13]). A more coherent understanding is that themes offer a way to organise your reading of your data, your sense-making activity, and provide the structure for the interpretative story you will tell. That story does not pre-exist the analysis, or reside in the data, but develops from you working to make sense of your dataset.

How a theme is conceptualised matters for a range of reasons, including what you understand data as giving you access to, what practical analytic processes you engage in, and methodological considerations you have to address. Take the notion that themes should accurately or faithfully represent the participant experiences conveyed in the data – a worthy idea, but one that is theoretically bounded, and needs unpacking. Do you imagine your analysis offers an accurate (or inaccurate) mapping of the data, or an analytic *interpretation* of the data? With the former idea, which overlaps with topic summaries and themes-as-diamonds, themes can be correctly or incorrectly identified; the allocation of data to themes through coding can be correct or incorrect. This post-positivist framing means processes to ensure accuracy – such as someone else checking/validating that data have been correctly interpreted – become necessary. Other practices that fit with post-positivist logic are realist/concrete measures of (theme) frequency and calculations to determine 'sample' sizes (e.g. [14]).

With shared-meaning-based interpretative story themes, the idea that themes might be correct or incorrect makes no sense. Because of the inherent subjectivity in the analytic process, themes cannot be validated as correct or incorrect by anyone else. However, just because themes are conceptualised as stories the researcher has produced, based on their analytic engagement, this does not mean anything goes. Themes cannot be right or wrong, but they can be stronger or weaker, with greater or lesser interpretative depth. And what we can say is always bounded by the dataset [1].

The thematic analysis family: a tripartite typology

Methods of thematic analysis get us to themes in quite different ways. We have developed a typology of approaches based around these procedural differences – reflecting 'textbook' characterisations of thematic analysis methods, rather than the messier reality of these methods as used and reported in practice. We call these coding reliability, reflexive and codebook approaches to thematic analysis. The procedural differences overlap, but imperfectly, with whether themes are analytic outputs (and interpretative stories) or analytic inputs (and topic summaries).

Coding reliability thematic analysis
Coding reliability thematic analysis falls at the scientifically descriptive [2], small q end of the spectrum. Informed by a post-positivist paradigm, a central concern is establishing the accuracy and reliability of data coding (e.g. [15, 16]), and the analytic process is designed for this purpose. Themes tend to be conceptualised as topic summaries, and developed early in the analysis, alongside a coding frame

or codebook, which is then used to guide the allocation of data to themes. The coding frame consists of a definitive list of codes. For each, there is a label, definition, instructions on how to identify the code, details of any exclusions, and examples [15]. Themes are typically described as 'found' and 'identified' evoking a 'diamonds in the sand' conceptualisation. In coding reliability thematic analysis, coding is primarily about *process*, rather than generating a specific product (codes); themes and codes are not clearly distinguished, and the terms are often used interchangeably. A typical code/theme would be 'negative experiences of GPs' mentioned earlier – coding would identify all instances of such experiences in the data, and then this data would be summarised and reported as a 'theme'. Multiple coders (some ideally naïve to the topic) would independently apply the coding frame, to avoid assumptions and expectations, or 'bias'. The level of coder agreement is calculated, with high levels of intercoder agreement, determined by standard statistical tests, treated as evidence the coding was reliable and accurate. The reassurance of objectivity that coding reliability approaches appear to offer may hold appeal to clinical education students who have been taught to value objectivity and avoid bias, and where commonly deployed quality criteria (e.g. [17]) can reinforce such notions. To us, in terms of the qualitative insights they can produce, such approaches are limited by their conceptual and procedural commitments (see also [2]).

Reflexive thematic analysis
Reflexive thematic analysis – including the approach we have developed [1, 18] – is firmly Big Q and artfully interpretative [2]. In reflexive thematic analysis, themes are conceptualised as meaning-based, interpretative stories. Themes are 'developed' or 'generated' by an active and ideally reflexive researcher, after thorough familiarisation and coding processes. Coding is radically different both conceptually and in practice, to coding reliability thematic analysis. Codes are a *product* of the process of coding – conceptualised as 'things' produced during the analytic process. Rather than the broader coding categories characteristic of coding reliability thematic analysis (e.g. 'negative experiences'), necessary to facilitate high levels of intercoder agreement, codes in reflexive thematic analysis tend to be more nuanced, capturing your analytic 'take' on the data as well as summarising meaning you consider to be analytically relevant. Code labels are typically pithy phrases (e.g. 'I know my body' evoked the ways participants in the pernicious

anaemia study claimed experiential authority on their bodily experience), rather than one or two words capturing the topic. The coding process itself is open, organic (evolving) and does not involve a (fixed) codebook or coding frame. As coding progresses, codes can and should evolve to better capture your deepening insight into your data (e.g. coding labels can be tweaked; the boundaries of a code refined; two or more codes collapsed together; a particularly complex code split into two or more codes to better parse out different meanings). Potential themes are explored through clustering codes, considering the stories they capture and convey about the dataset, and re-clustering and refining until a robust, meaningful, and important story of the dataset has been developed. As a subjective, iterative process, there is no right or accurate way to code, no correct themes to 'identify'; any analyst could bring different understandings. A single researcher is common. We hope to convey to clinical education researchers the value of the rich, nuanced, unexpected insights that Big Q/reflexive thematic analysis can generate and that this can support resistance to the post-positivist traditions delimiting research in some clinical disciplines (e.g. [19]).

Codebook thematic analysis

Codebook thematic analysis is located somewhere between coding reliability and reflexive approaches and encompasses methods often developed for applied research, such as template analysis [20] and framework analysis [21], which may make these particularly useful for some of the research questions and contexts clinical education researchers work on. For example, framework analysis was developed for applied social policy research, to help researchers, working as teams, often including qualitative novices, analyse large datasets to tight deadlines, and to produce analyses that addressed very focused research questions (e.g. what are the barriers to or facilitators of successful implementation of a policy?). In order to meet pragmatic demands, codebook thematic analysis tends to offer relatively structured analytic procedures, using some kind of codebook (template, framework, etc). This compromises on the open-ended and exploratory character of Big Q, even as qualitative research values are still embraced. In codebook approaches, in contrast to coding reliability approaches, the intent of using a codebook is to chart or map the developing analysis, rather than to determine the accuracy or reliability of coding. Where a team of coders is used, as is often the case with framework analysis, this is

typically to divide the labour of analysing a large dataset to a tight deadline, not to determine the accuracy of coding. As with coding reliability thematic analysis, the themes produced through codebook approaches tend to be topic summaries, developed early on – an input orientation – though some variants, like template analysis, do allow for the possibility of developing themes from and through coding.

These procedural variations also more subtly shape the nature of the components of the developing analysis. For instance, as previously noted, in coding reliability thematic analysis, a prioritisation of coding agreement necessitates having codes/themes that are relatively broad or coarse and often focused on relatively superficial meaning [22]. For similar reasons, codes tend to be relatively descriptive and concrete; a code/theme might be designated as latent because the participant does not use particular words, even though the ideas they are explicitly expressing are captured by the code/theme. The open organic approach of reflexive thematic analysis, where coding quality is not judged by consensus or agreement between coders, means that codes are often more fine-grained, nuanced, and interpretative. In reflexive thematic analysis, the notion of latent codes designates the assumed, the unspoken, the inferred, rather than the explicitly stated, which semantic codes capture.

The role of the researcher in thematic analysis

Researcher subjectivity – what we bring to the analytic process, and how that (potentially) shapes analysis – is treated very differently in different thematic analysis methods. The post-positivist foundations for coding reliability thematic analysis, which idealise objectivity, frame researcher subjectivity as 'researcher bias' [18]. Such subjectivity becomes a validity threat as it risks distorting the truth, and must be controlled for. Conceptually, such 'influence' is able to be managed and contained (through coding agreement procedures). In reflexive thematic analysis, situated in a non-positivist Big Q paradigm, the notion of 'influence' itself is problematic, as it conceptually evokes the research and the researcher as separable, with the latter only potentially acting on and shaping the former. In reflexive thematic analysis, these cannot be disentangled; the researcher *is* the research. Researcher subjectivity is positioned not just as inherent and inescapable, but as an asset, as valuable. This position reflects a non-positivist take on knowledge generation as inherently subjective and situated (see [21]), and researcher subjectivity as not something to be afraid of. Reflexive thematic analysis invites us – requires us – to interrogate our subjectivity, our generative role in the research, and to reflect on and articulate this in our research and research reporting. However, centring research subjectivity does not mean 'anything goes'. The practice of *reflexivity* is key to good quality practice for Big Q qualitative research. Helpfully, there are many resources around reflexivity (e.g. [23, 24, 25]), including an excellent example of reflexivity when doing reflexive thematic analysis [26]. We offer a brief reflexive account of researcher subjectivity as an asset in the pernicious anaemia study in Box 18.3.

BOX 18.3   Subjectivity in the pernicious anaemia study

One of the aspects we engaged with reflexively in the pernicious anaemia study related to our positionality on the topic and our relationship to our participants – something that is also an ethical consideration! Basically, we might ask, am I an insider, sharing key aspects related to this project, or an outsider? (It is rarely this stark, we can be inside and outside in various ways, see [27].) In the past, only privileged outsiders were trusted to be 'objective' when researching socially marginalised groups. Thankfully, this has changed in many contexts, and the disability activist slogan 'nothing about us without us' captures the emphasis on working in partnership *with*, rather than doing research *on*, minoritised groups, especially when the researchers are outsiders. Valentina was an outsider in the pernicious anaemia study, as she did not have lived experience of pernicious anaemia or B12 deficiency. Victoria her supervisor did, and self-treated with B12 injections. Victoria's insider experience was highlighted in recruitment materials in an effort to build trust with potential participants and to convey a sense of Valentina and Victoria being broadly 'on their side', wanting to hear and do justice to their stories of diagnosis and self-treatment and any frustrations they experienced with standard treatment protocols.

Such positionality was also related to the *analysis* process – the ways their experience (or lack of experience) with B12 deficiency and self-treating shaped how they engaged with the data and was part of an ongoing dialogue from the 'noticings' in early familiarisation through interpretation of final themes.

Diversity of thematic analysis methods and questions of quality

Your approach to using (or managing) researcher subjectivity needs to conceptually fit with your approach to thematic analysis, and so is part and parcel of doing methodologically coherent, quality research. Unhelpfully, terms like 'researcher bias' and 'reflexivity' are often used interchangeably, including in quality criteria and reporting standards (e.g. [28, 29]), leaving us to navigate our way through a conceptual fog. This messy use makes it especially important that you build and gain conceptual and theoretical understanding of what you are doing, and why, when doing your research, starting with whether you are aiming to be a descriptive scientist or an interpretative storyteller [2]. Our top tip for doing good quality, methodologically coherent thematic analysis is to endeavour to strive to be what we term a *knowing* researcher. If you do not understand the philosophical/theoretical and conceptual differences across the approaches, and how these translate into procedural differences, thematic analysis can go very wrong (see [8]).

Common problems we encounter in published thematic analysis include some things we have already highlighted, including confusing topic summaries with shared meaning themes, and treating thematic analysis, and making claims about it, as if it were a single, homogenous method. Other problems are connected to theory, including treating thematic analysis as atheoretical, not specifying a theoretical framework, or treating the approach as inherently realist, essentialist or phenomenological, and/or descriptive/summative. Thematic analysis can indeed be these things. But reflexive (and codebook) thematic analysis hold the potential for more social/radical and interpretative/theoretically-informed research (see [1]). Theoretical consideration matters, not least because no analytic approach is ever atheoretical. You always make assumptions, whether knowingly or not, about what your data represent, and what constitutes meaningful knowledge. For quality, you need to ensure your research is theoretically and conceptually coherent (recognising that the landscape and language of this vary by disciplinary context, see [3, 4]).

That there is much variation across thematic analysis methods, and much design flexibility, especially within reflexive thematic analysis, is one of its advantages. Even just considering reflexive thematic analysis, there are multiple research questions that can be asked, from ones based in experience (as in the pernicious anaemia study) to ones unpacking how a topic is represented or constructed in a certain forum or context (see [1, 13]); multiple data types that can be analysed, such as the qualitative survey used in the pernicious anaemia study, or interviews, or policy documents; various interpretative lenses and frameworks that can be deployed, as well as ontologies and epistemologies used (see Chapter 3). This flexibility makes researcher knowingness (see Box 18.4) important because it is easy to produce philosophically and methodologically incoherent analyses unless theory, design, and analytic claims are considered as a package. Wider concepts of design coherence and methodological integrity (e.g. [13, 28]) are useful for guiding 'knowing' good practice.

In the pernicious anaemia study, we evidenced methodological integrity through different design elements 'fitting' together – theoretically, we adopted a critical realist ontology (we assumed the existence of a reality independent of human practices, but understood participants' experiences and representations of GP interactions were mediated by language and culture). This aligned with a research question exploring participants' experiences of diagnosis and self-treatment, but avoided a naïve experiential realism. The use of an online qualitative survey to gather self-report data from participants was appropriate to the research question and made sense for the participant community. Finally, our use of an inductively oriented reflexive thematic analysis approach, with mostly semantic (explicit) coding, cohered with the other design elements, and provided a robust approach for addressing our research question, while considering researcher subjectivity.

Ethical considerations are also part of the broader remit of knowingness and quality. Ethicality in thematic analysis is not just about adhering to professional ethics codes (see Chapter 7); being an ethical thematic analyst means reflecting on broader ethical issues, such as our social positioning in relation to our participants (as discussed in Box 18.3), and the ways the stories we tell about our participants might impact on the communities they are part of. Social power and privilege are part of research; ethical challenges will be nuanced by whether we have more social power and privilege compared to participants and in what ways this connects to our topics. Considering the impact of our stories is not just about whether individual participants might be upset if they do not like our analysis, but includes the potential for wider harm or other consequences we have not anticipated. Could our analysis inadvertently further stigmatise an already stigmatised group? Such considerations are especially important if our participants are vulnerable or socially

---

BOX 18.4   Becoming a knowing thematic analysis researcher

A *knowing* researcher is one who endeavours to 'own' their perspectives [30] – both personal and theoretical. Being a knowing researcher is about striving to research coherently from a clear values base, and being deliberative in your choices around, and practice of, thematic analysis. To do this (well), you need to develop a sense of 'who you are' as a researcher – and the values that inform your beliefs about research, and about life, the world, and so on. This is the case no matter what type of thematic analysis you are doing.

It also involves a questioning engagement with method – not simply doing something because someone tells you that is what good practice looks like, but considering the assumptions embedded in particular concepts and practices, and whether they align with your research values and thematic analysis approach. Take 'saturation' and 'member checking'. Both are widely touted and sometimes treated as (universal) quality measures for qualitative research (e.g. see [17]); other qualitative researchers argue that they are inherently post-positivist practices, and not coherent with all forms of qualitative research (e.g. [31, 32, 33]). Being 'knowing' involves working out whether a particular concept or practice is coherent with your research values base and methodological approach. Thankfully, qualitative methodologists enjoy thinking about such things, so much has been written about these and other concepts, to help us make these judgements.

Be(com)ing a knowing qualitative researcher will not happen overnight – especially if you are steeped in post-positivist values. Many of us are like the US psychologists described by Jeanne Marecek, who 'swim in the waters of logical positivism, empiricism, realism, and quantification without knowing they are wet' [34]. But knowingness is important, even for post-positivist forms of thematic analysis because values are inescapable and influential. We emphasise striving! Set being a knowing researcher as your goal, but give yourself time to become that, and do not stop asking questions, because knowingness is a way to travel, not a destination to reach.

marginalised. Ethics for Big Q thematic analysis/ qualitative research is not necessarily a place of tidy answers, hence the importance of reflexivity.

Summary

This chapter introduced you to the family of thematic analysis methods and highlighted some shared characteristics – producing a set of themes from data through processes of coding and theme development; the possibility of coding for semantic and latent meaning, and orientating to data inductively or deductively; and some degree of theoretical flexibility. We explored differences across the three main branches of the family – coding reliability, reflexive, and codebook approaches – in how themes are conceptualised, how coding and theme development are enacted, and the research values that ground analytic procedures. We discussed different ways researcher subjectivity is conceptualised – as problem or resource – and what that means for thematic analysis practice. Because of the diversity, which is often poorly recognised, we argued that researchers need to design coherent research, and to practice thematic analysis *knowingly*. This involves reflecting on and articulating your research values, selecting an approach that aligns with these, and using concepts and language that cohere with your research values and thematic analysis approach.

Common pitfalls

- Assuming thematic analysis is a single approach. Take time to develop understanding of different approaches when planning your research.
- Producing too many themes, rather than developing overarching patterns of meaning. Less is often more in the pursuit of interpretative depth and nuance.
- Justifying your choice of thematic analysis using generic characteristics (e.g. flexibility, accessibility), without explaining their specific value or relevance for your study. Make sure you provide a clear and coherent rationale for using thematic analysis (see [35]).
- Applying common quality criteria (e.g. saturation) without question. Consider which markers of quality are relevant for your chosen thematic analysis approach.

Ethical issues

- Reflect on your position in relation to your research participants. Are you an insider and/or outsider and where does power lie?
- Consider whether your analysis poses any risk of harm, particularly where marginalised groups are involved.

Top tips

- Strive to achieve philosophical and methodological coherence in your choice and process of thematic analysis.
- Clarify what you understand by a theme. Do you plan to develop topic summaries or shared meaning themes?
- Reflect on your role as analyst. Are you a descriptive scientist or an interpretive storyteller?
- Guide the reader through the structure of your analysis, with a clear overview of the themes and thematic structure that aligns with what is reported.
- Make sure your reporting style matches the thematic analysis approach you have taken. For reflexive thematic analysis, you need an analytic narrative to tell the reader what your interpretation is and why it matters, and a clear, overall story that brings everything together.

Further reading

Our TA website is a useful place to start your further reading and exploration of TA, as it links to all the resources we've created, as well as providing FAQs, reading lists and more: www.thematicanalysis.net.

For the definitive guide to doing reflexive TA, see: Braun, V. and Clarke, V. (2022). *Thematic Analysis: A Practical Guide*. London: SAGE Publications.

For a thorough discussion of design coherence in reflexive TA, see: Braun, V. and Clarke, V. (2022). Conceptual and design thinking for thematic analysis. *Qualitative Psychology* 9 (1): 3–26.

Two books that provide guidance on coding reliability approaches to TA are: Boyatzis, R.E. (1998). *Transforming Qualitative Information: Thematic Analysis and Code Development*. Thousand Oaks, CA: SAGE Publications.

Guest, G., MacQueen, K.M., and Namey, E.E. (2012). *Applied Thematic Analysis*. Los Angeles: SAGE Publications.

For guidance on template analysis (a codebook approach), see: King, N. and Brooks, J.M. (2018). Thematic analysis in organisational research. In: *The SAGE Handbook of Qualitative Business Management Research Methods: Methods and Challenges* (ed. C. Cassell, A.L. Cunliffe, and G. Grandy), 219–236. London: SAGE Publications.

For guidance on framework analysis (a codebook approach), see: Ritchie, J. and Spencer, L. (1994). Qualitative data analysis for applied policy research. In: *Analyzing Qualitative Data* (ed. A. Bryman and R.G. Burgess), 173–194. London: Routledge.

References

1 Braun, V. and Clarke, V. (2022). *Thematic Analysis: A Practical Guide*. London: SAGE Publications.

2 Finlay, L. (2021). Thematic analysis: the 'good', the 'bad' and the 'ugly'. *European Journal for Qualitative Research in Psychotherapy*. 11: 103–116.

3 Bergman, E., de Feijter, J., Frambach, J. et al. (2012). AM last page: a guide to research paradigms relevant to medical education. *Academic Medicine* 87 (4): 545.

4 Varpio, L., Paradis, E., Uijtdehaage, S., and Young, M. (2020). The distinctions between theory, theoretical framework, and conceptual framework. *Academic Medicine* 95 (7): 989–994.

5 Kidder, L.H. and Fine, M. (1987). Qualitative and quantitative methods: when stories converge. In: *New Directions for Program Evaluation* (ed. M.M. Mark and L. Shotland), 57–75. San Francisco, CA: Jossey-Bass.

6 Braun, V. and Clarke, V. (2013). *Successful Qualitative Research: A Practical Guide for Beginners*. London: SAGE Publications.

7 Braun, V., Clarke, V., Boulton, E. et al. (2021). The online survey as a qualitative research tool. *International Journal of Social Research Methodology* 24 (6): 641–654.

8 Braun, V. and Clarke, V. (2021). One size fits all? What counts as quality practice in (reflexive) thematic analysis? *Qualitative Research in Psychology* 18 (3): 328–352.

9 Braun, V. and Clarke, V. (2019). Reflecting on reflexive thematic analysis. *Qualitative Research in Sport, Exercise and Health*. 11 (4): 589–597.

10 Sandelowski, M. and Leeman, J. (2012). Writing usable qualitative health research findings. *Qualitative Health Research* 22 (10): 1404–1413.

11 Connelly, L.M. and Peltzer, J.N. (2016). Underdeveloped themes in qualitative research: relationship with interviews and analysis. *Clinical Nurse Specialist* 30 (1): 52–57.

12 Braun, V. and Clarke, V. (2016). (Mis)conceptualising themes, thematic analysis, and other problems with Fugard and Potts' (2015) sample-size tool for thematic analysis. *International Journal of Social Research Methodology* 19 (6): 739–743.

13 Braun, V. and Clarke, V. (2022). Conceptual and design thinking for thematic analysis. *Qualitative Psychology* 9 (1): 3–26.

14 Guest, G., Bunce, A., and Johnson, L. (2006). How many interviews are enough?: an experiment with data saturation and variability. *Field Methods* 18 (1): 59–82.

15 Boyatzis, R.E. (1998). *Transforming Qualitative Information: Thematic Analysis and Code Development*. Thousand Oaks, CA: SAGE Publications.

16 Guest, G., MacQueen, K.M., and Namey, E.E. (2012). *Applied Thematic Analysis*. Los Angeles: SAGE Publications.

17 Tong, A., Sainsbury, P., and Craig, J. (2007). Consolidated criteria for reporting qualitative research (COREQ): a 32-item checklist for interviews and focus groups. *International Journal for Quality in Health Care* 19 (6): 349–357.

18 Braun, V. and Clarke, V. (2006). Using thematic analysis in psychology. *Qualitative Research in Psychology* 3 (2): 77–101.

19 Newnham, E. and Rothman, B.K. (2022). The quantification of midwifery research: limiting midwifery knowledge. *Birth* 49 (2): 175–178.

20 King, N. and Brooks, J.M. (2018). Thematic analysis in organisational research. In: *The SAGE Handbook of Qualitative Business Management Research Methods: Methods and Challenges* (ed. C. Cassell, A.L. Cunliffe, and G. Grandy), 219–236. London: SAGE Publications.

21 Ritchie, J. and Spencer, L. (1994). Qualitative data analysis for applied policy research. In: *Analyzing Qualitative Data* (ed. A. Bryman and R.G. Burgess), 173–194. London: Routledge.

22 Morse, J. (1997). 'Perfectly healthy, but dead': the myth of inter-rater reliability. *Qualitative Health Research* 7 (4): 445–447.

23 Berger, R. (2015). Now I see it, now I don't: researcher's position and reflexivity in qualitative research. *Qualitative Research* 15 (2): 219–234.

24 Finlay, L. and Gough, B. (ed.) (2003). *Reflexivity: A Practical Guide for Researchers in Health and Social Sciences*. Oxford: Blackwell Science.

25 Lazard, L. and McAvoy, J. (2020). Doing reflexivity in psychological research: What's the point? What's the practice? *Qualitative Research in Psychology* 17 (2): 159–177.

26 Trainor, L.R. and Bundon, A. (2021). Developing the craft: reflexive accounts of doing reflexive thematic analysis. *Qualitative Research in Sport, Exercise and Health*. 13 (5): 705–726.

27 Hayfield, N. and Huxley, C. (2015). Insider and outsider perspectives: reflections on researcher identities in research with lesbian and bisexual women. *Qualitative Research in Psychology* 12 (2): 91–106.

28 Levitt, H.M., Motulsky, S.L., Wertz, F.J. et al. (2017). Recommendations for designing and reviewing qualitative research in psychology: promoting methodological integrity. *Qualitative Psychology* 4 (1): 2–22.

29 Levitt, H.M., Bamberg, M., Creswell, J.W. et al. (2018). Journal article reporting standards for qualitative

primary, qualitative meta-analytic, and mixed methods research in psychology: the APA publications and communications board task force report. *American Psychologist* 73 (1): 26–46.

30 Elliott, R., Fischer, C.T., and Rennie, D.L. (1999). Evolving guidelines for publication of qualitative research studies in psychology and related fields. *British Journal of Clinical Psychology* 38 (3): 215–229.

31 Braun, V. and Clarke, V. (2021). To saturate or not to saturate? Questioning data saturation as a useful concept for thematic analysis and sample-size rationales. *Qualitative Research in Sport, Exercise and Health.* 13 (2): 201–216.

32 Varpio, L., Ajjawi, R., Monrouxe, L.V. et al. (2017). Shedding the cobra effect: problematising thematic emergence, triangulation, saturation and member checking. *Medical Education* 51 (1): 40–50.

33 Smith, B. and McGannon, K.R. (2018). Developing rigor in qualitative research: problems and opportunities within sport and exercise psychology. *International Review of Sport and Exercise Psychology* 11 (1): 101–121.

34 Marecek, J. (2003). Dancing through the minefields: toward a qualitative stance in psychology. In: *Qualitative Research in Psychology: Expanding Perspectives in Methodology and Design* (ed. P.M. Camic, J.E. Rhodes, and L. Yardley), 49–69. Washington, DC: American Psychological Association.

35 Braun, V. and Clarke, V. (2021). Can I use TA? Should I use TA? Should I not use TA? Comparing reflexive thematic analysis and other pattern-based qualitative analytic approaches. *Counselling and Psychotherapy Research* 21 (1): 37–47.

19 Behind the scenes of qualitative analysis: learning from new researchers' struggles

Anne de la Croix, Malou Stoffels, and Jan Willem Grijpma

Learning objectives

By the end of this chapter, you should be able to:
- Anticipate common struggles in qualitative analysis.
- Develop strategies for navigating common dilemmas when undertaking qualitative analysis for the first time.
- Explain how ingrained post-positivist ideas can hinder the qualitative analysis process.
- Embrace subjectivity and refine ways of thinking about rigour.
- Deal with uncertainty when making analytic decisions.
- Select ways to talk about qualitative analysis with your team.

Introduction

We hope that the previous chapters on qualitative research have guided and inspired you to undertake qualitative clinical education research. However, our experience is that despite these excellent pieces of guidance, new researchers can still struggle when doing qualitative research. When we say 'struggle', we mean common and normal dilemmas or issues in the research process that you might worry about. These dilemmas arise as there are no one-size fits all descriptions of the exact analytic steps for your study. Every study is different, all data sets are different, all researchers are different, and all analytic approaches are different. Qualitative research is a labour-intensive, iterative process in which analysis is rarely done in a predetermined order or process and – even though it has developed so much in the last decades – it still goes against some strong post-positivist ideas that are ingrained in the image of 'doing science' (see Chapter 3). This means you will have to make many decisions, without the knowledge or confidence that is built through previous hands-on experience of working with qualitative data.

In this chapter, we follow Remi who is a first-time qualitative researcher (Boxes 19.1–19.6). We meet up with Remi just after the data collection phase of their study. Remi and the research team have followed procedures and knowledge obtained from this book. In a diary, Remi reflects on analytic struggles. We will use these experiences to analyse why new researchers might struggle ('what is going on here?') and offer further reading and strategies to cope ('what might help?'). The struggles Remi encounters include starting to create themes, embracing subjectivity and interpretation, revising research questions, and working with a diverse supervision team. We hope Remi's experience reassures you that you are not alone in your endeavours and that our suggestions support you in becoming a reflective and versatile researcher.

How do I get from data to themes?

BOX 19.1 Remi's diary entry 1

Dear diary,

I have finished coding the data, although I think I could equally have used more or fewer codes. Now I need to make themes. I read quite a few papers about research reports in which authors write that the 'themes emerged from the data'. I don't know. Nothing is magically happening right now. How will I ever get to themes from here. . . The software package that was recommended is not helpful either. . . Help!

Remi.

Starting Research in Clinical Education, First Edition. Edited by Eliot L. Rees, Alison Ledger, and Kim A. Walker.
© 2024 The Association for the Study of Medical Education (ASME). Published 2024 by John Wiley & Sons Ltd.
Companion website: www.wiley.com/go/clinicaleducation

What is going on here?

Manuals on qualitative data analysis describe how patterns or themes can be found after coding data. Many sources say that themes 'emerge'. Themes are patterns in the data that say something significant or interesting in relation to your initial research question. There are no clear rules or guidelines on how to get to them. The word 'emerge' seems to suggest the only job for you is to wait until these themes appear in front of you. Imagine that, sitting behind your laptop, waiting for magic.

Many new researchers think qualitative data analysis software (for example Atlas.ti, MaxQDA, or NVivo) will do the analysis for them, much like a statistical analysis package would do in quantitative analyses. However, these software packages – helpful as they might be for exploring your data in different ways – are really nothing but a fancy database that helps you organise the data. Unlike statistical analyses, it is impossible to write the syntax for analysis before the data has been collected. The step from codes to themes is a giant leap that involves a lot of work. It involves choices, not only considering your research question and data but also your target audience and the presumed originality of your findings. This can be overwhelming if you are struggling with the desire to make the 'right choices' based on this complex array of factors. This is particularly the case after you have been immersed in your data for a while, it is hard to see the bigger picture and to separate the wheat from the chaff.

What might help?

Themes do not emerge, it is *you* doing the work [1]. It is not a magical process on which you can just wait. It might become a more intuitive process, especially when you are more experienced as a researcher, or in your research topic. In that case, you might subconsciously integrate all these previous experiences which might lead you to suddenly 'see the light' or to see connections and relations that make sense to you because of your experience. This might actually feel like the themes emerging, and that feeling is not wrong, as long as you can substantiate your analysis.

Keep in mind an expert researcher may create *different* themes than you would, because of this experience, which is okay – we will dive into that struggle in the next section. Think of a sports game, during which you give a different interpretation to a professional sports commentator, which is equally plausible. In research, it is your job to reflect on how your interpretation was shaped by your experience and write reflexively when reporting your findings [2].

What can help you to gain experience, or to become conscious of the different possibilities to code, so you are able to make those hard decisions?

First of all: distance. Take a break from staring at your data. Imagine running into someone you went to university with, who asks you what project you are working on now. After explaining your research questions and methods, your friend asks, 'and, what did you find?' Try to answer this question in less than one minute. Do not overthink. Say the answer out loud. Try this every so often. Another way for creating distance is to create a visual representation (e.g. drawing, graph or mindmap) of your data, thought process, or conclusions.

Second: confidence. You are likely to have the best overview of the data given your role in data collection and analysis. Consider how long you have been thinking and reading about this topic, and how many people you have spoken to. Your brain has been doing a lot of work already. Using all that information you have (unconsciously) gathered along the process is not a bad thing and you can feel confident that your decisions on what is *really* going on in your data are not nonsensical (yet always need to be accounted for and/or discussed).

Third: Start with some guidance or a more structured approach. A simple way to start in your first qualitative project could be to choose a more deductive approach, in which a theory or model guides the analysis (see Chapter 18). Even in deductive work, one can still be open to new findings and codes. An example is directed content analysis [3]. After being immersed in your data, you might choose to use a theoretical model to guide your final codebook. This might save you from having to make hard decisions about codes. However, you do need to consider how your work might add to this theory and check if your research is still relevant and original. Also stay watchful that all elements (question, methodology, methods, and conceptual framework) are aligned in your study (see Chapters 3 and 4).

Fourth: Develop a variety of ways to look at your data in order to decide which elements of your data will make up the building blocks of your final report. Do not forget that qualitative analysis can be a team effort and not necessarily for the purpose of developing 'reliable' themes (see Chapter 18). Use your research team and work together with an analysis buddy to remain reflexive and develop your analysis. Also draw on the scientific community. Read qualitative research articles to see how other researchers have coded their data and created their themes. For example, you may find inspiration in the work of Gläser, who developed different coding families, which are ways to look at data and interpret relationships [4, 5]. However, pay close attention to the philosophies underpinning the analyses you read and follow examples that align best with your research question and paradigm (see Chapter 18).

How do I deal with subjectivity and interpretation?

BOX 19.2   Remi's diary entry 2

Dear diary,

Today, we had a team meeting to look at the data. One of my colleagues looked at my data and had observations that were very different to my own. It made me doubt myself. I went back to my notes, to the data, to the codes, and reflected on the themes and my analysis. But now I am wondering: how do I know my interpretation is right? Who am I to say that these are the results? Because if I make an interpretation, someone else could make a different interpretation, and we could both be right (or wrong). Was my colleague right in her observations? Is my analysis wrong? And shouldn't everyone who does the analysis find the same thing?

Remi.

BOX 19.3   Remi's diary entry 3

Dear diary,

Yesterday I presented a first draft of the results to the research team, but they thought the description of my results was too technical and seemed like a list of codes, rather than a cohesive story. So they suggested I rewrite them with the reader's perspective in mind. Initially, I was frustrated but this morning I converted my frustration into new energy and was inspired to write my results in a cohesive, attractive, elegantly simple way. My team was right, the previous version was terrible! I decided to take a fresh sheet of paper and write it in a single breath to keep a nice flow and maintain my sense of urgency. When I reread it, I was quite satisfied and so was my supervisor. Taking distance from my data allowed me to keep the reader in mind, but did I not just make up a story that the reader would like to hear? Was my story incomplete by leaving out 'obvious' findings? Of course, I will get back to my data to 'check', but to be honest I am relieved to have a nice story at least and don't feel like changing it another time. Neither will my research team.

What is going on here?

In diary entries 2 and 3, Remi worries about being held to account for incorrect inferences and also has a strong desire to do justice to the input of valuable participants. Choosing one frame over another feels like favouring one participant's story over another. You might feel like you are bluffing: Are there more stories? Why is this the one? Additionally, you might worry you are writing an analytic story that seems 'far away' from the data and the codes. This might feel unjustified and scary. However, just reporting a list of codes and themes is boring and not relevant to the reader.

Additionally, Remi suspects the results of the study might have been different if someone else had done the study. This feels strange, wrong, and subjective. They were previously taught that subjectivity is 'bad' in science. You too may hold a core belief that 'science must be objective'. Objectivity suggests there is one story to be found, one right result and you must try to uncover it with analysis. Therefore, it is reasonable to expect that you may struggle with subjectivity.

Without some sort of objectivity, how can we be confident in our findings? What does it mean that someone else can come to different findings, and you could potentially find different answers if you analysed the data again in the future? That is not 'scientific research', is it? Are validity and reliability no longer relevant? How else can we assure the integrity and quality of our study? And if you have the power to select or create the narrative in the results, how do you choose?

What might help?

Qualitative data does or should never claim a truth that is directly applicable to other settings. There is not *one* perfect model or overview of themes in the messy reality of thirty transcripts. So, the most important task for anyone doing qualitative research is to embrace subjectivity. Even though we are trained to fight and reduce it, 'your subjectivity is essential' [6]. The truth is that qualitative research is subjective by nature. There is no universal 'truth' or 'single best way' to cluster your data, no 'perfect story' that is inherently there and can be found by everyone.

It all comes down to making choices. The challenge in developing findings is to highlight some selected, but not all, patterns within that data and submit this to scientific debate. Which patterns are highlighted depends on the research question and, indeed, on you as the researcher. When you try to convey all the stories within a single paper, you can be sure that no one is going to read it. And yes, your story might be different from someone else's who works with the same data set.

However, this does not mean you can just make up a story based on your interviews and write it up. Subjective work is persuasive if you adhere to the rules of rigour. Think carefully about when and how you collect data to show *dependability*, be transparent about the context so readers can consider the *transferability* of findings to their own settings, reflect on the ways in which members of the research team might have interpreted data due to their *positionality*, and use quotes from the data to establish *credibility* [7, 8].

Furthermore, use your research question to help you tell your story. There is always much more in your data than you can convey, and you should choose a message which involves interpretation. As a new researcher, you might not have a full sense of what is already 'known' and what is novel when you start the research project and collect the data, but this should become more apparent the more you engage with your research topic. When finalising the story you wish to tell, go back to your research question to help you decide which findings are most relevant, original, and likely to impact on theory or practice.

Lastly, own your story. When writing up your results, it is important to explain your story and the way you arrived at this story. The use of quotes from your data is essential to support your story and establish your interpretation is credible. Your story can be your own, using 'integrated narration' to achieve 'rhetorical control' [9]. Make sure you have a critical research team around you who can challenge you to defend your interpretations. Know the data like the back of your hand, so you can rise to such challenge.

Is it possible to make changes along the way?

> ### BOX 19.4   Remi's diary entry 4
>
> Dear diary,
>   Today, I finished my results and discussion section. I found a nice theoretical framework to help me interpret my results and I think framing it like this will enable me to present it as a nice contribution to the literature. To create more alignment, I have now added this framework to the introduction section. However, knowing this, it makes sense to phrase the research question a little differently. It feels a bit strange to do that at this stage. Am I allowed to?
>   Remi.

What is going on here?

Those of us who are experienced in post-positivist research often expect the qualitative research process to unfold in a strictly linear way. However, these ideas – again – stem from a post-positivist research approach (see Chapter 3). They are amplified by the IMRaD (introduction, methods, results and discussion) format often used in research articles. The introduction and discussion are often written in the present tense, as they form 'the story', and methods and results are generally written in past tense and form 'the study' [10, 11]. The traditional way of thinking of chronology is start the 'story' with an introduction, then start the study with the methods. Then you write the results to close the 'study' part, which is the heart of the paper. Finally, the discussion ties back to the introduction and wraps up the story.

In post-positivist research, it is quite common to write the introduction and methods first. The results and discussion are later 'added on' when the analysis is finished and results are yielded. In quantitative research, this enhances transparency and makes sure theoretically substantiated hypotheses are tested. For this reason, 'going back' to a research question can feel wrong for those steeped in a post-positivist paradigm. However, the qualitative research process is often very different. It is much less straightforward and more interactive. There are some models and papers that can help us understand and embrace this.

What might help?

Joe Maxwell wrote a book about qualitative research in which he stresses the 'interactive' nature of qualitative research design, meaning that many elements are constantly in interaction and influence each other [12]. The central connecting element is the research question. This means all elements need to be figured out to finally come to a clear research question, which indeed can be *after* having gathered data or done a first round of analysis. Maxwell's book is a great resource to 'get people in the mood' for qualitative research work. It is rigorously and eloquently written with narrative power, metaphors, and a sense of humour.

Let us use a metaphor of building a table to ensure it is balanced and does not wobble. A strictly chronological approach would be to use a drill and screws to first solidly attach two legs on one end, and then use the equipment to screw two legs on the other end. The approach described above is more like building a table by loosely screwing in all the legs lightly, so they are in place but not yet firmly attached. This way, you can see if the legs are all aligned and the table is the right height. Then, when we feel that we have placed all the legs in the right place and it won't wobble, we screw them in tightly.

Another great source to help you through an evolving study is a paper by Jane Agee [13]. She offers strong support for adjusting or adapting your question, even during data collection and analysis: 'The development of new questions, especially sub-questions, often occurs during the inquiry process, sometimes during data collection and analysis. A researcher may find that the initial focus of the research question is too limited to fully address the phenomenon under study.'

It is not a problem to adjust elements of your study to align all elements and build a strong report. As you work to develop insight into complex phenomena, restricting yourself to predetermined questions may lead you to neglect important aspects or mechanisms.

How do I work with a diverse supervision team?

BOX 19.5   Remi's diary entry 5

Dear diary,
 I have received feedback from my supervision team on the draft of the paper. With some of the quotes I have included, they are asking me 'how often was something mentioned by the participants' and suggesting I add a table with frequencies. These are not comments fitting my paradigm. Counting does not prove anything. In my analysis, something was not more valid, or true because five people said it instead of one. But how do I have this conversation with the team?
 Remi.

What is going on here?

Most research teams are made up of people with varying degrees of practice and research experience. Quite often, you will work with colleagues who are more senior than you, but who have little to no experience with qualitative research. Supervisors who have progressed within a post-positivist research tradition may not be used to the more constructivist way of thinking. This might lead to comments and feedback about your study that do not suit the nature of qualitative research, often focused on making the study 'more objective', or 'more robust', for example by adding numbers. They may have different perceptions of quality. This poses a dilemma for you as a novice researcher. Do you try and find a middle ground? Or do you stick to your chosen approach, and if so, how can you convince your colleagues?

What might help?

First, for people to understand there are very different ontological and epistemological ideas behind the methods chosen (see Chapter 3), it could be valuable to have a 'meta-conversation' with the team about their own stance. You may find it helpful to refer to a BMJ paper, in which an expert in qualitative research converses with someone with less qualitative experience [14], and suggest discussing it in a supervision meeting to surface expectations. You could alternate between different stances across research projects, as long as you are aware of the stance you take and design your research accordingly.

Second, before starting the project, it might be an interesting exercise to let all the people in the team choose a qualitative article they like and take it to a supervision meeting. This, again, might lead to a conversation about perceptions of quality, relevance, originality, and rigour.

Third, it may help to discuss guidance about quality in qualitative research (e.g. [8]). Rigour in qualitative, constructivist research work contains different elements than post-positivist researchers are used to. It is therefore important to check the assumptions underpinning the guidance you read and to consider whether it matches your paradigm (see Chapter 18).

BOX 19.6   Remi's diary entry 6

Dear diary,
 I am done! It was a rough ride and I kept worrying I was not allowed to make the steps I ended up making. But I ended up with a story that feels like a great summary of what I heard participants discuss when it comes to my research question and study goals.
 Yesterday I presented my findings to my target audience, and they commented that they did recognise it, yet also had some real eye-openers.
 I was able to defend and explain my interpretation, and how my way of doing the analysis developed while doing the work. Actually, I was not able to write my plan of analysis in the 'method' section of my paper until after I had finished my analysis – the method developed during the process. And I now understand that that is okay, if I take into account the ideas around rigour.
 I am ready for the next qualitative study now – bring it on!
 Remi.

Summary

How qualitative analyses look on paper and in practice can be two different worlds. In this chapter, we explained common struggles in the data analysis phase, and how they relate mostly to post-positivist traditions about science and research learned during our health professional training. They influence our expectations with regard to analytic choices, interpretation, subjectivity, chronology, and collaboration.

It is common that new clinical education researchers struggle with the iterative, interpretive nature of qualitative research. You may feel like 'anything' is possible, just when you are seeking concrete tools to help you navigate the research process. This chapter offers some guidance about how to accept the uncertainty inherent in qualitative analysis, how to gain confidence, and hopefully start enjoying the freedom and creativity involved.

Top tips

- Open up a dialogue with supervisors about your paradigmatic stance. Clarify expectations with regard to rigour in qualitative analysis.
- Embrace subjectivity. Recognise the ways your experience shapes your interpretations.
- Dare to make choices. Know your data well and be prepared to explain your analytic process.

Common pitfalls

- Looking to guidance which does not align with your paradigm. Post-positivist markers of quality (e.g. objectivity, reliability) are not necessarily appropriate if you are interested in multiple interpretations of complex phenomena.
- Assuming themes will 'emerge' easily. Theme creation takes time and hard work on your part.
- Expecting qualitative analysis to unfold in a linear way. Remain open to refining your research question as you progress your analysis.

Ethical issues

- Subjectivity does not mean you can report any interpretation you like. Your interpretations are always bounded by what is in the data and you should consider the potential impact of your interpretations (see Chapter 18).
- Express and discuss any doubts with supervisors, collaborators, or peers.

References

1 Varpio, L., Ajjawi, R., Monrouxe, L.V. et al. (2017). Shedding the cobra effect: problematising thematic emergence, triangulation, saturation and member checking. *Medical Education* 51 (1): 40–50.

2 Olmos-Vega, F.M., Stalmeijer, R.E., Varpio, L., and Kahlke, R. (2022). A practical guide to reflexivity in qualitative research: AMEE guide no. 149. *Medical Teacher* 7: 1–11.

3 Hsieh, H.-F. and Shannon, S.E. (2005). Three approaches to qualitative content analysis. *Qualitative Health Research* 15 (9): 1277–1288.

4 Glaser, B.G. (1978). *Theoretical Sensitivity*. Mill Valley, CA: Sociology Press.

5 Böhm, A. (2004). Theoretical coding: text analysis in grounded theory. In: *A Companion to Qualitative Research* (ed. U. Flick, E. von Kardorff, and I. Steinke), 270–275. SAGE Publications.

6 Clarke, V., Braun, V., and Hayfield, N. (2015). Thematic analysis. In: *Qualitative Psychology: A Practical Guide to Research Methods*, 3e (ed. J.A. Smith), 222–248. SAGE Publications.

7 Korstjens, I. and Moser, A. (2018). Series: practical guidance to qualitative research. Part 4: trustworthiness and publishing. *The European Journal of General Practice* 24 (1): 120–124.

8 Levitt, H.M., Bamberg, M., Creswell, J.W. et al. (2018). Journal article reporting standards for qualitative primary, qualitative meta-analytic, and mixed methods research in psychology: the APA Publications and Communications Board task force report. *American Psychologist* 73 (1): 26–46.

9 Lingard, L. (2019). Beyond the default colon: effective use of quotes in qualitative research. *Perspectives on Medical Education* 8 (6): 360–364.

10 Lingard, L. and Watling, C. (2016). It's a story, not a study: writing an effective research paper. *Academic Medicine* 91 (12): e12.

11 Lingard, L. and Watling, C. (2021). *Story, Not Study: 30 Brief Lessons to Inspire Health Researchers as Writers*. Springer International Publishing.

12 Maxwell, J.A. (2012). *Qualitative Research Design: An Interactive Approach*. SAGE Publications.

13 Agee, J. (2009). Developing qualitative research questions: a reflective process. *International Journal of Qualitative Studies in Education* 22 (4): 431–447.

14 Pope, C. and Mays, N. (2009). Critical reflections on the rise of qualitative research. *BMJ* 339: b3425.

PART IV

Quantitative research

Kim A. Walker

Quantitative methods are widely used in clinical education research and are, perhaps, what most researchers including yourself are most familiar with. They are often used to evaluate the effectiveness of educational interventions, assess student performance, and measure outcomes. However, quantitative research can provide much more than simple outcomes. Advanced techniques and methodologies can help you and other researchers inform educators to make evidence-based decisions on future developments in clinical education. This part takes you on a quantitative research journey.

Chapter 20 describes best practice and principles for the design and conduct of surveys by providing you with a step-by-step approach. Chapter 21 explains experimental methods, which may be a new concept for you in clinical education research. It also uses a step-by-step approach on how to investigate causality with the elimination of bias. Quantitative research by its very nature generates numbers. Chapter 22 provides an introduction to statistical analysis including how to present your data. Chapter 23 provides an overview of how and where you can

access Big Data and details the benefits and challenges of working with large datasets. This is a new and expanding area of research.

Quantitative research may seem simple. However, a common thread in this part is the benefits and importance of collaborating with others. The support and help of a statistician and/or psychometrician and experts in the methodology you wish to use will also help you become a better quantitative researcher. This part will hopefully allow you to not only understand the basics of quantitative research but also alert you to other possibilities you may not have initially considered. Many of the chapters have provided further reading for supplementary information. You will also find some exemplary studies and figures on the companion website.

Quantitative research can be a powerful tool allowing you to identify patterns, trends, and correlations. However, it is important to use the right reliable data sources and the appropriate statistical techniques. Performed well, you can make informed decisions to drive your career forward.

Starting Research in Clinical Education, First Edition. Edited by Eliot L. Rees, Alison Ledger, and Kim A. Walker.
© 2024 The Association for the Study of Medical Education (ASME). Published 2024 by John Wiley & Sons Ltd.
Companion website: www.wiley.com/go/clinicaleducation

20 Survey research: uses and misuses

Patrick G. Corr, Radwa Aly, and Anthony R. Artino, Jr.

Learning objectives

By the end of this chapter, you should be able to:
- Explain the uses and misuses of surveys for research purposes.
- Describe how cognitive processes and motivation guide the way people understand and respond to survey questions.
- Identify well-written survey items.
- Apply a six-step process for survey design and development.
- Recognise the importance of conducting expert reviews and cognitive interviews.
- Address ethical concerns in survey research.

Introduction

Surveys are widely used for clinical, translational, medical, and health education research. From market surveys and election polling to patient satisfaction and other healthcare questionnaires, surveys continue to be one of the most widely used methods for collecting data from both small and large groups of individuals. For example, in medical education research, recent work indicates that surveys are the data collection method of choice in more than 50% of original research studies [1].

Surveys are employed to assess a variety of hard-to-measure phenomena in healthcare education and practice, like patient perceptions, trainee attitudes and opinions, and practitioner competence. Despite their widespread use, they continue to be poorly designed, ineffectively administered and analysed, inadequately reported, and generally misapplied in health-related research endeavours.

The purpose of this chapter is to introduce you to survey research, with a primary focus on surveys that use close-ended survey items and generate quantitative data. We provide an overview of how surveys can, and should, be used for research and programme evaluation together with a set of principles for developing high-quality surveys. We then describe a systematic approach to survey development that can help you avoid many of the common pitfalls in design and implementation. This approach includes guidance on how to write and pretest high-quality survey items, which are the foundation of any good survey. Ultimately, we hope this chapter will help you avoid some of the common mistakes that plague many surveys and increase the odds your own questionnaires are well designed and fit for research and programme evaluation purposes.

Survey uses (and misuses)

Surveys are used to gather information on individuals or to make generalisations about groups of individuals [2]. Although many data collection methods are informally referred to as *surveys*, we define a survey broadly as any instrument composed of pre-identified questions or items designed to produce statistical information about a specific portion of a population [3]. A *questionnaire* is simply a self-administered survey (as opposed to, for example, a survey administered by an interviewer over the phone). Surveys are best used to measure non-observable constructs such as respondents' attitudes, feelings, beliefs, opinions, and sometimes even behaviours. Although some surveys generate data that is amenable to qualitative analysis [4], we shall limit our attention to those attempting to *measure* something.

Beyond these basic considerations, survey research can be quite diverse. Surveys can be long or short. They can be conducted in person, by telephone,

---

Starting Research in Clinical Education, First Edition. Edited by Eliot L. Rees, Alison Ledger, and Kim A. Walker.
© 2024 The Association for the Study of Medical Education (ASME). Published 2024 by John Wiley & Sons Ltd.
Companion website: www.wiley.com/go/clinicaleducation

through the mail, or over the internet. Sometimes survey respondents are identifiable, whereas other times their responses are anonymous. Surveys can be about voting intentions, consumer preferences, social attitudes, health perceptions, medical practices, or virtually anything else you can imagine asking respondents about, so long as meaningful answers are likely to be obtained.

Although surveys are often appropriately used in health-related research and clinical education, they can also be misused. For instance, surveys are not the ideal way to gather information that can be observed directly or is already available from other sources. For example, a student's behaviour, such as their daily study habits, is more accurately recorded using a daily diary than a self-reported survey administered many days or weeks after studying has occurred. Similarly, data on patient discharge times are probably better obtained from a centralised electronic medical record than by asking individual doctors or nurses to self-report them. In addition, surveys are best when used to examine topic areas that are well enough understood to inform the design of the survey. In other words, before designing a survey, you should have a good sense of the full range of appropriate questions and their associated response options [5]. If not, it makes more sense to start your study with some exploratory, qualitative work to gather basic information about the topic of interest (e.g. by conducting interviews). Once this is done, a survey can then be created to further explore the research question by gathering survey data from a larger group (e.g. conducting a survey of all healthcare professionals in a practice).

Six principles of survey design

Designing a high-quality survey is challenging. Below we offer six key principles to guide the design and development of high-quality surveys to help you in your research and programme evaluation.

Principle 1: the questions shape the answers

How we frame our questions determines the answers we get. Schwarz made this point more completely when he noted 'self-reports of behaviours and attitudes are strongly influenced by features of the research instrument, including question wording, format, and context'. [4]. For example, an educator, asking the question, 'how would you rate the instructional quality of this

course?' could probably persuade a significant portion of their students to answer in a positive way by just offering an uneven set of response possibilities, such as outstanding, very good, good, and fair (three of the four options being positive).

However, ethical educators and researchers should not focus primarily on getting the results they desire when designing and administering a survey. Instead, it is important you adhere to evidence-informed best practices when creating survey items and arranging their visual design (see companion website). All respondents will be more likely to comprehend the survey questions and intent if you adhere to these and other principles.

Principle 2: a great deal of cognitive work is required to generate optimal answers

It takes a lot of mental energy on the part of respondents to be thoughtful when answering a survey. The response process model is the one used to describe the cognitive work associated with taking a survey [5]. It states that when respondents take a survey, they work through four cognitive processes. First, they must *comprehend* the question (i.e. they must interpret the meaning of the words on the page). Next, they have to *retrieve* the relevant information from their long-term memory and then integrate that information into a judgement. In some cases, they might also have to make an *estimation*. For example, respondents asked to report how often they gave blood in the last year might not remember all those instances and need to make an educated guess. Lastly, once respondents have an answer in mind, they want to *report* that answer in light of the response options available. Importantly, things can go wrong at any one of these processing steps. For instance, respondents might misunderstand the question because the visual layout is confusing or may not be able to make a good judgement because they do not have the necessary information to give an informed answer. When this occurs, response errors are likely, and answers provided will be difficult or impossible for you to interpret. Therefore, it is important the survey design and development process include pretesting to help assess these various response processes (see Principle 5 below).

Principle 3: respondents are generally unmotivated to take a survey

Respondents are often busy students, trainees, and health professionals who are not that motivated to sit down and complete a survey. Instead, respondents usually agree to take your survey out of the goodness of their hearts, because you have asked them nicely, or promised them a small incentive for their participation.

You can think of respondent motivation in at least two different ways. The motivation to even begin the survey, but also the motivation to answer the questions thoughtfully, accurately, and completely. Therefore, it is important you do everything possible to bolster respondent motivation. Designing a high-quality survey that is easy to understand and keeping the survey short can pay big dividends. Providing up-front incentives to potential respondents and obtaining sponsorship from a trusted person or organisation can also be helpful.

Principle 4: a survey is a conversation between you, the survey designer, and your respondents

A survey is a type of conversation; therefore, it is important to remember respondents will make assumptions when completing it based on conversational norms. There are four basic assumptions, all interrelated, sometimes referred to as Gricean Maxims, named after the linguist Paul Grice [6]. The first maxim is that of *quantity*. In a conversation, we assume the person speaking with us is providing the right quantity of information. Next is the maxim of *quality*. We assume that people are being truthful unless we have reason to believe otherwise. Next is *relevance*; we assume the person is giving us information relevant to the conversation at hand. And lastly, the maxim of *clarity* or *manner*. We assume the person is trying to communicate clearly. So, as survey designers in conversation with our respondents, we should try to honour these conversational norms. If, for example, you provide confusing or inconsistent information to respondents and then ask for their opinions about the information provided, you should not be surprised if you get strange answers. Likewise, if you provide respondents with a bunch of irrelevant information, you should not be surprised if their motivation to complete the survey begins to wane. After all, the person on the other end of the conversation – the respondent – is assuming the information you have provided is truthful, relevant, and clear, and so they will do their best to provide an appropriate answer.

Principle 5: pretest your survey to know how it functions

Practically speaking, this principle may be the most important one. Despite our best efforts in designing a high-quality survey using evidence-informed practices, we cannot know how well our survey will function until individuals attempt to complete it. We recommend two primary ways to pretest a survey: expert reviews and cognitive interviews. These two strategies are discussed in greater detail later in the chapter. Once completed, the results from expert reviews and cognitive interviews can be used as sources of validity evidence, which can bolster the survey's credibility as a useful measurement tool [7]. It is also important you report these pretesting efforts in any publications relating to your survey.

Principle 6: good decisions cannot be made from bad surveys

When we create a survey, we are usually trying to make a decision, based in part on the survey results. If you are surveying students completing a clinical experience, you are maybe trying to decide if they were satisfied with their educator. Or, if you are conducting an end-of-course evaluation, perhaps you are trying to decide if the learners felt the course achieved its learning objectives. In both cases, you are attempting to arrive at a conclusion (or make a decision). However, if the quality of the survey is low and the respondents do not understand the questions being asked, then the likelihood you have collected meaningful data to inform your decision is low, and your survey efforts will have been wasted. In the section below, we provide a step-by-step framework for designing, developing, and pretesting surveys to help yield credible results.

A six-step process for designing a high-quality survey

While surveys are widely employed because of their perceived ease of use and simplicity, they are often poorly constructed. At best, a poorly constructed survey provides little meaningful data; at worst, it results in a bad decision [8]. In this section, we describe a six-step process for developing high-quality surveys. This is one appropriate approach to designing a meaningful survey. See companion website for several of the best resources we have found.

Step 1: search the literature

The first step in developing a survey should include a review of existing literature that addresses issues similar to those you are studying [8–11]. This will provide important context and background to the topic under investigation.

A literature review plays two central roles. It helps to clearly define the scope of the question(s) [9, 10] and develop a clear definition of the phenomenon under study within the context of existing knowledge. It also aids in identifying what gaps your work will fill and ensures the language you are using aligns with existing literature.

It can also help you identify previously employed surveys with validity evidence in related contexts [10, 11]. Many researchers create their own survey tools when pursuing what they believe is a new line of inquiry. However, by thoroughly reviewing the literature, you can often identify existing questionnaires which have been used to address similar questions with similar populations. Further, previous research may have already collected validity evidence for the survey [10]. Therefore, you can often just request permission from the original authors to adapt their instrument for your new study. While the specifics of survey validation are beyond the scope of this introductory chapter, we recommend you collect some amount of validity evidence, even if you are using an existing, previously published survey instrument. For a more complete discussion of survey validation, please see the work of Cook [8].

Step 2: conduct interviews and focus groups

The next step is to gather qualitative data about the constructs you intend to assess with your survey, often, but not exclusively, by conducting interviews and/or focus groups with members of your target population [10]. This is critical to ensure the theoretical understanding you developed during your literature review aligns with the experiences and understanding of your prospective participants. It also allows you to appreciate how a lay person makes sense of a particular phenomenon. For example, if you are collecting data from a group of students to understand how they address perceived mistreatment from faculty, a focus group can help you determine whether the average student recognises and can identify when they experience professional mistreatment. Conducting a focus group prior to writing new survey items also helps you determine what background information participants need before they are able to complete the survey, which can then help you better craft understandable survey questions.

Step 3: write survey items

This step, our third, is often where new researchers mistakenly begin. It is during this phase of the development process that you must ensure all facets of the construct are being addressed by your survey items; you must also confirm your questions are clear and specific. In addition, you should check your answer options are well labelled, and any

visual cues are clear to the population under study (e.g. ensuring all answer options appear on a single line or a single column, not mixing numeric responses and text-based responses, etc.) [9].

It is important you consider the types of questions you plan to include in your survey and determine the best response options. There are many ways to design survey questions. Some common item types are listed below [12].

Close-ended items. These are the most common in surveys; they can have different formats and allow for quantitative analysis.

- *Nominal.* Nominal questions present multiple options but only allow respondents to select a single response. For example, the item: 'Select your clinical site from the following: site X, site Y, site Z'. LaRochelle and Artino note that nominal options 'are useful when no hierarchical relationship exists between the options . . . the options do not have implicit numeric values' [13].
- *Dichotomous.* Dichotomous options are employed when you are asking a question that can only elicit two possible answers [14]. For example, 'Do you consent to take part in this survey research?' The only available options for participants are yes or no. If yes, they will be directed to the start of the survey; if no, they will be directed to close the survey.
- *Ordinal.* Ordinal items contain a list of options with a natural order and are used to measure gradations of opinions, attitudes, or attributes. For example, 'How effective was the course?' (response options: not at all effective; somewhat effective; moderately effective; quite effective; extremely effective).
- *Item-specific response options.* Ordinal items that ask respondents to consider statements and then rate their level of agreement on a scale are known as Likert items or a Likert scale. Although commonly used, recent research suggests that Likert items are not the most effective way to elicit high-quality survey responses. Instead, most survey design experts recommend items that use 'item-specific' response options. That is, response options that are 'written to directly ask about their underlying response dimensions using response categories tailored to match the response dimension' [15]. Therefore, instead of asking respondents to agree or disagree with the statement 'I am confident I can take a complete history on a paediatric patient', you might ask, 'How confident are you that you can take a complete history

on a paediatric patient?' and then use a set of item-specific response options that focus on confidence (e.g. not at all confident; somewhat confident; moderately confident; quite confident; extremely confident).

- *Ranking*. Ranking items ask participants to rank a set of items from, for example, most to least desirable. Ranking items can be especially useful when you want respondents to directly compare a group of highly desirable options, because you force them to make hard choices between the various options. That said, ranking tasks can be cognitively challenging for respondents and, generally, you should never ask respondents to rank more than about five or six items [13].

Open-ended items. These items are useful when you cannot be certain of all the best possible responses to a particular prompt. For example, if you ask about the subjective experiences of a student in a particular clinical rotation, providing close-ended questions may not sufficiently capture the essence of the student's experience [13]. However, contextual characteristics of open-ended questions may influence the qualitative data obtained. For example, if you provide very limited space for an open-ended question (e.g. limited to 50 characters), you

may only elicit very short responses. As stated earlier, however, caution needs to be applied when using open-ended items in a survey.

Some examples are shown in Box 20.1 and Table 20.1. The results of your literature review and interviews/focus groups will inform your survey. Your goal in item writing is to draft clear and concise questions that all respondents interpret the same way (and in the way you intended) and which are structured in a natural, conversational manner. Item clarity at this point will allow a smooth transition into step four.

Step 4: pretest the survey and survey items through expert reviewer

Prior to fully administering a survey, you need to first determine whether the individual survey items meet your needs and address all the important components of your research construct(s) [18]. Pretesting a survey usually begins with expert reviews, sometimes loosely referred to as 'expert validation'. This is a process where experts in the subject matter under study (and/or survey design experts) assess the degree to which your draft items are well written and well aligned with the topic under study [13]. However, the definition of 'expert' can vary widely. Experts typically have

---

BOX 20.1   Good survey design [10]

Provide a textual label for each response option

When providing response options, particularly for Likert-type items, each possible answer should have a corresponding text label. By labelling each response option, you reduce potential confusion from respondents and consequently collect more accurate data.

Example:

	Not at all helpful	Not very helpful	A little helpful	Quite helpful	Extremely helpful
How helpful was your clinical preceptor during your most recent rotation?	O	O	O	O	O

Maintain equal spacing between response items

By maintaining equal space between each possible response, you remove the perception that any one answer has greater significance than another. Additionally, equal spacing between response items reinforces that there is equal 'distance' between each response (i.e. in the example below, there is a consistent difference between *almost nothing* and *a little bit* as there is between *a lit bit* and *some*) which can reduce response bias.

Example:

	Almost nothing	A little bit	Some	Quite a lot	A great amount
How much did you learn during today's food as medicine workshop?	O	O	O	O	O

Source: Adapted from Artino et al. [10].

Table 20.1 Common errors in survey design [5, 16, 17]

1 Asking leading questions	Example: *How important do you think it is to include patients in medical decision making?* Improved: *How important or unimportant do you think it is to include patients in medical decision making?*
2 Asking double-barrelled questions	Example: *To what extent was your instructor knowledgeable about course material and effective in their teaching style?* Improved: *To what extent was your instructor knowledgeable about the course material?* *To what extent was your instructor effective in delivering course content?*
3 Asking vague questions	Example: *How was your clinical training experience?* Improved: *Please rate the quality of your clinical preceptor's supervision* *Please rate the diversity of patient cases you saw during your clinical placement*
4 Including negatively worded questions	Example: *How often did you neglect to start your interviews on time?* Improved: *How often do you begin your interviews on time?*
5 Including acronyms or unfamiliar terms	Example: *Please rate the efficacy of the Big Sibs programme in supporting MS1s through first year exams* Improved: *Please rate the quality of the student mentoring programme in supporting first year medical students during their exam period*

Source: Adapted from Gehlbach and Artino [5], Sullivan and Artino [16], and Artino [17].

detailed content knowledge on the topic under study, some may also have expertise in survey design and statistical analysis. In educational environments, experts often include other clinicians and/or PhD-trained faculty members. Furthermore, the number of experts needed depends on the nature of the survey and its intended purpose (i.e. you may want more experts for a high-stakes survey or research project), but often 6–12 expert reviewers is sufficient. In addition, it is often useful to have a statistician involved at this stage to help you consider the analysis plan that corresponds best to the survey items being developed.

Typically, expert reviews will include a complete evaluation of the survey to determine whether questions are clearly written for the intended audience and relevant to the subject under study. Experts can also assess whether or not there are any questions that should be added or deleted. In seeking expert reviews, you should consider developing a rubric or feedback form to share with reviewers. See companion website for additional resources.

Step 5: employ cognitive interviewing

Cognitive interviewing, sometimes referred to as cognitive testing, is an under-utilised approach to survey pretesting that can pay huge dividends [8, 10–15, 18]. Willis defines cognitive interviewing as 'the supplementation of the participant's answers to the survey questions through the collection of verbal reports obtained by either think-aloud or probing procedures' [18]. In cognitive interviewing, you specifically recruit a sample of participants and conduct qualitative interviews to determine whether your items are understandable and meet their intended purpose [19]. Since this is primarily a qualitative approach, cognitive interviewing projects are typically small in scope and may involve as few as 5 or as many as 30 participants. For small-scale education-related survey projects, five or six participants may be enough to provide actionable information to improve the survey items and overall instrument. Care should be taken, however, to ensure you are sensitive to the potential for bias when only a small group of interviews are conducted.

The think-aloud approach encourages participants to verbally state their thoughts as they read each survey item and the associated response options. This process allows you to determine whether the survey items are clearly understood by participants. There are a number of limitations associated with the think-aloud process including the significant burden of analysing the reams of qualitative data gathered through this process. The verbal probing approach allows you to gather specific information from sample participants through the use of a predefined list of probing questions that you ask as participants review each survey item and response option (concurrent probing) or after they complete an independent review of the entire survey or portion of the survey (retrospective probing). Ultimately, conducting a series of cognitive interviews is extremely useful for both verifying expected issues and discovering unanticipated problems with your survey items and overall questionnaire [13–15, 18, 19].

Step 6: pilot test the survey

The final step in developing a high-quality survey is to conduct a pilot test with members of the population under study. Pilot tests are distinct from cognitive interviews in that they provide a representative sample of participants who take the actual survey under realistic conditions. Pilot testing is useful when designing a new survey as it allows you to test items that have been developed and further refined through expert reviews and cognitive interviews [10]. Small pilot studies can also assist you in further refining your items to ensure they are appropriate for your population [20]. While there are no specific requirements as to the number of participants who should be included in an initial pilot, it is often good practice to use approximately 10% of your eventual sample [21, 22]. Ultimately, the size of the pilot study will depend in part on the purpose of the survey. A survey used as part of a national study will require a much more substantive pilot study than one used for a small, course evaluation project.

Survey administration

The choice of administration method is often dictated by the sample size and study timeline. The most common methods include the following:

- *Electronic.* Online surveys are the most popular, as you can reach many people for little to no cost using a professional format. Surveys can be sent, for example, via email, through electronic health records, or via other online software programmes.
- *In person.* Educational surveys may be completed in person directly with respondents. In a classroom, students may be given a set amount of time at the beginning or end of a class period to complete a survey and drop it in a centrally located box. For clinical research, a survey may be administered in a waiting room during a clinic visit.
- *Mail.* 'Snail-mail' surveys are sent and returned by traditional mail. Mailing your survey presents several challenges, including high costs, difficulty in tracking who received it and who did not, whether you have correct/current addresses, and whether recipients are reading the survey or just throwing it away.

Each of these administration options comes with different ethical considerations (see Chapter 7). See companion website for resources which discuss survey administration in further detail.

Reporting results

Once your survey is completed, including the analysis, you will want and sometimes need to disseminate your findings. This could be via your thesis, a report, and/or a peer-reviewed paper. The goal is to convince your audience that your survey instrument and results are credible [8]. Whether your audience is your degree supervisor(s), members of a journal's editorial review board, or stakeholders within your organisation, it is important you carefully consider the content you need to deliver and the most appropriate way to highlight the salient components of your survey and survey data [23]. Using a set of established reporting guidelines is a good way to ensure you have thoroughly reported the most important parts of your design and data collection efforts (see companion website and Chapters 27 and 28).

Summary

Surveys are pervasive in clinical, translational, medical, and medical education research. When done well, surveys can answer questions no other research method can. Using the existing and ever-emerging literature of survey design, this chapter is intended to introduce you to the science of survey research. Using our six principles and systematic design process, we hope you now have the tools needed to begin developing a survey that can reliably capture your respondents' thoughts, opinions, attitudes, and experiences.

Top tips

- Adhere to evidence-informed practice. This is particularly the case where Likert scales are concerned.
- Do your research to gather basic information about your topic before you begin designing your survey. Search the literature and undertake preliminary qualitative work to define your phenomenon.
- Pretest and pilot your survey. Use cognitive interviewing techniques such as think aloud and verbal probing.

Common pitfalls

- Using a survey when other methods are more appropriate because it seems easier. Only use a survey when observational methods or existing data are not available to you.
- Assuming survey respondents will be motivated. Craft your survey so it is reader-friendly and invites participation.
- Devising questions to get the responses you think you want. Offer an unbiased set of response options, so as not to lead participants in a particular direction.
- Pretesting or piloting with participants who are unlike your study population. Try to gain a range of views, even when the number of participants is small.

Ethical issues

- Ensure informed consent is obtained and documented.
- Inform participants that taking part in your survey is voluntary.
- Only ask questions that are needed to answer the research questions.
- Be careful with the use of incentives. These should match the amount of work of completing the survey.

Further reading

Dillman, D.A., Smyth, J.D., and Christian, L.H. (2014). *Internet, Phone, Mail and Mixed-Mode Surveys: The Tailored Design Method*, 4e. Hoboken, NJ: Wiley.

Phillips, A.W., Durning, S.J., and Artino, A.R. (2022). *Survey Methods for Medical and Health Professions Education: A Six-Step Approach*. Philadelphia, PA: Elsevier.

References

1 Phillips, A.W., Friedman, B.T., Utrankar, A. et al. (2017). Surveys of health professions trainees: prevalence, response rates, and predictive factors to guide researchers. *Academic Medicine* 92: 222–228.

2 Frechtling, J. (2002). Section IIIa. An overview of quantitative and qualitative data collection methods: some tips and comparisons. In: *The 2002 User Friendly Handbook for Project Evaluation* (ed. J. Frechtling), 43–49. Arlington, VA: The National Science Foundation.

3 Cleland, J.A., Poobalan, A., and Durning, S.J. (2022). Needs assessment. In: *Survey Methods for Medical and Health Professions Education: A Six-Step Approach* (ed. A.W. Phillips, S.T. Durning, and A.R. Artino), 5–19. Philadelphia, PA: Elsevier.

4 Schwarz, N. (1999). Self-reports: the questions shape the answers. *American Psychologist* 54 (2): 93–105.

5 Gehlbach, H. and Artino, A.R. (2018). The survey checklist (manifesto). *Academic Medicine* 90 (3): 360–366.

6 Grice, P. (1975). Logic and conversation. In: *Syntax and Semantics*, Speech Acts, vol. 3 (ed. P. Cole and J. Morgan), 41–58. New York, NY: Academic Press.

7 Tourangeau, R., Rips, L.J., and Rasinski, K. (2000). *The Psychology of Survey Response*. New York, NY: Cambridge University Press.

8 Cook, D.A. (2022). Establishing evidence. In: *Survey Methods for Medical and Health Professions Education:*
A Six-Step Approach (ed. A.W. Phillips, S.T. Durning, and A.R. Artino), 37–53. Philadelphia, PA: Elsevier.

9 Phillips, A.W. and Artino, A.R. (2017). Lies, damned lies, and surveys. *Journal of Graduate Medical Education* 9: 677–679.

10 Artino, A.R., La Rochelle, J.S., Dezee, K.J., and Gehlbach, H. (2014). Developing questionnaires for educational research: AMEE guide no. 87. *Medical Teacher* 36 (6): 463–474.

11 Gehlbach, H. and Brinkworth, M.E. (2011). Measure twice, cut down error: a process for enhancing the validity of survey scales. *Review of General Psychology* 15: 380–387.

12 Younas, A. and Porr, C. (2018). A step-by-step approach to developing survey research. *Nurse Researcher* 26 (3): 14–19.

13 LaRochelle, J. and Artino, A.R. (2022). Survey construction. In: *Survey Methods for Medical and Health Professions Education: A Six-Step Approach* (ed. A.W. Phillips, S.T. Durning, and A.R. Artino), 19–36. Philadelphia, PA: Elsevier.

14 Burrell, Nancy A., and DeAnne Priddis (2017). *The SAGE Encyclopedia of Communication Research Methods* Vol. 4. Thousand Oaks, CA: SAGE Publications, Inc.

15 Dykema, J., Schaeffer, N.C., Garbarski, D. et al. (2022). Toward a reconsidering of the use of agree-disagree questions in measuring subjective evaluations. *Research in Social and Administrative Pharmacy* 18 (2): 2335–2344.

16 Sullivan, G.M. and Artino, A.R. (2017). How to create a bad survey instrument. *Journal of Graduate Medical Education* 9 (4): 411–415.

17 Artino, A.R. (2017). Good decisions cannot be made from bad surveys. *Military Medicine* 182 (1–2): 1464–1465.

18 Willis, G.B. (2016). Questionnaire pretesting. In: *The SAGE Handbook of Survey Methodology* (ed. S. Wolf, D. Joye, T. Smith, and F. Yang-chih), 359–381. Los Angeles: SAGE Publications.

19 Willis, G.B. and Artino, A.R. (2013). What do our respondents think we're asking? Using cognitive interviewing to improve medical education surveys. *Journal of Graduate Medical Education* 5 (3): 353–356.

20 Abu Hassan, Z., Schattner, P., and Mazza, D. Doing a pilot study: why is it essential? *Malaysian Family Physician* 1 (2–3): 70–73.

21 Thabane, L., Ma, J., Chu, R. et al. (2010). A tutorial on pilot studies: the what, why and how. *BMC Medical Research Methodology* 10 (1).

22 Connelly, L.M. (2008). Pilot studies. *Medsurg Nursing* 17 (6): 411–412.

23 Mavis, B.E., Phillips, A.W., and Durning, S.J. (2022). Data analysis. In: *Survey Methods for Medical and Health Professions Education: A Six-Step Approach* (ed. A.W. Phillips, S.T. Durning, and A.R. Artino), 65–82. Philadelphia, PA: Elsevier.

21 Experimental methods: more than simply testing hypotheses

Peter Yeates and Rebecca Edwards

Learning objectives

By then end of this chapter, you should be able to:
- Justify the use of experiments in clinical education research.
- Explain when it is appropriate to use experimental methods.

- Follow a step-by-step approach to design valid experiments.

Introduction

In this chapter, we will discuss what an experiment is, why you may (or may not) want to use them, and the fundamental components of experimental design. By the end of this chapter, you should be able to design a basic experiment and understand the key limitations of this approach.

What is an experiment?

An experiment can be defined as 'an operation or procedure carried out under controlled conditions in order to discover an unknown effect or law, to test or establish a hypothesis, or to illustrate a known law' [1]. Each word of that definition is critical, and we will unpack it throughout this chapter.

Experiments are a useful research methodology which, when employed diligently, are able to answer questions and provide insights that are otherwise unavailable by alternate means. However, ensuring that your experiment provides valid results is not straightforward. Many new researchers have fallen into the trap of assuming that an experiment will be simple: 'I'll just compare what happens when I give this intervention to some people and not others'. What could be simpler? Yet, well-conducted experiments are almost never simple; poorly conducted experiments can produce results which offer an illusion of truth which is far from fulfilled. So, whilst experiments are not usually

complex, conducting them well is complicated as they rely on intricate attention to detail across numerous potential sources of bias. This is defined as any intentional or unintentional tendency or action that prevents unprejudiced consideration of a question and potentially leads to false conclusions. This may occur at any stage of research, including design, data collection, data analysis, interpretation, or publication [2, 3].

To experiment or not?

Experiments investigate *causality*, the relationship between variable(s) and an outcome, whereby a change in variable A (or combination of variables) leads to a change in outcome B. They can be a way of demonstrating that A causes B, rather than A and B being related or co-occurring (e.g. 'good sleep causes better memory retention in learners, rather than people with good memories also happen to sleep well'). Experiments also allow you to quantify the magnitude of effects: this amount of A will cause that amount of B. Or, perhaps more usefully, A and B both cause C to increase, but A has a larger influence on C than B. For example, surgical students learning with computerised virtual patients showed a 30.6-point increase in test scores versus students experiencing small-group teaching, who showed a 9.7-point increase [4]. Lastly, and perhaps most importantly, experiments enable researchers to measure the influence of effects which people either

---

Starting Research in Clinical Education, First Edition. Edited by Eliot L. Rees, Alison Ledger, and Kim A. Walker.
© 2024 The Association for the Study of Medical Education (ASME). Published 2024 by John Wiley & Sons Ltd.
Companion website: www.wiley.com/go/clinicaleducation

have no insight into or cannot reliably report. For example, if you want to know whether examiners score candidates fairly, regardless of their ethnicity, it is unlikely that just asking them will be sufficient; they may believe they score fairly, but still have unconscious bias. As a result, a carefully conducted experiment is required to determine this effect [5]. Numerous influences on our thinking, learning and behaviour operate beyond our conscious awareness and consequently experiments are the only way to determine how they operate.

There are also shortcomings to experiments. First, their artificiality. In order to isolate, control, and compare, it is usually necessary to remove the object of study from its natural environment and simulate or replicate it in a controlled environment. As a result, we end up with high certainty that A causes B . . . in a laboratory setting. This requires researchers to argue why the effects they have observed in the laboratory will be generalisable to the real world. Triangulating findings with observational data from practice can help, but the lack of implicit generalisability of laboratory experiments remains their biggest limitation, especially given that context is so important in education [6].

Secondly, experiments are a poor means to research complexity. Educational settings usually involve the interaction of a myriad of ill-defined variables which produce a richly complex environment. Experiments necessarily isolate a few of these and study their interaction. Therefore, experiments tend to be reductionist in the answers they give.

As a result, we assert that experiments are best used within a programme of research which explores related phenomena through several means. Realism (see Chapter 10) offers an accommodating philosophical perspective by which to blend such findings, although philosophical pragmatism [7] will also happily blend findings from post-positivist and constructivist approaches.

Seven steps to designing experiments

Through the rest of this chapter, we will take you through a step-by-step approach to designing valid experiments.

Step 1: hypothesis

All good quality research relies on a well-constructed research question (see Chapter 2), developed by identifying the gap in what is already known and using theory to postulate how the phenomenon of interest might operate. Experiments go a step further in that they answer one or more precise hypotheses.

A hypothesis is a precise prediction which your experiment will test.

Hypotheses are traditionally expressed with a direction – 'flipped classroom teaching will cause students' grades to increase', as opposed to 'flipped classroom teaching will influence students' grades'. The direction of your hypothesis should be based on your theory (derived from literature) but you should still consider the potential for the opposite outcome and run a two-tailed test [8].

More precisely, you should include your comparator – 'The magnitude of B will be greater in the presence of A than the absence of A'. For example, 'Physiology exam scores will be greater for students who have ingested two cups of coffee than those who have avoided caffeine'. This makes it absolutely clear how the causal relationship will be determined.

Hypotheses can also express interacting relationships of causality: 'A's tendency to increase B will be greater when C is present than when C is absent', i.e. 'The increase in physiology exam scores produced by caffeine versus no caffeine will be greater in the presence of sugared snacks than the absence of sugared snacks'. In this example, the hypothesis is testing what is known as a *factorial relationship*, or the synergistic impact of two interventions combined. Hypotheses tend to be phrased in a future tense, as predictions, which are at the heart of the hypothetico-deductive method. Theory is used to develop predictions, expressed in the form of hypotheses; empirical evidence is obtained to confirm or refute the prediction.

An experiment can test several hypotheses simultaneously. A number of interacting hypotheses within the same experiment can often provide much more detailed theoretical insight into a phenomenon than a single hypothesis. Similarly, a sprawling mass of weakly theorised hypotheses provides a mess which is unlikely to be informative. It is critical you have a strong theoretical basis as to why you have posed your hypotheses. You will exert a lot of effort testing them and it would be helpful if the answer will have importance regardless of what you find. A good hypothesis emerges from a position of equipoise: there are equally good reasons why the hypothesis may or may not be true. This might be because competing theories offer opposite predictions which need to be empirically resolved, confirm assumptions when there is important need to do so, or usefully contradict assumptions in a way which would alter understanding. Regardless, spend time carefully developing your hypotheses so that you can clearly and rigorously answer your research question(s).

Step 2: control

The ability to compare participants exposed to the intervention with those in the control group is the crux of experiments. The control condition is equal to the intervention group in all meaningful ways other than the presence of the intervention. This equality enables you to logically conclude that any difference observed between the intervention and control groups is most likely caused by the intervention. If the control and intervention groups are not functionally equivalent, then any observed difference may be *confounded*, that is the difference may be due to differences between the groups rather than the effect of the intervention. As a result, the test of the hypothesis will be invalid.

As humans, we are pre-disposed to spuriously attribute causality to all manner of uncontrolled observations, a tendency known as 'illusion of causality' [9]. In an educational setting, you may find people making assertions along the lines of 'we used (for example) virtual-reality based simulation, and the students scored very highly in their assessments'. Our implicit tendency is then to assume the virtual reality simulation caused this strong performance, but it is important to remember that the co-occurrence of two variables does not necessarily mean a causal relationship is present (you may have previously heard the phrase 'correlation does not equal causation'). Logically, we can see this group of students may simply have been very capable and would have performed strongly without virtual reality simulation, or, further, perhaps might have performed better still had other teaching methods been used. Possibly virtual reality simulation reduced their performance. Without a control group for comparison, we cannot tell which explanation is correct. Moreover, education differs from other general interventions in that learners will almost always learn something, regardless of intervention efficacy [10]. Therefore, the simple demonstration of learning following an intervention can be meaningless, as almost any education intervention will show some effect. This makes it vital, in an educational setting, to ensure the presence of a realistic control group for comparison to clearly establish intervention efficacy.

The control needs to be equal to the intervention group and unless you have exactly the same individuals at the same moment in time, under exactly the same conditions, then your control is arguably different to the intervention group. As achieving this is impossible, the best way to achieve this is for the control group to be identical in all meaningful ways. In practical terms, this relies on making a judgement about which parameters might plausibly confound

the observation and ensuring they are equal. As a field evolves, disciplines gain a clearer sense of the parameters which must be controlled, but for a new area, it is your responsibility to spend time thinking carefully about what effects could be present, and how these can be controlled.

In educational settings, historical control groups (i.e. comparing against previous year groups) are rarely effective because variation due to different groups of individuals, or variation due to the effects of time, are both frequently capable of confounding the effects of interest. So, a better way is required to allocate individuals to intervention and control groups.

Step 3: randomise

Allocating people to two groups (intervention and control) has the potential to create groups which are, in fact, unequal and will therefore confound the test of the hypothesis. If participants self-select, then those with a preference for the intervention will volunteer, perhaps because they are already capable of the task in question. As a result, they may naturally outperform those who opt for the control group. If you pick those who arrive first, you may select those who are most motivated, again confounding your observation. If you pick alphabetically, you may inadvertently allocate people of different race or social class to your different groups [11]. If a teacher selects students to participate in an intervention which they believe will be beneficial, then they may select those they like (who may be more capable) or those who they think are most in need (and therefore potentially less capable), or unconscious biases that they are unaware of may influence their choices. However they pick, it is unlikely to be neutral, and therefore likely to confound. All of these confounds are examples of what we might term *confounding by indication* [12], namely whilst it appears that being in the intervention group caused an observation, it was actually the reason why they were in the intervention group which caused the observation.

The only way to avoid these biases is through randomisation [13]; in all other cases, there will be some level of bias in group allocation which will likely confound (see Chapter 6).

Randomisation ensures the absence of systematic reasons for anyone to be allocated to one group rather than another, but does that necessarily ensure that your intervention and control groups will be equal? Unfortunately, not. Randomness can, and does, produce clusters. This can potentially result in imbalance between your groups in any of the characteristics you consider important (a feature we will return to later) although with larger sample sizes this rarely occurs in practical terms. Additionally, and more often problematically, randomness can cause uneven group sizes (for example, 65% of participants randomised to the control group and only 35% randomised to the intervention group). This will have significant impact on your analysis.

The way to avoid this depends on how participants are recruited. If all your participants are available before you start, then after randomly allocating them, you can simply check that the group sizes are roughly equal, and, if needed, repeat the randomisation before the study begins. If (as is often the case in experiments or trials) participants are recruited sequentially and randomised at the point of enrolment, then there is a real possibility of randomly allocated groups becoming uneven over time. This will (at best) affect the power of your study or can even introduce a time-series bias if the majority of participants in the intervention group were enrolled either early or late in the study.

To avoid group imbalance, researchers often use 'block randomisation' [14, 15] in which participant allocation is initially random but is forced to balance by a specified number of participants (i.e. a block). This avoids both significant imbalance in groups sizes and time-series biases. Similarly, if you have good theoretical grounds to suspect that one subset of participants will behave differently to another subset (for example, graduate students versus undergraduate), then you may opt to use stratified randomisation in which you first allocate new participants to groups based on the relevant characteristic (i.e. whether undergraduate or postgraduate) and then randomise participants separately within each strata. This avoids the potential situation where 80% of the participants who received the intervention also turned out to be postgraduate students. Notably, with block randomisation and large numbers of participants, the latter is unlikely to occur.

Randomness can and does produce clusters. This should be assessed before you analyse your results, by determining how important 'baseline characteristics' (i.e. values which describe relevant parameters which are not the main focus of the hypothesis, but which could produce confounding effects) compare between your intervention and control groups. Typical baseline characteristics for students include demographic data, prior educational attainment, socioeconomic status, or any other factors that are considered important to ensure groups are equal at baseline. For example, if you are using an experiment to compare how a new web-based study platform influences end of year exam scores compared with traditional learning in pharmacy undergraduates in a rural campus, you should probably gather prior educational attainment and quality of internet access as baseline data since both could confound your observation if they are unevenly distributed between groups. In an ideal world, baseline characteristics would be compared after randomisation and before the intervention is administered. Practically, this is rarely feasible, so baseline characteristics are typically compared prior to analysis. By this stage, it is too late to repeat the randomisation if groups are unequal, but it may be possible to adjust for any differences which are observed. The important thing is to have specified and collected the relevant characteristics.

Step 4: sampling and power

Before you can randomise individuals to groups, you need to recruit them. As with all research, you should define the population of interest, determine how you wish to sample that population, and define a strategy to recruit people based on your sample (see Chapter 6). Whilst in most research, sampling aims to maximise the representativeness of your sample to the wider population, sample size in experiments is focused more on whether you have sufficient participants to be able to reliably measure differences between your intervention and control groups, with external representativeness secondary (although still important).

It is important to make sure your study is likely to find an effect if one exists in the target population. The number of participants you need is determined by an established relationship between a small number of variables, based on *statistical power*.

To calculate your required sample size for a simple two group design, you will need:
- The minimally important difference expected for your study.
- An estimation of variance or standard deviation.
- Desired power.
- Desired error rate.

The latter two are the easiest to establish. Power is the likelihood of finding an effect in a sample if it indeed exists in the population. As a general rule, most studies opt for the conventional power level of 80% [16], and generally there is no need to alter this. Error rate relates to your desired level of statistical significance when you conduct your analysis. The conventional choice for error rate tends to be 0.05 [16, 17]. Therefore, practically, you usually only need to know two things to do a power calculation: minimally important difference between your groups and the likely standard deviation of your sample.

Minimally important difference and estimation of variance will require a little more effort. First, you need to establish a reasonable estimate of how much variability you would expect in your measurements (e.g. standard deviation). Existing literature may be able to guide you here (if available), otherwise you may need pilot data.

Ultimately, you need to determine how big or small of a difference you wish to detect (or the minimally important difference). In education, there is often no preagreed difference, so it requires judgement. This may be based on knowledge and experience with the topic, prior literature, or pilot data.

As an additional note, the type of statistical test you wish to use will also impact the power calculation, as this calculation is an estimation of how the test is likely to perform [17]. Therefore, it is important to decide at this early stage how you intend to analyse your data (see Chapter 22).

Unfortunately, more complex designs (repeated measures, crossover, or hierarchical designs) do not conform to this formula, and estimating power requires statistical simulation which can be complex. Sometimes researchers will use a rule of thumb, based on a simpler design, although this is likely to underestimate the power of the study (or conversely, require you to recruit more participants than was strictly necessary). In practical terms, it would be unusual to be able to complete a valid experiment with less than 20–30 participants, even if you are only trying to find a moderate to large difference, and it may require hundreds or even thousands of participants to find small differences. The complexity of the design has an important bearing on this, and whilst factorial experiments (such as the caffeine/sugar snacks example above) can be theoretically very informative, they tend to require very large sample sizes. The pragmatic experimentalist, having found an interesting hypothesis, will judge whether they are likely to be able to obtain a sufficient sample size (having estimated a standard deviation and minimally important difference) before deciding whether it is a study they have the means to pursue. For all new researchers, we would advise working with a statistician on these issues.

Step 5: manipulate or (administer)

Having constructed two randomly allocated groups, who are equivalent in all meaningful ways, the next step of an experiment is to manipulate (or administer the intervention to) the intervention group.

To ensure that you test your hypothesis in a valid manner, ensure participants in the intervention group receive the intended intervention (the correct 'stuff', rather than something a bit different), in the correct dose (enough of it, not too much), that they actually receive or experience the intervention in the intended manner (they do not somehow avoid it) and the exposure to the intervention lasts for a sufficient duration to be able to measure its influence whilst its effect is still present. Generally, researchers will need to devise a valid means of manipulation which addresses all of these elements, unless a method has already been devised by similar, or previous research. As a result, planning how to manipulate participants in the intervention group of an experiment can be the most difficult but often the most fun and creative element of designing and conducting experimental research.

There are several measures you can take to help you get this right. First, pilot the manipulation. Try out repeated versions of different approaches and measure the influence on the intended construct with each. You will need to obtain ethical approval prior to this kind of experimentation on human participants. This pilot work is immensely valuable but is often omitted for reasons of time or to avoid using up members of a limited potential participant pool. Pretesting, perhaps using informal interviews, can support the construct and explore potential unintended consequences prior to conducting the main study. Piloting may be omitted if you are confident the manipulation will work but you should include a 'manipulation check' within the study. This is some measure or demonstration that participants engaged with or received the manipulation in the intended manner and (ideally) it did indeed induce the intended cognitive, emotional, or physiological state. A successful manipulation check greatly adds to the validity of the study and should be included wherever practical. Caution may be needed though, as sometimes a manipulation check can have the perverse consequence of diminishing or neutralising the effect that it has measured (see example in Box 21.1). In this instance, you may be better to pilot the intervention separately and rely on the pilot to assert that the manipulation is likely to be effective.

A frequent concern within experiments is how knowledge of the manipulation may influence participants' behaviour. This can make them either suppress or exaggerate particular behaviours, whether deliberately for reasons of social desirability, or due to the Hawthorne effect (where observation of people's behaviour changes how they act [19]). This may then confound the experiment. For this reason, it is often beneficial to conceal information about the intervention to prevent this effect. Sometimes this can be simply achieved by withholding information (i.e. by not telling participants which intervention they have received). Often

BOX 21.1   Example of a manipulation check going wrong

A (never published) study, which one of the authors contributed to, involved manipulating whether examiners felt happy or sad before they judged students' performances. The aim was to determine the effect of different emotions on their judgement. Having obtained ethical approval, examiners were successfully manipulated through an 'autobiographical writing task' which involved writing about previous experiences which were either happy or sad in order to induce that emotional state [18]. They then completed an emotion questionnaire as a manipulation check. This (as expected) showed a clear difference in emotional state between the 'happy' and 'sad' groups of examiners, but the survey seemed to cause the examiners to reflect on their mood and neutralise it, as a repeat version of the survey later in the study showed no difference in emotional state between the two groups. As a result, it was unclear whether participants in the happy or sad groups really were happy or sad whilst they scored the test performances and so it wasn't clear whether the intended construct had been manipulated and (by extension) the hypothesis tested. This could have occurred because the manipulation check gave the game away, or because the manipulation was not strong enough or wore off for another reason. Either way, as the study failed to successfully manipulate the hypothesised construct, the hypothesis remained untested.

though, the manipulation is self-evident and then more elaborate strategies may be needed to effectively conceal the intervention. One means of achieving this is through deception, in which participants are told that researchers are studying one thing, whereas they are actually studying another. For example, in a study testing, the influence of students' ethnicity on examiners' judgements, we deceived examiners by simply telling them we were researching aspects of the way that examiners make judgements [5]. The deceptive premise often serves to occupy participants' focus, such that they do not realise the true premise, so avoids confounding.

Generally deceptive premises are considered ethical as long as: their use is adequately justified; the procedures aren't harmful; and participants receive a structured debrief which includes the chance to withdraw their consent once they know the true premise. The debrief should include a stage where participants are asked what they think the study is

testing (to see whether they guessed the true premise), they are then told the true premise and purpose of the study, including reasons for deception, and then their further consent is sought. Guidelines for using deceptive premises in research should be followed [20].

You may opt to maximise the strength of the manipulation in the first study you conduct, to maximise the chance of finding an effect, if the manipulation is not expected to be harmful, before looking for subtler (possibly more realistic) effects in follow up work. Conversely, if the manipulation could be harmful, then the opposite strategy must be employed, with the minimal feasible dose and gradual escalation. Importantly, a control that consists of nothing at all is rarely realistic in educational settings; it is usually much more meaningful to compare the intervention against a realistic alternative (for example the existing method of teaching) [21]. More generally, experimental control does not need to be 'intervention' versus 'nothing'; it can be option *A* versus option *B*. In this case in which there is no neutral control, there is a controlled comparison of the relative effect of two different interventions.

It is also important to consider the influence of workload of your intervention on your potential participants during manipulation design, and how this may impact your study overall. For example, when working with clinicians it is important to consider the high intensity and time constraints of their role, so a lengthy intervention would likely discourage participation or cause a high drop out by these individuals. It is therefore important to balance the time and effort required of your participants with the efficacy of your manipulation of choice.

Step 6: measure

Having successfully manipulated the intervention group, you then need to measure the relevant construct (i.e. the 'thing' that you have hypothesised that the intervention will influence) in each member or instance of both the intervention and control groups. This will provide the data which you will compare to finally answer your hypothesis. Measuring the intended construct can be very simple or very difficult. Many constructs in education are abstract and rely on a proxy measure, which the researchers assert is a valid representation of the construct of interest. For example, if researchers wish to compare the influence of an intervention on the growth of knowledge, they may use a multiple-choice knowledge test as their measure. Scores on the test are a proxy for actual growth of students' knowledge and as a result the success of the measure relies on how well the test actually measures knowledge. Many potential experiments fail to get going because researchers cannot think of a means to operationalise a measure of the construct they want to compare.

Where possible you should use measures or scales whose psychometric properties are already known. This reduces the need to justify the validity of the measurements you make. If no such measure exists, then you must support the validity of the measure. This may be through scale development work, pre-testing, think-aloud methods, or showing they are already used in the anticipated way by the participant population. Think about how any measure you develop can be analysed, for example whether it will produce categorical, ordinal or interval data [22] and what implications this will have.

Consider where error may arise in the measurement process and how you can either limit its extent, or, alternatively, ensure that it balances across groups. This is particularly important if the measure relies on judgements by third-party raters or judges (i.e. people whose role is to make the measurement of participants rather than to participate in either the intervention or control groups). Try to keep judges or raters from knowing which condition they are judging (intervention or control group), so this knowledge does not bias their judgement. Devise procedures to balance the influence of individual judges (or groups of judges) across intervention and control groups. For example, you might video students from both the intervention and control performing a task, and then ask a judge to score an even mix of performances from both groups in random order, whilst concealing which group each performance came from. This will keep the judge from knowing the study condition and ensure that any systematic tendency this judge has to give either high or low scores will balance evenly across both groups, thereby avoiding a confound. The process of presenting stimuli in a balanced order is known as *counterbalancing*. If the measure you choose has low reliability (i.e. there is a lot of additional noise around the signal it produces), this will add to the sampling requirements or reduce your statistical power, so trying to select a fairly reliable measure is always helpful.

Step 7: compare
You have your study data and are finally ready to make the comparison which will answer your hypothesis. However, there are final checks you should consider to avoid further potential sources of confounding (see Figure 21.1).

Cleanse your data (i.e. remove incomplete, corrupted, or duplicate data), and then compare baseline

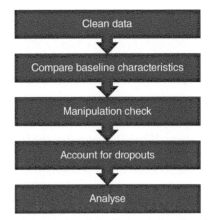

Figure 21.1 Process of final checks for confounds prior to formal comparisons within experimental design.

characteristics of the participants to ensure your intervention and control groups were indeed equivalent at baseline in the ways you specified. If they are not, this complicates things, but you may be able to account for substantial differences through covariate analyses to determine whether or not they confounded any observed differences.

On examining your manipulation check, does it show the intended pattern of response in the intervention group and their absence in the control group. This should provide the confidence your groups were indeed manipulated as intended.

It is vital you account for dropouts. Ensure that you have a record of all the participants at each stage of the study: who was screened, volunteered, enrolled, randomised, received the intervention/control, and completed the study (see part 13 of the CONSORT guidelines [23] for a fuller description of accounting for participants). Whilst it is normal for some participants to drop out of the study (i.e. withdraw or fail to complete), uneven participant dropouts can confound your study. Imagine a situation where randomisation creates two even groups, but many of the less able participants then withdraw from the intervention. The high average ability of the remaining more-able participants will confound the observation. You should compare dropout rates between groups and, where necessary, look at baseline characteristics of those who dropped out. If your study aims to determine the effectiveness of an intervention, then consider using an 'intention-to-treat' analysis, which accounts for those who did not complete when determining overall effectiveness [24]. Only once you have completed these baseline checks should you go on to compare your main hypotheses.

Statistical methods will be used to compare the measurements between the intervention and control group, determined by a mixture of elementary statistics (categorical, ordinal or interval data, parametric or nonparametric) and the experimental design you have chosen (see Chapter 22).

Summary

This chapter has briefly outlined the principles of conducting experiments and when it is appropriate to use them. It has also included the fundamental principles of good experimental design, including the key components of: hypothesis construction; control; randomisation; sample size; variable manipulation; outcome measurement and how to compare groups characteristics. You should now have the tools to design a basic experiment. On the companion website, we offer a series of practical recommendations based on our own experience of successful (and not so successful) experiments in clinical education, including a discussion and demonstration of conducting experiments over the internet, an example of sample calculation using G*Power, a practical demonstration of randomisation, and description of several different experimental designs and description of their pros and cons.

We hope that this will provide useful practical advice to take these principles forward.

Top tips

- Enlist the help of a statistician especially in a complex design experiment. The sooner the better.
- Deploy pilot work prior to conducting an experiment. This helps to ensure the experiment runs well.
- Employ measures or scales whose psychometric properties are already known. This means you can refer to previous work.

Common pitfalls

- Improper use of, or lack of control group. Where possible, check that your intervention and control group are similar on important baseline characteristics, before introducing your intervention.
- In education, a realistic alternative may be better than no control.
- Lack of an operationalised measure of your construct. Where possible, use a measure that has been previously tested.

Ethical issues

- Ensure use of deceptive premises are justified and guidelines followed.
- Use of manipulation must be controlled.
- Ethical approval is required, even for piloting.

References

1 Merriam-Webster (2021). Experiment. Merriam-Webster.com dictionary: Merriam-Webster Incorporated. https://www.merriam-webster.com/dictionary/experiment (accessed 10 May 2023).

2 Simundić, A.M. (2013). Bias in research. *Biochemia Medica* 23 (1): 12–15.

3 Pannucci, C.J. and Wilkins, E.G. (2010). Identifying and avoiding bias in research. *Plastic and Reconstructive Surgery* 126 (2): 619–625.

4 Seifert, L.B., Socolan, O., Sader, R. et al. (2019). Virtual patients versus small-group teaching in the training of oral and maxillofacial surgery: a randomized controlled trial. *BMC Medical Education* 19 (1): 1–10.

5 Yeates, P., Woolf, K., Benbow, E. et al. (2017). A randomised trial of the influence of racial stereotype bias on examiners' scores, feedback and recollections in undergraduate clinical exams. *BMC Medicine* 15 (1): 179.

6 Regehr, G. (2010). It's NOT rocket science: rethinking our metaphors for research in health professions education. *Medical Education* 44 (1): 31–39.

7 Moon, K. and Blackman, D. (2014). A guide to understanding social science research for natural scientists. *Conservation Biology* 28 (5): 1167–1177.

8 Ringwalt, C., Paschall, M.J., Gorman, D. et al. (2011). The use of one- versus two-tailed tests to evaluate prevention programs. *Evaluation & the Health Professions* 34 (2): 135–150.

9 Matute, H., Yarritu, I., and Vadillo, M.A. (2011). Illusions of causality at the heart of pseudoscience. *British Journal of Psychology* 102 (3): 392–405.

10 Cook, D.A. (2012). If you teach them, they will learn: why medical education needs comparative effectiveness research. *Advances in Health Sciences Education* 17: 305–310.

11 Cauley, A. and Zax, J.S. (2018). Alphabetism: the effects of surname initial and the cost of being otherwise undistinguished. SSRN: https://ssrncom/abstract=3272556 or http://dx.doi.org/10.2139/ssrn.3272556 (accessed 10 May 2023).

12 Kyriacou, D.N. and Lewis, R.J. (2016). Confounding by indication in clinical research. *Journal of the American Medical Association* 316 (17): 1818–1819.

13 Altman, D.G. and Bland, J.M. (1999). Treatment allocation in controlled trials: why randomise? *BMJ* 318 (7192): 1209.

14 Altman, D.G. and Bland, J.M. (1999). How to randomise. *BMJ* 319 (7211): 703–704.

15 Sedgwick, P. (2011). Block randomisation. *BMJ* 343: d7139.

16 Hickey, G.L., Grant, S.W., Dunning, J., and Siepe, M. (2018). Statistical primer: sample size and power calculations – why, when and how? *European Journal of Cardio-Thoracic Surgery* 54 (1): 4–9.

17 Jones, S., Carley, S., and Harrison, M. (2003). An introduction to power and sample size estimation. *Emergency Medicine Journal* 20 (5): 453.

18 Mills, C. and D'Mello, S. (2014). On the validity of the autobiographical emotional memory task for emotion induction. *PLoS One* 9 (4): e95837.

19 McCarney, R., Warner, J., Iliffe, S. et al. (2007). The Hawthorne effect: a randomised, controlled trial. *BMC Medical Research Methodology* 7: 30.

20 Oates, J., Carpenter, D., Fisher, M. et al. (2021). *BPS Code of Human Research Ethics*. British Psychological Society.

21 Cook, D.A. and Beckman, T.J. (2010). Reflections on experimental research in medical education. *Advances in Health Sciences Education* 15 (3): 455–464.

22 Streiner, D.L., Norman, G.R., and Cairney, J. (2015). Scaling responses. In: *Health Measurement Scales: A Practical Guide to Their Development and Use*, 38–73. USA: Oxford University Press.

23 Moher, D., Hopewell, S., Schulz, K.F. et al. (2010). CONSORT 2010 Explanation and Elaboration: updated guidelines for reporting parallel group randomised trials. *BMJ* 340: c869.

24 Hollis, S. and Campbell, F. (1999). What is meant by intention to treat analysis? Survey of published randomised controlled trials. *BMJ* 319 (7211): 670–674.

22 Statistical analysis: unpacking uncertainty

Christy K. Boscardin, H. Carrie Chen, and Justin L. Sewell

Learning objectives

By the end of this chapter, you should be able to:
- Distinguish between descriptive and inferential statistics.
- Identify and select the appropriate descriptive statistics to summarise and present your data.
- Describe and select the appropriate statistical methods associated with inferential statistics.
- Define the sources of error and how to minimise bias in statistical analysis.

Introduction

As you conduct research, you gather empirical data for analysis. Statistics is the science that pertains to the collection, organisation, analysis, interpretation, and presentation of your data.

It is rarely practical or feasible to research the entire population of interest (see Chapter 6). Therefore, a sample of the population of interest is usually taken (Figure 22.1). Data are then collected from the participants in the sample. There are two major types of statistics that can be used to analyse and report these data; *descriptive statistics* summarise and describe the data in the sample and *inferential statistics* enable you to make inferences about the whole population of interest based on the data from your sample group. These inferences cannot be certain, and so with these statistics a probability is calculated to find if the inference is true. The challenges of uncertainty are particularly relevant in clinical education research which often involves greater randomness and unquantifiable influences than, for example, laboratory experiments. This chapter will discuss statistics with this in mind, providing recommendations for addressing uncertainty, including reporting measures of imprecision (e.g. standard errors and confidence intervals) and considering not only statistical significance (e.g. *p*-values) but also the range of likely values for the true values when determining the significance of an intervention. Statistical support, be it from a statistician or supervisor with relevant experience, is

invaluable at every phase of the process, including study planning, statistical analysis and interpretation, and results presentation.

Descriptive statistics

The purpose of descriptive statistics is to provide a summary of the data on one group without necessarily drawing conclusions based on comparisons or relationships between/among groups. This summary can be in the form of numerical descriptions such as means and percentages or in the form of visual or graphic representations such as histograms and box plots. More simply, it involves the analysis and description of a single variable (univariate analysis) or multiple variables (multivariate analysis). We will explain the different types of data researchers collect and how individual variables can be described (univariate analysis), including descriptions of frequency, central tendency, and dispersion, together with common graphic representations of these descriptions.

Types of data
Data collected can be of two types: quantitative or categorical. The procedures for describing and graphically depicting these data differ. Quantitative data (e.g. number of participants, time, age, and exam score) can be discrete or continuous. Discrete data have gaps between values and typically come from counts such as the number of objects. One can

---

Starting Research in Clinical Education, First Edition. Edited by Eliot L. Rees, Alison Ledger, and Kim A. Walker.
© 2024 The Association for the Study of Medical Education (ASME). Published 2024 by John Wiley & Sons Ltd.
Companion website: www.wiley.com/go/clinicaleducation

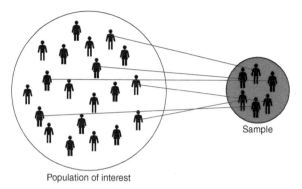

Population of interest

Figure 22.1 Sample of a population of interest.

have 11 or 12 books but not 11.5 books. Continuous data can assume any value between two values within a dataset and typically come from measurements. A bag of books can weigh 3 or 4kg or any amount in between such as 3.6kg. All quantitative data allows the meaningful subtraction of one value from another (12−11 books=1 book, or 4−3.6kg=0.4kg). In practice, many researchers treat both discrete and continuous quantitative data as continuous data in the analysis.

In contrast, categorical data describe attributes or properties of an object that can be categorised (e.g. gender, institution, and faculty rank). At times, these categories may be assigned numeric values, but the numeric values themselves hold no meaning (for example three different institutions assigned numeric values of 1, 2 and 3 for the analysis, but these values hold no intrinsic meaning). Categorical data may be *nominal* or *ordinal*. Nominal data cannot be ordered (e.g. institution in the above example). Ordinal data can be put in meaningful order (e.g. faculty rank or grades). Some ordinal scale data, such as data from the commonly used Likert scale (see Chapter 20), are often treated as continuous quantitative data for analysis [1]. While this is increasingly accepted practice in clinical education research and in some disciplines [1, 2], there is disagreement in the broader literature whether or not this is appropriate [1] and other fields have been slow to adopt this approach [3].

Frequency

The frequency distribution is a summary of the frequency of individual values or ranges of values for that variable. This can be reported in a frequency table for either quantitative or categorical data. Frequencies can be presented as absolute frequencies (e.g. number of respondents identifying as male) and/or relative frequencies (e.g. percent of respondents identifying as male). In general, relative frequencies can be more useful and

most researchers report both (e.g. 36 [45%] respondents identified as male).

Central tendency

Central tendency provides information about the centre of the distribution of values for a quantitative variable. There are three main measures: mean, median, and mode. The mean is the average of all values in the distribution – the sum of all values divided by the total number of values. The median is the middle point of the distribution – the value that divides the distribution into two equal halves or the 50th percentile. In a distribution with an odd number of values, it is the middle value. In an even number of values in the distribution, the median is the average of the two middle values. The mode is the most frequently occurring value in the distribution.

For example, in a sample of 10 students with the following exam scores: 70, 75, 76, 79, 80, 80, 82, 83, 86, 90, the mean, median, and mode are all 80. When they are all the same, the data is *normally distributed* (i.e. symmetric bell-shaped distribution of data where most values cluster towards the middle). In this instance, the best measure of central tendency is the mean.

However, if the sample of the same students had exam scores of 29, 70, 75, 76, 79, 81, 82, 82, 86, 90, the mean is 75, the median is (79+81)/2=80, and the mode is 82. The score of 29 is a datapoint that differs significantly from the others; this is known as an 'outlier'. The distribution is described as *asymmetric* (skewed), and the median can be a better measure of central tendency. Skewness can be best appreciated by viewing a frequency plot; if the plot does not reveal a bell-like structure or has a longer tail on one side, the data are likely to be skewed. When reporting on the central tendency of a single item measured with a Likert-type scale (e.g. 1=strongly disagree to 5=strongly agree), median or mode is commonly used. However, if several Likert-type items are combined to create a composite (sum of all responses) score (e.g. 5 item composite with 5-point Likert-type scale can range from 5 to 25), then mean is an appropriate measure of central tendency.

Dispersion

Dispersion refers to the spread of, or variation, in values for a quantitative dataset. Common measures of dispersion include range and standard deviation. The range is the spread between the highest and lowest values. In the previous example of exam scores where the distribution was not normal, the range is 90−29=61. Since the range is very sensitive to the presence of outliers in the dataset, a more useful measure is the interquartile range. To calculate the interquartile range, the data distribution is broken into four equal parts or quarters. The interquartile range is the range of data falling between the 25th and 75th percentiles. The interquartile range of the exam scores would be from 75 to 82 or 7. Reporting the spread of exam scores as having a range of 61 and interquartile range of 7, it signals that while there was a large spread in scores, half of the scores fell into a much narrower span.

Standard deviation quantifies how distant each value is from the distribution mean. In the exam score dataset, the mean was 75. The deviation from the mean is 46 for the first value (75 − 29) and 15 for the last value (90 − 75). Deviations for all values in the dataset can be calculated, squared (squaring allows adding of positive and negative deviations), and then divided by the total number of values to obtain the variance. Taking the square root of the variance results in the standard deviation (SD), which therefore provides information on the average deviation of the dataset from the mean. In a normally distributed dataset, 68% of values lie within one SD of the mean, 95% within two SDs, and 99.7% within three SDs.

Graphic presentations

When presenting your research (see Chapters 26 and 27), you must decide whether to display data numerically, graphically, or even both. Graphical presentations can effectively and succinctly portray data and are therefore often used for data most critical to the study. They can be particularly helpful in showing information that may be difficult to describe in text or as a simple table of numbers.

For instance, histograms (further described below) can rapidly demonstrate how a dataset is symmetrically distributed – whether it is symmetric or skewed and if it is unimodal (clustered around one peak) or multimodal (clustered around two or more peaks).

Histograms, bar, and pie charts show the frequency and distribution of data. Histograms are used to display continuous quantitative data. Here, data are divided into bins based on values or value ranges, and the frequency of data points in each bin is plotted on the *y*-axis against the bins on the *x*-axis (Figure 22.2). A 'density histogram' can also be used to depict relative frequencies rather than absolute frequencies. Bar and pie charts are used to display the frequency and distribution of categorical data. Whereas information in a pie chart shows relative frequencies (all segments of the pie adding up to 100%), information on a bar chart can show either absolute or relative frequencies.

A box plot or box and whisker plot depicts central tendency and dispersion information for quantitative data. It shows the median, the interquartile range, and the minimum and maximum values in the dataset. A box is drawn to indicate the interquartile range and a line is drawn through the box at the point of the median (Figure 22.3). Box plots convey how tightly data are grouped (interquartile range), whether the distribution is symmetrical (location of the median and interquartile range), and if not symmetric, how the data are skewed. A histogram can provide similar information visually. The boxplot more explicitly displays the values for the median and the ranges and does so in a more compact visual

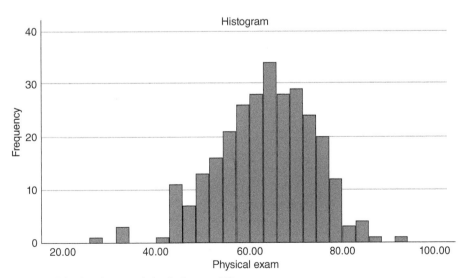

Figure 22.2 Histogram of the distribution of physical exam skill scores.

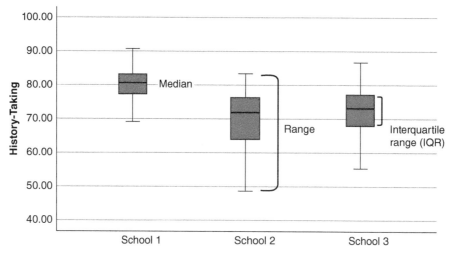

Figure 22.3 Boxplot comparing history-taking skills among three schools.

allowing representation and comparison of several datasets in one graphic. For instance, the histogram in Figure 22.2 could only represent the physical exam skills scores from one school, while the box plots in Figure 22.3 concisely represent the history-taking skills scores from three different schools in relation to each other.

These are the main types of graphic presentations, but there are always other methods being developed, for example the Violin plot [4]. This combines information from a box plot with a density histogram and has the advantage of showing the density of data points at each given value. For further information on types of presentations, please see the companion website.

Inferential statistics

Inferential statistics help you to accomplish two primary goals: (i) compare two or more groups with respect to outcomes of interest and (ii) identify relationships between or amongst groups. For example, in the early 1900s, bleeding was advocated as the primary treatment for most illnesses until Pierre Louis, a French clinician, used inferential statistics to show that bleeding, contrary to popular beliefs, made his patients worse rather than better [5]. He compared the outcomes of patients who were treated with bloodletting in early phase versus late phase of the disease and concluded the treatment had no effect and, in some cases was detrimental to patients' health. In this section, we will discuss statistical tests for comparing variables and those for identifying relationships amongst variables

Making comparisons
Independent and dependent variables

Inferential statistics require variables to be selected which will be used to group participants or observations for comparison, i.e. predictor variables, also called independent variables. This selection is based on characteristics critical to the study question and are often categorical (e.g. training level, gender). In clinical education research, common predictor variables may include stage in training, level of experience, different educational interventions, amongst others. For example, in a study of cognitive load during colonoscopy training, the research question was to identify how certain participant characteristics were associated with cognitive load. Therefore, the predictor/independent variables included year in training and prior number of procedures completed [6, 7].

Next, you must define outcome variables (also called dependent variables). Outcome variables are those that will be compared among one or more groups. The types (e.g. categorical, ordinal, continuous) will determine which inferential statistical tests should be used (e.g. Chi-square test, Student's *t*-test, and others discussed below). Analysis can be *univariate* (i.e. analysing individual outcomes without controlling for potential covariates) and/or *multivariate* (i.e. controlling for potential covariates). In the study mentioned earlier, cognitive load was the dependent variable.

Determining statistical significance

A primary value of inferential statistics is to determine whether differences between groups are likely to reflect reality, or whether the differences observed could be due to chance alone. This is determined primarily by the *p*-value. Before you do your analyses, you must determine what level of probability you will consider to be statistically significant (this threshold is called the alpha [α] value) The most commonly selected α value for statistical significance is 0.05, meaning there would be a 5% or lower likelihood that findings are due to chance [8, 9]. If your *p* value is less than your α value you would reject the null hypothesis (that there is no difference between the groups). If $p \leq 0.05$, it means there is a 95% or higher likelihood that your findings represent a 'true' difference in the study sample. Importantly, the *p*-value is only one measure of 'meaning' for a statistical test; theoretical plausibility and practical significance are equally important. For the former, the question is whether results make intuitive or theoretical sense; a statistically significant finding that does not make intuitive or theoretical sense may be spurious. It is important you consider whether the results will have meaningful impact [10, 11]. For example, an intervention that saves learners five minutes of total study time per semester might be statistically significant but is not considered practically significant.

Choosing inferential statistical tests to compare groups

Which test you use depends on the type of outcome variables and the number of groups being compared. The most common tests used to compare outcome variables for two or more participant groups are described below [12–14].

The *Chi-square* test is used to compare categorical outcome variables. They are often used to compare relationships between one categorical (i.e. nominal or ordinal) predictor variable and one categorical outcome variable. The test can be used to compare additional predictor or outcome variables, though interpretation can become challenging. The Chi-square test produces a test statistic and *p*-value that is related to the number of rows and columns (i.e. degrees of freedom). In the study mentioned earlier, we compared the gender of participants with the gender of the remainder of US gastroenterology trainee population to assess generalisability of our sample (see Table 22.1) [6].

The Chi-square statistic for this analysis is 0.014, which corresponds to a $p=0.90$, confirming no statistical difference in gender between our sample and the overall US gastroenterology trainee population.

The *Student's t-test* (also simply called *t-test*) is used to compare means of continuous outcome variables between two (and only two) groups. The *t*-test can be performed with one or two *tails*. The former is used when the directionality of the difference in means is definitively expected (e.g. we know for certain that the mean for group A will be higher than group B), whereas the latter is used when directionality cannot be assumed and is more commonly used. *t*-Tests can be unpaired (i.e. compare outcome variables between two groups of unrelated participants) or paired (i.e. compare outcome variables in the same group of participants under two different conditions such as before and after an intervention). The *t*-test calculation produces a test statistic that corresponds to a *p*-value. In the study noted above [6], we compared mean age in the sample population (32.4 years) to the overall US trainee population (32.3 years); this produced a test statistic of $t=0.65$, which corresponds to $p=0.51$, indicating no statistical difference in age of our sample and the overall US gastroenterology trainee population.

To compare continuous outcome variables among three or more predictor groups, you should use an *ANalysis Of VAriance* (ANOVA) test. It tests whether all groups plausibly have equal means and if not, identifies the strongest pairwise differences. An *F* statistic is produced, which corresponds to a *p*-value depending on the degrees of freedom. For the study mentioned above [6], we used ANOVA to compare intrinsic cognitive load across three groups based on year in training. Mean intrinsic cognitive load was 3.14 for first-year trainees, 1.78 for second-year trainees, and 1.21 for third-year fellows. The *F*-value was 58.02, corresponding to $p < 0.001$. This result indicates only a significant difference exists somewhere amongst the multiple groups but does not indicate which groups differ. To determine exactly where differences exist, posthoc tests must subsequently be performed. These involve multiple individual *t*-tests comparing groups pairwise and using a *p*-value threshold that has been corrected for the number of *t*-tests performed (see 'Multiple Comparisons' section). For the cognitive load analysis, all pairwise comparisons between groups had $p < 0.001$.

Multiple comparisons

It is important to be aware when conducting multiple comparisons, every additional statistical test increases the likelihood of finding a difference that is not true (i.e. type 1 error) in an additive fashion

Table 22.1 Example of Chi-square table

	Our sample	Overall United States
Female	166 (34.8%)	503 (34.5%)
Male	311 (65.2%)	955 (65.5%)

(as seen in Table 22.2). Therefore, if you perform 20 different statistical tests, there is a 100% probability that you will incorrectly identify a 'statistically significant' difference that does not reflect reality. Type 1 error is generally considered to have greater potential harm than type 2 error (failing to detect a difference that exists in reality), as it can lead to incorrect claims and assertions.

There are three primary ways to reduce the likelihood of committing type 1 error. The first (and most important) is to select your statistical tests carefully. Most analysis should be planned a priori, based on a theoretical framework with secondary analysis selected with caution. It can be tempting to perform numerous statistical analyses not directly related to your research question especially when you have a rich dataset containing multiple variables. Be aware of the risk for type 1 error and make thoughtful decisions directly informed by your research question. Second, the α value threshold for statistical significance can be corrected based on the number of tests performed, such as use of a post-hoc test in the ANOVA above. One such method is the *Bonferroni correction*, in which the threshold α value is divided by the number of statistical tests (see Table 22.2). While the Bonferroni correction greatly reduces the likelihood of type 1 error, its use remains debated [5].

Identifying relationships

We will now focus on how to describe relationships between variables (e.g. investigating the association between a doctor's communication skills and overall patient satisfaction with the consultation) using statistical methods. In inferential statistics, we use the term association to describe a relationship between two or more variables. Two variables are associated if knowing the value of one of the variables tells you something about the value of the other variable. Described below are the major statistical methods for investigating relationships including correlation, linear regression analysis, and logistic regression analysis.

Table 22.2 Impact of multiple comparisons on type 1 error

Number of statistical tests	Expected number of type 1 errors	α Value with Bonferroni correction
1	0.05	N/A
5	0.25	0.01
10	0.50	0.005
20	1.0	0.0025
50	2.5	0.001

Correlation

Correlation (r) is the numerical measure that summarises two important aspects of an association: the direction (either positive or negative) and the strength. Positive correlation signifies that as the value increases in one variable, there is also an increase in the other variable. For example, the correlation between amount of studying (i.e. time increases) and improvement in exam performance (i.e. higher scores). A negative correlation is the opposite, where the increase in one variable results in a decrease in the other variable. For example, the level of anxiety (measured through a scale) increases in correlation with a decrease in exam performance (score). The value of the correlation ranges from −1 (perfect negative correlation) to +1 (perfect positive correlation) representing the strength of the association. Values closer to −1 or 1 signify stronger association. In clinical education research in general, correlations less than ±0.2 are considered weak, those between ±0.3 and ±0.5 are considered moderate, and correlations between ±0.5 and ±1.0 are considered strong [15]. A scatter plot (Figure 22.4) helps to visualise the direction and strength of association between two quantitative variables. The values of one variable are shown on the horizontal axis and the values of the other variable are shown on the vertical axis. The individual dots or points in the graph represent the scores or values of a particular case or sample.

For example, in a study examining the relationship between standardised patient overall satisfaction rating (ranging from 50–100) and performance ratings on communication skills score (ranging from 60–100), the communication skill ratings had a strong positive correlation ($r = 0.70$) with standardised patient overall satisfaction. As shown in Figure 22.5, as communication skill scores increases the overall standardised patient satisfaction ratings also increases.

Regression

Regression analysis is a statistical technique used to examine the relationship between two or more variables, which appear to be linearly related and can be useful for two primary purposes: to make predictive or causal inferences based on the relationship between variables, and to determine how much of the variability in one variable is explained by another variable.

In regression analysis, we 'fit' a line to the data that best describes the relationship. Once the linear relationship is determined through regression analysis you can predict (estimate) the value of the outcome (dependent) variable (Y) based on the value of

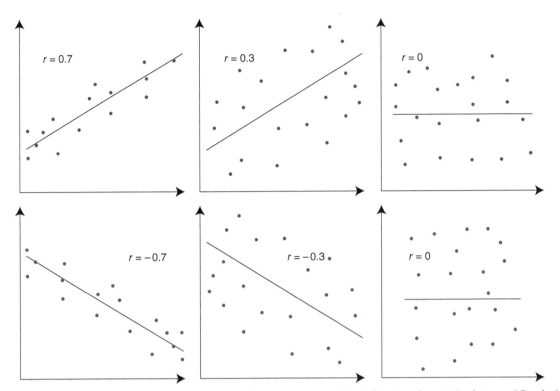

Figure 22.4 Scatter plots of correlation between two variables ranging in strength and direction of association between 0.7 and −0.7.

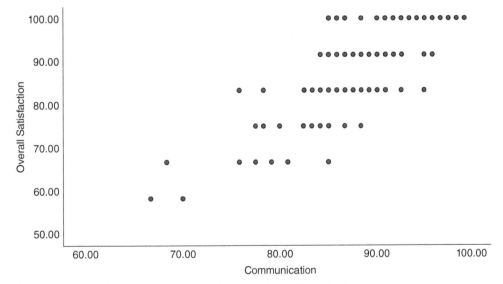

Figure 22.5 Scatter plot of correlation between communication and overall satisfaction score.

the predictor (independent) variable (*X*). The points along the regression line are the predictions (estimates). Based on the value of one variable, you can predict the value of another variable by looking at the corresponding value on the regression line. How well the regression line fits the data is determined by the amount of distance or discrepancy (often referred to as residuals) between the predicted points on the line and actual observed data points. Greater distance (residuals) between the points along the line (estimates) and the actual data points indicates greater uncertainty of the predictions. As shown in Figure 22.4, the scatterplot corresponding to *r* = 0.7 (signifying a strong association between the two variables) has a much shorter distance between the points on the line and the other data points. This shorter distance leads to more certainty in the prediction. In contrast, the plot with $r = 0.3$ has more variability along the line with greater distance between the points along the line and the observed data points. This leads to much less certainty in the estimates (prediction) based on the regression line. Accordingly, correlation is closely connected to the regression analysis. In simple linear regression, a squared correlation (*r-square*) is the amount of variance that is explained by linear regression of one variable on the other variable.

When you want to examine the relationship between two or more explanatory variables with the outcome of interest, multiple linear regression models are used to fit the data. Similar to simple linear regression, in multiple regression analysis, the outcome variable (Y) is explained by more than one predictor ($x_1, x_2, \ldots, x_p$) variable instead of just one as in simple linear regression. Instead of one slope in simple linear regression, in multiple regression analysis, you have multiple slopes (amount of change in relation to the variables) to represent the association between the multiple predictor variables and the outcome variable. For example, using the study above, when we first examine the relationship between student gender and overall score on the clinical skills exam, we find that female students significantly outperformed male students by 3% (89% versus 92%). To determine how both gender and communication skills are related to the overall clinical skills performance, multiple regression analysis can be conducted. Based on the multiple regression analysis, the communication skills variable is statistically significantly associated with the clinical skills performance score. However, the association between gender and the clinical skills scores is no longer significant in the multiple regression analysis (Table 22.3). This analysis reveals the initial three percentage point difference between female versus male students was confounded by the higher percentage of female students with higher communication scores compared to male students. In other words, the analysis suggests the reason female students performed better is because female students had better communication skills than the male students. You could also say that once

controlled for communication skills performance, there was no longer any difference in overall scores between female and male students.

There are several elements to consider when interpreting regression analysis results. The annotated description of the table is presented below:

B. These are the values for the regression equation for predicting the dependent variable from the independent variable. These are called *unstandardised coefficients* because they are measured in their natural units which make the interpretation of the coefficients much more intuitive. For example, based on the table, we can say that for one unit increase in communication skills score, we can expect a 1.01 unit increase in clinical skills performance score. However, since the coefficients are in their natural units, these cannot be compared with one another (e.g. gender) to determine which one is more influential in the model because they are measured on different scales.

Standard error. The standard errors can be used to form a confidence interval for the coefficient (parameter estimate), as shown in the last two columns of this table. This provides one measure of precision in the estimates.

Beta. These are the standardised coefficients. By standardising the variables, putting all of the variables on the same scale, you can compare the magnitude of the coefficients in the model to see which one has more of an effect. You will also notice that the larger betas are associated with stronger associations. In this example, beta for communication skills is much larger than gender.

Sig. This is the *p*-value. For example, if you chose α to be 0.05, coefficients having a *p*-value of 0.05 or less would be statistically significant at the 0.05 level.

Lower and upper bound CI. These are the 95% confidence intervals for the coefficients. The confidence intervals are related to the *p*-values such that the coefficient will not be statistically significant at $\alpha = 0.05$ if the 95% confidence interval includes zero. These intervals provide another measure of precision in the estimates by providing perspective on the range of possible predictive values.

Table 22.3 Regression analysis examining the relationship among gender, communication, and clinical skills exam score

	B	Standard error	Beta	Sig	Lower bound CI	Upper bound CI
Intercept	0.03	0.04		0.41	−0.05	0.11
Male (gender)	−0.01	0.01	−0.04	0.23	−0.02	0.01
Communication skills	1.01	0.05	0.67	0.00	0.92	1.10

Logistic regression

Similar to linear regression, logistic regression is used to examine the relationship between predictor (independent) variables and the outcome (dependent variable). However, logistic regression is used for categorical outcome variables. The most common is binary logistic regression, where the outcome is a binary event (e.g. 1 or 0; yes or no; pass or fail). Consider a simple example analysing the outcome variable of pass/fail (0 = fail and 1 = pass) as it relates to the categorical predictor variable of gender (0 = male and 1 = female). The probability of pass (y) is a function of gender (x) and can be expressed mathematically as

$$\text{Logit}\left(\text{Pr}\left(y = \frac{1}{x}\right)\right) = a + bx$$

To make sure the predicted probability falls within 0 to 1, transform the regression equation to the logit (or natural log of the odds) of being in one outcome category ($\hat{Y}$) versus the other category ($1 - \hat{Y}$). Instead of beta coefficients, in logistic regression, the strength of the predictor variable's contribution to the outcome is presented as an odds ratio (OR). For example, the OR associated with gender is 1.5, meaning the odds of passing the exam are 1.5 times higher for female students compared to male students. If the predictor variable is continuous, you must determine a meaningful unit of measurement to best express the degree of change in the outcome associated with that independent variable (e.g. hours spent on studying for the exam might be expressed in increments of 10 hours). For this example, for every 10 hours spent studying, the odds of passing the exam increases by 1.5-fold.

Uncertainty and bias

As noted in the introduction, everyone interprets, uses, and makes decisions on data within the context of uncertainty and potential errors. In statistics, this is usually described as the proportion of variance in the outcome explained by the model and the level of precision (error) in the estimates derived from the analysis.

First, the proportion of variance explained (explanatory power of the model) is expressed as r-squared (r^2) in regression analysis. This is a goodness-of-fit measure for linear regression analysis that summarises how much the variables in the model explain the variance observed in the outcome variable. In the example with the clinical skills exam, the regression model with communication ratings and student gender as predictors had an r^2 of 0.45, meaning those two predictor variables accounted for about 45% of the variance in clinical skills exam scores. This number quantifies the explanatory power of the regression model, but the overall interpretation should be considered in the context of your data and your research question. Logistic regression analysis also produces goodness-of-fit measures, there are pseudo-r^2 type measures and the c-statistic to quantify the amount of variation that is explained by the model.

Second, the level of precision in the estimates provides a good indication of how much uncertainty there is in your data analysis. The standard error and the typically reported 95% confidence intervals (CI) are important indices for the level of uncertainty in your data analysis. The wider the confidence intervals, the less precision in your estimates of the associations between the predictors and the outcome variable.

In terms of bias, one important aspect to consider is the potential for confounding variables. These are predictor variables associated with both the outcome and other predictor variables in the analysis. Consider the following hypothetical example: you notice based on your regression analysis, there is a strong association between shoe size and the performance on a reading assessment. Without consideration for potential confounding variables, you may erroneously conclude that shoe size is highly predictive of reading ability. However, upon further review, you realize that age and shoe size are also highly correlated. Once age is added to the model, shoe size is no longer predictive of reading ability.

There are several potential strategies to avoid these misspecifications in the analysis and minimise confounders. These include making sure the models are theoretically and hypothesis driven rather than 'fishing' for statistically significant findings, using a literature review to check and identify any potential confounding variables, and checking for collinearity (high correlation among two or more predictor variables) by examining correlations among the predictor variables prior to building the final model.

Similarly, there may exist measured or unmeasured factors associated with both predictor and outcome variables (i.e. confounders) that contribute to uncertainty. Confounding bias occurs when erroneous inferences are made caused by a 'mixing of effects'. Confounding variables often obscure and obfuscate the true relationship between variables due to the omission of an important factor in the data analysis. The impact of random contributors to uncertainty can be mitigated to some degree through participant selection and adequate sampling (see Chapter 6), good experimental design (see Chapter 21), assessment of data for skewness, and analyses that control for potential confounders.

Thoughtful interpretation of statistical results can also counteract uncertainty and bias. Statistical results should be interpreted through a realistic lens grounded in a theoretical framework. An unexpected statistical difference between two groups may be a novel finding, but more likely represents bias or confounding. The discussion section of a dissertation or manuscript should address potential contributors to uncertainty and provide suggestions for the holistic interpretation of study results.

Statistical test

It is important to select the appropriate statistical tests. Table 22.4 provides more detail on this with examples related to clinical education research.

There are various statistical packages available to support you to undertake statistical tests. The many different options include both commercial products and open source [13, 14, 16].

Summary

Statistical analyses are used to transform raw data into comprehensible results that can be communicated to others to promote ongoing evolution and transformation in the education and training of current and future healthcare professionals. By extension, statistical analysis has substantial power to impact not only the education of healthcare professionals but also the care their future patients will receive. It is therefore critical that statistical analysis is thoughtfully designed, carefully and expertly executed, and thoroughly and clearly reported. This chapter has provided introductory guidance for you to conduct your first statistical analyses. Following this guidance under the mentorship and/or the support of a statistician or researcher in your team with the relevant experience will promote your growth, development, and lead you to contribute to the ever-changing field of health professions education.

Table 22.4 Commonly used statistical tests with corresponding research questions and variable types

Statistical test	How test is used	Example research question	Variables and type
Chi-square	To compare one or more categorical outcome variables for two or more groups	Is there a difference in the proportion of female versus male students between intervention and non-intervention groups?	Predictor: gender (categorical) Outcome: intervention versus ion-intervention (categorical)
t-Test	To compare one continuous outcome variable for two groups	Is there a difference in the exam performance between students at rural versus urban sites?	Predictor: rural versus urban sites (categorical – two groups or dichotomous) Outcome: exam performance (continuous)
ANOVA	To compare one continuous outcome variable for three or more groups	Is there a relationship between types of curricula, (lecture based didactic, problem-based learning, and team-based learning) and student performance on exams?	Predictor: curriculum type (categorical) Outcome: exam performance (continuous)
Linear regression	To investigate the relationship between continuous outcome variable with one or more predictor variables	What factors are associated with clinical skills performance score?	Predictor: gender (categorical) History-taking skills (continuous) Communication skills (continuous) Outcome: overall clinical skills performance score (continuous)
Logistic regression	To investigate the relationship between categorical outcome variable with one or more predictor variables	What factors are associated with whether the students have concerns raised in their multi source feedback?	Predictor: gender (categorical) Attendance at classes (continuous) Communication skills (continuous) Outcome: concerns raised or no concerns raised (categorical)

Top tips

- Determine the types of data (e.g. continuous, categorical) in your dataset and preplan which statistical tests to perform.
- Use graphical displays to facilitate interpretation and maximise impact of the data.
- Consider both statistical and practical significance and check for correlations among the predictors when interpreting statistical analysis.
- Seek advice from supervisors and statisticians at every phase of the process, including study planning, statistical analysis and interpretation, and presentation of results.

Common pitfalls

- Performing statistical analysis without theoretical plausibility or that are too ambitious for the sample size. Investigate associations that will have practical relevance and avoid inadequately supported assertions.
- Forgetting to look for outliers. This can lead to skewed and inaccurate statistical results, so plot your data to check.
- Omitting the step of investigating potential confounding variables. In statistical analysis, it is essential that possible sources of bias are ruled out.
- Conflating association with causation. Do this with caution unless you have employed a robust experimental design.

Ethical issues

- Post hoc analyses should be performed with caution as these may be construed as trying to find a preconceived outcome.
- Ensure the models are theoretically and hypothesis driven rather than 'fishing' for statistically significant findings.

Further reading

Acock, A.C. (2008). *A Gentle Introduction to Stata*. Stata Press.

Dawson, L.G., Moore, D.S., and McCabe, G.P. (2005). *Introduction to the Practice of Statistics Excel Manual with Macros*. Macmillan.

Field, A. (2013). *Discovering Statistics Using IBM SPSS Statistics*. SAGE Publications.

Field, A. (2017). *Discovering Statistics Using IBM SPSS Statistics*, 5e. London: SAGE Publications.

Huang, J.Z. (2014). An introduction to statistical learning: with applications in R by Gareth James, Daniela Witten, Trevor Hastie, Robert Tibshirani, Daniela Witten. *Journal of Agricultural, Biological and Environmental Statistics* 19: 556–557.

References

1 Sullivan, G.M. and Artino, A.R. (2013). Analyzing and interpreting data from Likert-type scales. *Journal of Graduate Medical Education* 5 (4): 541–542.

2 Mircioiu, C. and Atkinson, J. (2017). A comparison of parametric and non-parametric methods applied to a Likert scale. *Pharmacy (Basel)* 5 (2): 26.

3 Boone, H.N. and Boone, D.A. (2012). Analyzing Likert data. *Journal of Extension* 50 (2): 1–5.

4 Tanious, R. and Manolov, R. (2022). Violin plots as visual tools in the meta-analysis of single-case experimental designs. *Methodology* 18 (3): 221–238.

5 Morabia, A. (2006). Pierre-Charles-Alexandre Louis and the evaluation of bloodletting. *Journal of the Royal Society of Medicine* 99 (3): 158–160.

6 Sewell, J.L., Boscardin, C.K., Young, J.Q. et al. (2016). Measuring cognitive load during procedural skills training with colonoscopy as an exemplar. *Medical Education* 50 (6): 682–692.

7 Sewell, J.L., Boscardin, C.K., Young, J.Q. et al. (2017). Learner, patient, and supervisor features are associated with different types of cognitive load during procedural skills training: implications for teaching and instructional design. *Academic Medicine* 92 (11): 1622–1631.

8 Kennedy-Shaffer, L. (2019). Before p < 0.05 to beyond p < 0.05: using history to contextualize p-values and significance testing. *The American Statistician* 73 (Suppl. 1): 82–90.

9 Baker, M. (2016). Statisticians issue warning over misuse of P values. *Nature* 531 (7593): 151.

10 Betensky, R.A. (2019). The *p*-value requires context, not a threshold. *The American Statistician* 73 (Suppl. 1): 115–117.

11 Laber, E.B. and Shedden, K. (2017). Statistical significance and the dichotomization of evidence: the relevance of the ASA statement on statistical significance and p-values for statisticians. *Journal of the American Statistical Association* 112 (519): 902–904.

12 Freedman, D., Pisani, R., Purves, R., and Adhikari, A. (2007). *Statistics*. W. W. Norton & Company.

13 Field, A. (2013). *Discovering Statistics Using IBM SPSS Statistics*. SAGE Publications.

14 Field, A., Miles, J., and Field, Z. (2012). Discovering statistics using R. *Choice Reviews* 50 (04): 50–2114.

15 Moore, D.S., Notz, W.I., and Flinger, M.A. (2013). Scatterplots and correlation. In: *The Basic Practice of Statistics*, 6e, 102–104. New York, NY: WH Freeman and Company.

16 Acock, A.C. (2008). *A Gentle Introduction to Stata*. Stata Press.

23 Big Data: where to start and what to expect

Milou Silkens, Asta Medisauskaite, and Chris McManus

Learning objectives

By the end of this chapter, you should be able to:
- Describe what is Big Data, why big datasets are useful and how they can be problematic.
- Identify the key features of planning and preparing big data research and analysis.

- Recognise strengths and limitations of big datasets.
- Appreciate the volume and complexity of work involved and the need for collaboration.

Introduction

In a world where data are collected from people everywhere, big datasets are ubiquitous. Big Data, as a concept, was said to have been introduced in the 1990s by John Mashey [1] who realised that faster computers, cheaper memory, and greater internet connectivity meant organisations collected and stored ever more data, which often arrived in real time. As a result, Big Data refers to datasets that are very large and complex, typically driven by automatic data collection and characterised by high volume, high velocity, and high variety [2]. Data available in clinical education are now far bigger than educational data from two decades ago, but still minuscule compared with, say, the five petabytes of data hoovered up each day by Facebook.

Big datasets are often (though not always) administrative data, which means the data are routinely collected, and can vary in whether they are:
- *Structured*, meaning they are stored and organised in relational databases. These are typically quantitative data (e.g. prescriptions or hospital activity analyses);
- *Semi-structured*, meaning the data are not stored in a relational database but still have some structural properties or underlying organisational framework. These are usually qualitative data organised by, for example subject or topic (e.g. patient notes or discharge summaries);
- *Unstructured*, meaning they are not stored and organised in relational databases. These are commonly qualitative data or images (e.g. portfolios or digitised X-rays).

Each type of big dataset offers powerful opportunities for studying clinical education and training as well as posing unique challenges for education researchers. This chapter provides a general introduction to big datasets in clinical education, discussing the processes of working with big datasets, including appropriate preparation, cleaning, and analysis of big datasets, the reporting of research, and an illustrative case study. The emphasis is mostly on big datasets that are *quantitative*, although there are studies of big datasets that are *qualitative* (such as text from Twitter or other social media, see Chapter 13). Most Big Data research is *secondary* analysis, the researchers themselves not having collected the original, *primary*, data. Inevitably, there are technical terms, and Table 23.1 provides the most important definitions supporting this chapter.

Big Data in clinical education

Big Data research can address some of the limitations of other more common research methods in clinical education. Most clinical education research is *cross-sectional*, with study subjects being investigated at one point in time. Although these are relatively quick and inexpensive to conduct and can easily answer a range of descriptive questions, they cannot easily study change and are not best suited for investigating causal relationships [6].

Starting Research in Clinical Education, First Edition. Edited by Eliot L. Rees, Alison Ledger, and Kim A. Walker.
© 2024 The Association for the Study of Medical Education (ASME). Published 2024 by John Wiley & Sons Ltd.
Companion website: www.wiley.com/go/clinicaleducation

Table 23.1 Table of definitions

Bootstrapping	A computationally intensive statistical technique which makes no assumptions about data having normal or other distributions
Code/syntax	The set of instructions that computer programs use for carrying out tasks
Data dictionary	A text file of meta-data which describes the variables, their origins, the codes used in them, and their interpretation. Sometimes missing for older datasets and have to be inferred
De-anonymisation	The process by which users may attempt to find out the real identity of anonymised or pseudonymised individuals. Most data holders regulate against it and work hard to prevent it
GDPR	General Data Protection Regulation. The EU/EEA and UK law regulating data protection and privacy, particularly of personal data
Ibry chart	A graphical representation showing a project schedule, indicating what types of data were collected and when [3]. See Figures 23.1 and 23.2 for examples
Meta-data	Data, often textual, describing numerical data in a structured way, which helps to sort and identify attributes the information it describes. Similar to a Data Dictionary. Data without meta-data can sometimes be very hard to analyse, requiring inferences about what numeric values might mean
Missing data imputation	A process for 'filling in' missing values in datasets with plausible estimates of what the values might have been. Missing data is ubiquitous in large studies, which is a problem for most statistical analyses, particularly if listwise deletion is used
Porting	Transferring data from one program or statistical package to another
Profile paper	A paper that does not provide statistical analyses, but describes the process of data collection, etc., and can be referenced in later statistical analyses and research papers without the need for repetition of details
Safe haven (secure environment)	A secure computing environment, where sensitive data can be stored safely and made available only to those with permission for particular analyses. Sometimes safe havens are physically secure, with access only in particular buildings or places, and not via the Internet
Structured data	Data which have a clear structure, as for instance with examination data and results and stored in a database. Unstructured data can be free text, such as student comments, and are much harder to analyse, and often are voluminous

Longitudinal studies address the shortcomings of cross-sectional studies by following study subjects over time, measuring multiple variables on multiple occasions across the study timeframe. Longitudinal studies allow the possibility of *causal inference*, meaning they are most suited to study the relationships between independent variables and one or more outcomes [6] (see Chapter 22). The *prospective cohort study* is the most well-known type of longitudinal study. A good example in education and healthcare is the UK National Child Development Study (NCDS) which looked at 17,415 people born in England, Scotland, and Wales in one week of 1958 (https://cls.ucl.ac.uk/). Studied firstly at birth, the participants were followed up eleven times over 60 years. As the study progresses some participants will be exposed to particular events, and some will show particular outcomes. This enables researchers to infer whether earlier events caused the outcome (i.e. to identify causality). In clinical education, events may include particular forms of teaching, exposure to different clinical disciplines, and examination successes and failures. Study outcomes may include qualifications gained, experiences of burnout, or drop out from courses. It is important to note that cohort studies are strictly observational rather than experimental (interventional),

meaning that researchers have no influence on who will be 'exposed' to the events and who will not. Cohort studies can however sometimes act as a base for randomised controlled trials (RCTs).

In many ways, longitudinal prospective cohort studies can often answer questions the original organisers never anticipated, particularly as new data are collected at each *follow-up* or *wave*. However, they are inevitably time consuming and expensive, particularly given the large samples required [6]. Such challenges, as well as data security and survey fatigue, can potentially be overcome by researching big datasets which are already collected. Big datasets often have large numbers of variables collected over time, allowing researchers to explore several research questions and to study causal relationships. Multiple researchers can also interrogate the data, increasing transparency, reproducibility, and productivity.

Within clinical education, the concept of using Big Data is still relatively new, but is now well developed within healthcare research, with the development of 'health data warehouses' which are centralised repositories for healthcare organisation's data which are retrieved, processed, and structured for analytical querying and reporting [7]. Moreover, the availability of big datasets in clinical education is rapidly increasing providing growing

Table 23.2 Examples of Big Data and other data sources in clinical education.

Dataset	Country	Description
The UK Medical Education Database: UKMED	UK	A dataset collating data on the background, training, performance and career tracks of UK medical students and UK trainees
National Training Survey (NTS)	UK	A survey administered each year by the General Medical Council (GMC) to all doctors in training. Data available in UKMED
The List of Registered Medical Practitioners (LRMP)	UK	The GMC's list of all registered doctors in the United Kingdom, showing dates of registration, training, and revalidation status
GMC Data Explorer	UK	A dataset hosted by the medical regulator in the United Kingdom, showing, for example doctors' revalidation and fitness to practise data
National Health Service (NHS) Staff Survey	UK	One of the largest workforce surveys in the world including experiences within the NHS of all staff, including doctors
Dutch Institute for Clinical Auditing: DICA	Netherlands	A dataset on clinical outcomes and the quality of patient care. These data facilitate the linkage of educational data and patient outcome data
Accreditation Data System	USA	A dataset collected by the Accreditation Council for Graduate Medical Education, detailing accreditation data and trainee/faculty surveys
Data sources		
University data		Data collected by universities or medical schools on, for example applications, acceptance, progression, and background characteristics
Quality data for teaching/ training programmes		Data collected for quality improvement purposes, including students' or trainees' experiences
Postgraduate training programme data		Data collected by Royal Colleges on, for example the number of trainees and doctors registered and their training status
Patient records		Patient information including clinical outcomes
Quality of care data		Data collected for quality improvement purposes, including patient satisfaction and outcomes

opportunities for interested researchers to utilise such data. Table 23.2 provides examples and sources of big datasets in clinical education; the rapid growth of Big Data means every country, jurisdiction, and organisation may have their own big datasets with different variables collected so listing and discussing the many potential sources of data is therefore an impossible task. Access to a big dataset is through an application to the data holder (usually an organisation) who will have their own governance structures regarding the access and use of their data. The largest big dataset freely available in clinical education is the UK Medical Education Database (UKMED) [8].

Working with big datasets

This section will discuss the steps involved in working with Big Data: the preparation and planning required, considerations on the linkage of multiple datasets, software and coding which may come in useful when working with big datasets, data cleaning, exploration, and analysis including the handling of missing data. The principles and steps are mainly similar to working with smaller datasets (see Parts II–IV). However, research with big datasets

faces unique challenges and the major differences are discussed in each section below.

Preparation and planning

The first step in any research is to formulate an appropriate (set of) research question(s) (see Chapter 2). However, with big datasets, where the data have already been collected, the research questions are necessarily limited by what data are actually available, rather than in primary research where the questions decide what data should be collected. This is exemplified in the illustrative case study (Box 23.1). However, due to the sheer quantity of measures and participants, it can allow quite subtle research questions to be tested. So, it is important you think carefully *what* data you need and *why* to answer the research questions for your Big Data project. Just looking at anything and everything, so-called 'dustbowl empiricism', is rarely successful. It is tempting when applying for access to a big dataset to ask for as much information as possible, but datasets are usually huge and data holders may worry that your study is unfocused if you require all variables available. More variables mean more time for organising and cleaning, and more difficulty in gaining an overall perspective. If needed, it is better to go back and ask for additional data if required.

The following steps can be helpful when deciding on your research question(s) and what data is needed to answer these questions:

- *Discussion with expert practitioners.* Teachers and trainers know the intricacies of the relevant processes the data are saying something about, know the problems of interpreting many of the measures and can help formulate worthwhile research questions that are relevant to practice, and more crucially, are answerable. They are also likely to know what data are collected and who the data holders are. Students and those in training will describe many of the problems, processes as seen from their perspective, which can be helpful too.

- *Discussion with expert researchers.* Experienced researchers who have worked with particular big datasets know the unique challenges the data pose. Administrative data for instance may be collected in very different ways than you might think. Experts can often help you to better understand the true potential and challenges of big datasets particularly in relation to the richness of the measures available. They can also help avoid reinventing the wheel, as for instance when they point to previous research, both in terms of using the data but also how to clean and analyse data, sometimes using previously used code saving you work.

- *Use the data dictionary.* Data holders will most likely provide (publicly or on request) information about their data, often as a *data dictionary*. Ideally, this should include some *meta-data*, which can be helpful in understanding what data are available and to better understand what the data looks like (e.g. meta-data might show the variable 'ethnicity' is included in the dataset and that the variable is coded using two answer options: white/Black, Asian, and Minority Ethnic). However, meta-data are often limited, particularly with older datasets.

- *Approach data holders.* Data holders will best know their data and its potential, making them well positioned to advise on what research questions can or cannot easily be answered. They are a useful source of advice and support and probably have interesting hypotheses of their own on what is happening.

- *Understand the limits of datasets.* Datasets often have measures for only subsets of participants for particular years, which can produce problems for longitudinal explorations. Plotting available data against time slots using tables, diagrams, or charts, can be helpful in understanding what data are available, when, and what questions can be asked of the data. Of particular use is an *Ibry chart* [3], which graphs progression through various career stages, in relation to academic or calendar year, so that separate cohorts can be visualised. Figure 23.1 shows a simple example from 1985 [4], and Figure 23.2 a more recent, more complex, example from a published paper using UKMED data [5] in which not all data are available for all cohorts for structural reasons.

Accessing big data

Once you know what dataset and what variables you require to answer your research questions, you

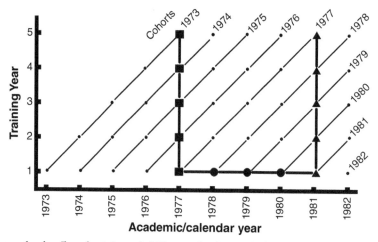

Figure 23.1 A simple example of an Ibry chart. An early UK example of a simple Ibry chart used in a study of medical students in Birmingham between 1977 and 1981 [4]. Academic/calendar year is shown horizontally, and training year in medical school (1–5) is shown vertically. The black squares show a cross-sectional study in 1977 of students in all five years. The diagonal lines show the successive cohorts, so for instance the 1973 entrants were in year 1 in 1973, year 2 in 1974, and so on to year 5 in 1977. Simple surveys of first-year students were also carried out in 1978, 1979, and 1980 (black circles). Finally, in 1981 a second cross-sectional study was carried out of students in all five years (black triangles). As a result, a series of longitudinal analyses could be carried out, e.g. of the 1977 cohort in year 1 and in year 5, the 1978 cohort in year 1 and year 4, and so on. Secular trends could also be assessed by comparing the fifth (and fourth, third, and second) year students in 1973 and 1977. The Ibry chart makes the design clear, distinguishing training years, academic years, and entry cohorts. *Source:* Adapted from McManus [4].

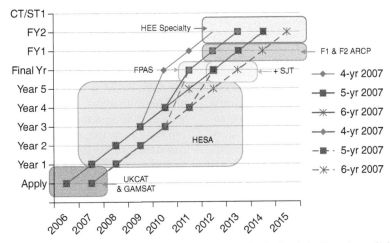

Figure 23.2 Ibry chart showing 2006 and 2007 graduate entrants to UK medical school. An Ibry chart, slightly redrawn from the original, for a UKMED study of graduate entrants to UK medical schools [5]. The horizontal axis shows academic/calendar year, and the vertical axis shows course progression from application to postgraduate training. The study looked at two successive cohorts, shown as diagonal lines, who took the UKCAT/GAMSAT selection tests in 2006 and 2007. Cohort lines branch as students could be on four, five, or six year courses. Some students also delayed due to exam failure, intercalated degrees, etc. but are not shown. Data sources are shown by boxes. Data from HESA were available for all participants. However, for final year students, FPAS scores were only available from 2011 onwards, and SJT scores from 2012 onwards. ARCP results were only available from 2012 onwards, as were HEE specialty selection scores. As an example of structural limitations, 2006 applicants on four-year courses had neither FPAS nor ARCP outcomes, but did have HEE specialty selection scores. Note: UKCAT, United Kingdom Clinical Aptitude Test (now UCAT); GAMSAT, Graduate Australian Medical School Admission Test; HESA, Higher Education Statistics Agency; FPAS, Foundation Programme Application System; SJT, Situational Judgment Test; ARCP, Annual Review of Competency Progression; HEE, Health Education England; F(Y)1/2, Foundation Year 1/2; CT, core training; ST, specialty training. *Source*: Garrud and McManus [5] / Springer Nature / CC BY 4.0.

will need to obtain access to the dataset(s). This process of gaining access will differ greatly between data holders. Some will require a detailed *research protocol* including the research questions, aims and methods to tackle the data, and often researchers are not allowed to explore outside of their stated protocol. There may also be an access fee. As an example, the UKMED has two data application periods a year, with an online form which is reviewed by the research sub-group. In order to be successful, it is important to only ask for data which are currently in the database, not be too ambitious (i.e. requesting all the data), or too narrow (asking for only two or three variables), use the correct statistical procedures (see Chapter 22), and particularly important, the team must have relevant experience. In contrast, access to the General Medical Council's (GMC) List of Registered Medical Practitioners, which is published as a statutory requirement, is open to anyone and only requires filling in a form and paying a relatively small fee.

The process for gaining access to big datasets can be tedious, so never underestimate the amount of time needed. 'Everything takes longer (and costs more)', as says one of the many variants of Murphy's Law of Research [9]. A *Gantt chart* is helpful for planning a realistic workload and timescale (and

some data holders will require it) (see Chapter 25). Other important points to consider include:

- *Gaining access to datasets.* Approval for access takes time. This is partly at your end whilst reviewing literature and writing applications to access data, and partly because the data holder usually works within their own time windows for review and approval.

- *Setting up access to data.* Data access often involves contractual arrangements such as data sharing agreements, which may involve your university or employer. Data holders often require evidence of training on data protection legislation such as the General Data Protection Regulation (GDPR), confidentiality, and ethical approvals.

- *Work environment.* Data is usually accessed through a *secure environment* or *safe haven*, which includes restrictions on the location at which one can work on the data, the devices that can be used, and the platforms on which the data are held. Sometimes a safe haven can be accessed remotely, through special software, but some data holders require access only in a strictly controlled physical location, typically in a major city, which can add another layer of complexity to planning, e.g. software, travel, device/platform speed. Some data holders will not allow numerical data to be let out of a safe haven or will require release to be approved, hence having experienced team members who are familiar with this process is crucially important.

- *Pseudonymisation.* Most data holders provide *pseudonymised data*, where individuals cannot easily be identified, but identification might still be possible for a determined user. Preventing *de-anonymisation* and access to personal information is a major security concern for providers, and safe havens are a reassurance to data holders and to participants in databases. Data holders rightly regard any infringement as a serious professional issue, with likely disciplinary action by regulatory bodies.

Linking multiple datasets

One dataset may not include all the information necessary to answer your particular research question. *Data linkage* of several datasets can offer new opportunities for analysis, but linkage is often not easy and some data holders may not approve or sanction linking or require it to be done via an independent third party. There are many issues to consider: unique identifiers across datasets, different and incomplete identifiers, names differ in their spelling, and, in large databases, identifiers, such as dates of birth, are far from unique, meaning false linkages are sometimes created. Data linkage always raises ethical issues, and participants must have been informed and consented to their data being linked and shared with other researchers. Expert advice is needed when merging databases and is probably not something you should try in your first project with a big dataset.

Software and coding

Although the principle of analysing data is the same as for smaller datasets, actually doing it is a very different matter. A common error is to assume data can be analysed in a spreadsheet. However, they never, ever, should be used for handling big datasets. Statistical packages such as Statistical Package for the Social Sciences (*SPSS*) have elegant front ends with point-and-click drop-down menus, and a broad range of standard statistical methods, and are a good starting point for *exploring* data and for basic multivariate statistical analyses (see Chapter 22). However, like any package, it has limitations reformatting and combining data from multiple files. The statistical functions are fairly advanced but limited in range. Nevertheless, a good starting point for basic analyses of big datasets is packages such as *SPSS*, *Stata*, or *SAS*.

For more advanced analysis, powerful open-source programming languages such as *R* or *Python* become necessary. *R* is the more popular, with its thousands of contributed software packages providing a huge range of analytic methods (see https://cran.r-project.org/). We recommend that the best way to learn *R* is with a mentor, a buddy, or a course.

A practical strategy for you would be to use *SPSS* (or *Stata* or *SAS*) for exploring and cleaning data, and basic analyses, and then for more complex analyses port *SPSS* data into *R* using the *haven* function (an *R* package that enables *R* to read and write various data formats used by other statistical packages) in *tidyverse* (https://haven.tidyverse.org/). The workflow of the entire process can be recorded by saving both the *.spx* syntax file in *SPSS* and the *.R* program file in *R* (see Figure 23.3).

Data cleaning and exploration

The first step on accessing a dataset is to familiarise yourself with the variables and how they relate to your research questions. During this process, you will continually be making decisions on how to use the variables and how to optimise the data analysis. Big datasets are often so large it is hard to keep track of these discoveries, decisions, and changes to variables. Therefore, it is important to keep an accurate *research log*, writing down all the discoveries, discussions, decisions, and actions applicable to the dataset. A paper notebook (or an electronic version of a lab notebook) is always useful, noting by date what worked or did not, what problems occurred, and how they were solved or circumvented. This is not only important for yourself but also for data holders and/or reviewers that may request logs to check and learn from the work. Journals often require authors to deposit programme or syntax files (and sometimes raw data), in repositories such as the Open Science Foundation (https://osf.io/). Reviewers and other researchers then know exactly what was done and can replicate and extend analyses.

Hand in hand with a log goes *version control* of datasets and software: every change to the dataset should be logged and subsequently the dataset and program files should be saved with new file names so that changes are traceable. For complex datasets with multiple researchers, version control can be implemented by specialised software such as Git and GitHub (https://github.com/) [11].

When exploring a dataset, it can help to chunk the dataset into smaller datasets, cleaning the dataset in sections and later merging the separate, smaller, datasets into one overall dataset for analysis. Looking at a large dataset with possibly thousands of subjects and variables can be overwhelming, confusing, and very slow in computing time, so breaking up the dataset into smaller pieces can make the process more manageable, particularly

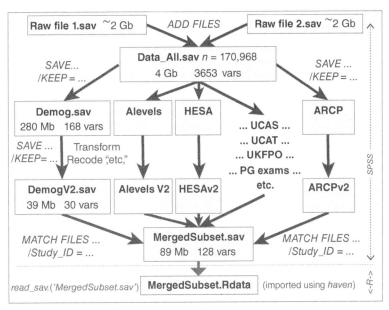

Figure 23.3 Dataflow for a large UKMED project, using SPSS and R.

Figure 23.3 shows a schematic *dataflow* for analysing a large UKMED dataset [10], which makes clearer the process of the various analyses. Typical code is shown in italics, with SPSS for basic data cleaning and exploration, and R for more complex analyses. The data arrived in the safe haven as two *SPSS* .sav files, each two gigabytes in length. Using SPSS, the two merged files contained 3653 variables from 170,968 participants. Such a file is very unmanageable (and is only a small subset of UKMED). Variables on different topics were extracted, so that the 168 variables describing demographics went into *Demog.sav*. Cleaning, transformation, recoding, and selection then resulted in a reduced, smaller file, *DemogV2.sav* with 30 key variables. Similar analyses were then carried out for other chunks of the data, such as A-level results, progression data (HESA and ARCP), etc., with smaller files created for each. The reduced files were finally merged to give a file, *MergedSubset.sav* with just 128 variables, which was still large, but more convenient for statistical analysis. Finally, the file was ported from SPSS into *R* using the haven package as *MergedSubset.Rdata*. A diagram such as that in Figure 23.3 makes the dataflow clearer to users. *Notes.* HESA, Higher Education Statistics Agency; ARCP, Annual Review of Competency Progression.

when combined with version control. The example shown in Figure 23.3 illustrates the analysis of a large UKMED dataset [10] with 4 GB of data. Data are split into smaller sections which are then cleaned, transformed, and reduced in size in SPSS, before being merged together once more, and then ported into *R* for analyses.

A good principle for large datasets is that the raw dataset itself should never be altered but written into further files by software (e.g. using *syntax* when working in SPSS or code in R). Sometimes an error is found in coding, which means that entire data files need rebuilding from scratch, and good software should allow that straightforwardly. Data can also sometimes be updated by the provider, if variables were cleaned, errors found, or an additional year of data provided. If updated raw files are provided, then it should be possible to automatically re-run the entire analyses using the various program files, and this should be straightforward if all software has been kept.

Besides keeping a log, it is important to check the dataset in detail. Considering the size and complexity of big datasets, working on such sets inevitably is prone to unexpected errors. Working in a team allows for swapping work, sharing code with other users, and checking that everyone can understand what the others did. For high profile analyses which may impact on policy decisions and accuracy is essential, two or even three people should separately code the same data and reconcile code until the same answers are obtained. At all stages, it is worth looking at frequency tables, scattergrams, and other descriptive measures to identify data errors that have inadvertently occurred and to provide reassurance to the whole team.

Once the dataset is ready for analysis, initial exploration should include calculating basic statistics, assessing the numbers and reasons for missing values, and looking for unusual values in frequency distributions as a part of data cleaning checks. Big datasets are often collected for administrative reasons, and missing data or data errors are common, which can impact the quality of variables needed to answer research questions. Depending on the situation, research questions or strategies may need amending, or introducing the need for methods such as imputation of missing data. It may surprise you that the majority of your time will involve restructuring and reorganising data to make it suitable for statistical analyses, which should then be relatively straightforward. Since the data cleansing and sorting is so important, it is crucial that you seek help from more experienced researchers. In addition, with a hundred thousand cases and many variables, it is sensible to collaborate with data scientists. Educationalists understand well what the raw data mean, where they come from, and what the questions are that need answering. However, data scientists have the experience and tools for processing such data, hence the importance of collaboration.

Statistical analysis

Statistical methods are described more fully in Chapter 22. However, one of the key differences when dealing with big datasets is considering significance levels, since most statistics are designed for small sample sizes where sampling variation matters. With an N of 100,000 almost all statistical comparisons on real data are significant with $p < 0.05$, and therefore it may be better to set a more robust significance level of about $p < 0.000001$ [12]. In general, it is better to use parametric statistics, with effect sizes expressed in the units of the measures themselves, as well as standardised effect sizes such as Cohen's *d*. A major difference with big datasets is that variables are not normally distributed due to the very large number of cases. To compensate, you could use a parametric analysis with a bootstrap, which makes no assumption of normality [13].

Missing data

Missing data are inevitable in big datasets, sometimes in substantial amounts, and need handling in a principled way. Keeping only cases with complete data can lead to very small sample sizes compared to the original dataset. Therefore, when working with large datasets, missing data can be 'imputed' (replaced with plausible estimates) so that a dataset becomes complete. There are several methods for this, but *multiple imputation* is now seen as the best approach, using functions in *R* such as *mice* (multiple imputation by chained equations); van Buuren [14] provides an accessible and clear introduction to this. In general, impute all missing data, not just the measures needed for a particular analysis, and include dependent variables in imputations. The more variables in an imputation, the more likely that patterns behind the missingness will properly be taken into account. In some instances, it may be useful to do a multiple imputation and a parallel analysis on the listwise deleted data to help in understanding the inadvertent biases and the loss of power resulting from listwise deletion. Again, this is an area where it is important to collaborate and use the expertise of others.

Reporting and dissemination

Studies reporting big datasets can be boring, mainly because of endless tables packed with numbers. The human brain is bad at reading tables, and readers therefore try to visualise what is happening. Grab the attention of the reader by providing a graph which shows what is actually happening. Graphs for big datasets are frequently quite clear as sampling errors are smaller and patterns easier to see. Advances in technology have made this much easier since software for drawing graphs has improved immensely in recent years, although not in *SPSS* which is frustrating as you may have used this for your statistical analysis. The most versatile and powerful is probably *ggplot2* in *R*. Although it has a steep learning curve, the end products can be very impressive. Big datasets allow the plotting of raw data, so that distributions, as scattergrams, histograms or 'pirate plots' (a type of graph displaying raw data in addition to summary statistics), can be appreciated and emphasise the richness of the data.

The final dissemination of the study results will depend on the purpose of a study and on the agreement with data holders (see Chapter 28). You may be asked to present your preliminary findings in the form of an oral presentation or a written report prior to sharing the results more widely (e.g. peer-reviewed articles). As an example, the UKMED research subgroup reviews interim reports before preliminary findings are presented at conferences and final reports are submitted for publications. It is therefore important to consider the time which might be required to obtain the necessary permissions before submitting for conferences, etc. Reporting restrictions often apply to tables and graphs from external data from UKMED, Office for National Statistics (ONS), High Education Statistics Agency (HESA), and other external bodies.

As working with big datasets involves many decisions and space to publish these is limited, a tip is to use supplementary material to provide more details. You might also want to publish more than one article which means repeating the description of data preparation. One way around this issue is to publish so-called profile papers describing in detail what data were picked and why and how they were prepared for the analysis. Such a paper can then be cited in other papers without each time needing to describe the process of data preparation in detail. Finally, preprints, in journals such as *medRxiv*, are useful both for putting out results quickly and getting critical comments before final publication (but should be cleared as necessary with data holders).

BOX 23.1   Illustrative case study of progression in UK psychiatry trainees

The Royal College of Psychiatrists together with Higher Education England funded a research project to help them better understand career choices in psychiatry. The funder had identified attrition during training was the key problem. Therefore, it was hoped the research project would inform mental health workforce policy to reduce attrition in psychiatry training [15, 16]. To reach these goals, the research team proposed a mixed methods study and identified three research objectives:

1 Identifying and exploring attrition rates according to trainees' attributes (researched using UKMED).

2 Identifying factors that contribute to psychiatry trainees leaving or intending to leave their training, or not progressing through their training (researched using a questionnaire).

3 Exploring in-depth how and why these (and other) factors contribute to attrition or retention (researched using interviews).

Why big data?

The research team chose to apply for the UKMED datasets to access comprehensive longitudinal data collected nationally about UK medical trainees each year. This allows follow up of trainees and assessment of training progression. Demographic data enabled researchers to investigate differences between different groups of trainees.

Challenges

- *No attrition variable.* After exploring the data, it became clear that investigating the original research objective would not be possible. Although there is a clear general understanding of what attrition is, the nature of UKMED posed many challenges in analysing the career paths of psychiatry trainees (and attrition) (e.g. trainees move a lot, they go through career paths that deviate from traditional career paths, relevant information is not provided or is contradictory in UKMED). There was no simple variable that would indicate with confidence that a trainee had left training and therefore the only option was to follow up trainees. The original research objective was amended from focusing on *attrition* to *progression*: 'Explore rates of and reasons for trainees' progression with and without delays'.

- *Limited time window for investigation.* Psychiatry training takes six years (without trainees taking breaks) and with data recorded from 2012 in the UKMED database, there is a limited time span for which trainees can be followed up. Considering the limitation of how far back UKMED data can go, the researchers also investigated List of Registered Medical Practitioners data to give an overview of how long on average in the past it has taken trainees to enter the Specialist Register as psychiatrists, with some delays of course reflecting interruptions in training, e.g. maternity leave, gap year, transferring from other specialties, and so on.

- *No explanation.* There is limited information on the reasons *why* trainees are not progressing through training without delays, reflecting the fact that UKMED is primarily an administrative database. The mixed methods approach uses interviews and survey data to complement the UKMED data for understanding trainees' reasons and motivations.

Outputs and findings

Statistical modelling used a survival analysis and showed that the probability of completing psychiatry training in six years (which is minimum years of training in the United Kingdom) was 17.2% [16]. This probability varied between groups of doctors: 4.8% for non-UK graduate females to 29% for UK graduate males. Based on the List of Registered Medical Practitioners data, the study revealed that 76.3% of UK graduates on the psychiatry specialist register are registered within 12 years after medical school qualification (approximately four years of delay) with some doctors taking up to 27 years to get on the register [15, 16].

Summary

Big Data offers many opportunities for research in clinical education, but it also offers challenges, both technical and methodological. Techniques used for smaller datasets are not always appropriate, statistically or computationally, so new approaches may need to be learned. However, there are many opportunities to undertake longitudinal studies which would normally take years for primary data collection. The secondary analysis of Big Data can be very informative for the future direction of both research and policy.

Top tips

- Work with a team so you can make informed decisions and do quality checks.
- Take advice from data scientists who may have more experience working with Big Data.
- Keep extensive research logs and record version control.
- Invest in skills such as SPSS. Acquiring more advanced options such as *R* are undoubtedly worthwhile but require help.
- Use pre-prints, supplementary materials, and profile papers to properly describe the data and how you have prepared the data for analysis.

Common pitfalls

- Asking for more data than you need. This may lead to an unsuccessful application.
- Using inappropriate software for complex analyses. Sometimes more advance statistical packages are required.
- Misjudging how much time it takes to undertake a Big Data project. Due to the amount of data, it often takes longer to clean and prepare the data compared with the actual analysis.
- Producing results only in lengthy tables or uninformative graphics. This makes the information and the data unclear to readers and reviewers.

Ethical issues

- Be aware of the possibility of de-anonymisation.
- If you are linking datasets, ensure participants have provided the relevant consent.
- Data holders will often ask for previews of papers, results, or reports prior to publication or dissemination of results at conferences.

Further reading

Chahine, S., Kulasegaram, K.M., Wright, S. et al. (2018). A call to investigate the relationship between education and health outcomes using Big Data. *Academic Medicine* 93 (6): 829–832.

Ellaway, R.H., Pusic, M.V., Galbraith, R.M., and Cameron, T. (2014). Developing the role of big data and analytics in health professional education. *Medical Teacher* 36 (3): 216–222.

Holmes, D. (2017). *Big Data: A Very Short Introduction*. Oxford: Oxford University Press.

Manocha, S. and Saini, P. (2022). Insights of Big Data analytics in education—challenges & opportunities: a review paper. *International Management Review* 18: 20–26.

Salganik, M. (2018). *Bit by Bit: Social Research in the Digital Age*. Princeton: Princeton University Press.

Wilhite, J.A., Altshuler, L., Zabar, S. et al. (2020). Development and maintenance of a medical education research registry. *BMC Medical Education* 20:199.

References

1 Diebold, F.X. (2019). On the origin(s) and development of "big data": the phenomenon, the term, and the discipline. https://www.sas.upenn.edu/~fdiebold/papers/paper112/Diebold_Big_Data.pdf (accessed 8 May 2023)

2 Jin, X., Wah, B.W., Cheng, X., and Wang, Y. (2015). Significance and challenges of Big Data research. *Big Data Research* 2: 59–64.

3 Wainer, H., Harik, P., and Neter, J. (2013). Visual revelations: Stigler's law of eponymy and Marey's train schedule: did Serjev do it before Ibry, and what about Jules Petiet? *Chance* 26 (1): 53–56.

4 McManus, I.C. (1985). Medical students: origins, selection, attitudes and culture. MD thesis. University of London. http://www.ucl.ac.uk/medical-education/publications/md.

5 Garrud, P. and McManus, I. (2018). Impact of accelerated, graduate-entry medicine courses: a comparison of profile, success, and specialty destination between graduate entrants to accelerated or standard medicine courses in UK. *BMC Medical Education* 18 (1): 1–16.

6 Coggon, D., Barker, D., and Rose, G. (2009). *Epidemiology for the Uninitiated*. Wiley.

7 Madhusoodanan, J. (2022). Health data for all. *Nature* 605 (7908): 182–183.

8 Dowell, J., Cleland, J., Fitzpatrick, S. et al. (2018). The UK medical education database (UKMED) what is it? Why and how might you use it? *BMC Medical Education* 18 (1): 6.

9 Spark, N.T. (2006). *A History of Murphy's Law*, 68. Lulu. com.

10 McManus, I., Woolf, K., Harrison, D. et al. (2021). Predictive validity of A-level grades and teacher-predicted grades in UK medical school applicants: a retrospective analysis of administrative data in a time of COVID-19. *BMJ Open* 11 (12): e047354.

11 Tsitoara, M. (2020). *Beginning Git and GitHub*. Springer.

12 Raftery, A.E. (1995). Bayesian model selection in social research. *Sociological Methodology* 25: 111–163.

13 Chernick, M.R. and LaBudde, R.A. (2011). *An Introduction of Bootstrap Methods with Applications to R*. Hoboken, NJ: Wiley.

14 van Buuren, S. (2018). *Flexible Imputation of Missing Data*, 2e. New York: CRC Press.

15 Medisauskaite, A., Rich, A., Silkens, M. et al. (2020). Understanding career choices in psychiatry. *Consultant* 60: 96.

16 Silkens, M.E., Sarker, S.-J., and Medisauskaite, A. (2021). Uncovering trends in training progression for a national cohort of psychiatry trainees: discrete-time survival analysis. *British Journal of Psychiatry Open* 7 (4): E120.

PART V

Succeeding in clinical education research

24 Maximising opportunities and overcoming challenges

Susil Pallikadavath and Simon Gay

Learning objectives

By the end of this chapter, you should be able to:
- Appreciate how to maximise the opportunities and rise to the challenges offered by a research project.
- Recall top tips for research project success.
- Avoid common pitfalls in research.

Introduction

Clinical education research projects are becoming ever more popular. PhDs, master's degrees, student selected components, intercalated degrees, and standalone projects have all expanded significantly in number in recent years. Taught courses culminating in research, the formalisation of credentialisation for certain educational roles, and efforts to improve the quality of support for educational research have all promoted wider participation in educational research projects.

This chapter draws on experiences of undertaking, supervising, and assessing educational research projects to offer guidance for those embarking on their first projects. While some of the advice is specific to those of you undertaking clinical education research as part of a degree course, much of it is transferable to any small project. The guidance has been structured into three key phases of the project: preparation, design, and conduct.

On your marks: preparing for your research project

> By failing to prepare, you are preparing to fail
> Benjamin Franklin

Preliminary sources of information

There are many useful sources of information to consider before embarking on your own research project. If you are doing your project as part of a degree course, your university will usually have detailed handbooks, in print, and/or online. These usually outline most of what you need to know about how to position and conduct your study within the relevant educational research landscape. If you are conducting your project as part of another pre-structured research opportunity, for example a summer studentship, there may be similar information available. If it is a standalone project, you may still benefit from consulting the information provided by supervisors and research ethics committees before commencing your project.

Before investing significant time and energy into your project, ensure you have read and understood any requirements from your course handbooks. It can be helpful to recognise that research projects which are part of degree courses are designed to develop your skills and experience in education research. This is an opportunity to take your time and make sure you are doing things well. The learning is from the process as well as the outcome.

Knowing what is expected of you is essential in order to logically plan your project and maximise your learning and development as an education researcher. Beyond understanding the guidance offered for the conduct of the research, it is also really useful to familiarise yourself with course regulations. This is because, even in the best of worlds, things will not always go as planned. Work pressures may mount, or life events may occur. Understanding what adjustments can be made in these exceptional circumstances can help you to consider how to respond and what the implications might be for your project. Furthermore, it is important to know about the availability of such adjustments before they are

---

Starting Research in Clinical Education, First Edition. Edited by Eliot L. Rees, Alison Ledger, and Kim A. Walker.
© 2024 The Association for the Study of Medical Education (ASME). Published 2024 by John Wiley & Sons Ltd.
Companion website: www.wiley.com/go/clinicaleducation

needed. If the time comes to require them, there is often already enough pressure arising from the inter-current event. This is one of the reasons why it can be helpful to develop a risk register early in your project planning (see Chapter 25). Time tends to be a precious and scarce commodity, and it is better to choose your action plan from a list of pre-identified alternatives rather than opt for the only solution you can find in a stressful moment.

Choose your supervisor wisely

If you are new to clinical education research, it is essential to get a supervisor to support you in your project. This will always be the case for degree students, but it can be extremely helpful for those doing independent projects (including those who have significant clinical research experience but are new to education research). First and foremost, having a supervisor offers the opportunity to learn more about the research process and will help you to avoid many of the potential pitfalls lurking in the detail of any research project.

The project supervisor role is pivotal to the success of the project and your development as a researcher. It is important this educational relationship works well. Consequently, giving some thought to whom you would like your supervisor to be is as important as considering what you are interested in working on. Think about the potential supervisors you have come into contact with in the past whether as tutors on a course or researchers. Were there any you developed a particular connection with? Were any conducting research in areas that were particularly interesting for you? Draw up a shortlist of potential supervisors and then find out about them. Look at their online profiles on university or other websites. Look at their experience of supervising students and of conducting their own research. If possible, speak to past students and other new researchers they have supervised – find out what their supervisory style is like and consider whether that is what you are looking for. For example, do they put their students or research fellows as first authors on subsequent publications or do they tend to simply acknowledge them or place them as mid-list authors?

Don't feel that you need to pick one person and then commit to them. It is perfectly acceptable to arrange informal discussions with multiple academics to discuss areas of interest before committing to one. As long as you are clear about this, they will not be offended if you ultimately ask someone else to supervise you. We will discuss working with your supervisor later in the chapter.

Methods versus subject expertise

It is worth considering whether you are seeking a supervisor who is a research method expert or a supervisor who is an expert in the subject matter to be studied. Both options have their merits. It is important to remember, regardless of which you choose, if you have selected wisely, they are very likely to have much more experience than you in education research in general.

It is also not uncommon for research projects to have more than one supervisor, particularly where projects are more substantial and long term such as a PhD study. In this event, you would then have co-supervisors who may be a mix of subject and method experts. The inclusion of co-supervisors in such situations opens up a wide range of expertise possibilities.

Finally, in the same way that most potential supervisors will not be offended if you ultimately ask someone else to supervise you, it is also important you do not take offence if a particular supervisor decides not to supervise you. The decision not to supervise can be for a whole host of reasons, many of which will be absolutely nothing to do with you. Causes could include the wider pressure of work, already having reached their maximum learner supervising capacity, or discovering a potential conflict of interest.

Developing a proposal

Once you have identified a supervisor, you should finalise the topic you intend researching (see Chapter 1) and turn this into a clearly articulated research question (see Chapter 2). From here you can start to develop it into a research proposal considering which methodological paradigm is most appropriate (see Chapter 3) and whether there are any relevant theories you could draw on to inform the design and conduct of your research (see Chapter 4). We recommend engaging with relevant stakeholders early in this process to enable them to have meaningful input in to both the final research question and the design of your research project (see Chapter 5).

Project approval

Once you have assembled a final draft of your research proposal, it is time to seek formal approval of your plans. Depending on the context in which you are conducting your study, you may need to obtain various forms of approval. Whilst this is not an exhaustive list, the approvals needed could include

1 Your supervisor(s)
2 Your course or programme director, or their nominated deputy, if your research project is taking place as part of a course of study that you are enrolled upon.

3 Anyone responsible for the provision of the educational activity in which your study is situated. For example, a medical school year lead, or a course or programme director.

4 The relevant research gatekeeper – most educational / clinical institutions will have some sort of research gatekeeper even if they are not given this precise title. The gatekeeper's role is to ensure only good quality research projects take place in their institution, and any new research projects do not overlap with projects already approved and taking place. This helps to reduce the interference of one project with another and prevents the overburdening of potential research participants with requests to participate in research.

5 A relevant research ethics committee (see Chapter 7).

The above list also represents the typical order in which it would be wise to seek the above formal approvals as, for example, the gatekeeper is unlikely to approve a project without the prior approval of your supervisor and the other responsible educators connected with the study or its environment. Similarly, the research ethics committee would expect to see supervisor and research gatekeeper approvals.

As you might anticipate, formal approval is usually provided in writing. However, even that can range from a simple signature or email from your project supervisor or research gatekeeper through to a formal letter of approval complete with project reference number from the research ethics committee.

Research ethics committees

In essence, research ethics committees exist to protect the rights and well-being of research participants and to promote the progression of good quality, ethical research (see Chapter 7). Their membership is made up of people with a broad mix of experience of research. Research ethics committees also often have at least one lay member who is viewed as representing both society as a whole and the potential participants.

In clinical education, there is often more than one potential research ethics committee available to review a research project. Some institutions have special ethics committee specifically for student projects or educational research. It is also sometimes possible to submit your proposal under a 'low-risk' route (as the risks for educational research are often low compared with clinical trials, for example, and the proposal may not need the same degree of scrutiny). The decision about which to use is often important and your supervisor ought to be able to help clarify which research ethics committee is best suited to your project.

Another thing to be aware of with regard to research ethics committees is the value and power of the committee Chair. The Chair can in certain circumstances make a quick decision without that decision needing to be considered by the rest of the research ethics committee. This can be useful, for example, if you want to conduct a two-centre research project and you have already received ethical approval from the research ethics committee at one of the centres but also need to seek approval from the other centre. An ethics committee Chair alone could give this 'second' approval. Ethics committee chairs can also advise if your project does not require ethical approval (i.e. is considered exempt). Having this in writing is useful when it comes to submitting your work for publication.

Research ethics committees are often viewed with a great deal of trepidation by those seeking approval for a research project, and it is certainly true ethics committees have the power to inhibit or stop a research project progressing before it has even begun in earnest. However, if, when preparing your research proposal for submission to a research ethics committee, you are fearful of applying for ethical approval for your research project then we would encourage you to reframe that perception because research ethics committees are almost always really your friend. They are especially the friend of new researchers because they:

- Are usually particularly supportive of early career researchers as members may remember what it is like to be a new researcher and be keen to help people to produce good research.
- Are often happy for a member of the committee to meet with new researchers prior to ethics application submission, talk through your project, and alert you to common pitfalls of that research type.
- Provide an important point of focus in the preparatory stage of a research study.
- Encourage, facilitate, and support a good standard of study documentation, such as the project proposal, consent forms, and participant information sheets.
- Offer an opportunity for your research project proposal to be reviewed by people with a lot more research experience than you.
- Provide impartial, constructive feedback on how to strengthen your research project.
- Can help researchers to focus more closely on the key elements of the research project.
- Often prevent ethical problems arising later on in the project.

- Improve the chances of publishing the study once it is completed. If ethical approval would normally be required to publish a particular study, then it is quite rightly, extremely difficult to publish it if prior ethical approval, obtained before the study was started, does not exist.

If your project has obvious flaws at this initial stage, it is better that you are made aware of them. Most flaws are correctable and research ethics committees usually provide feedback which helps you make those corrections. However, even if an identified flaw is insurmountable (and that situation is very uncommon if you have carefully thought about and planned your project with appropriate input from your supervisor), it is still much better to know that before you have invested any more time and effort into the project and perhaps still have time to come up with an alternate project.

These days application for research ethics approval is usually via an online system which often makes application relatively streamlined and straightforward. However, some institutions still operate a paper-based system through a named administrator.

Get set: designing your research project

Get the research question right

The importance of crafting the research question cannot be overstated (see Chapter 2). The research question you develop will underpin your whole project design; getting it right is imperative. Mattick et al. [1] describe three fundamental features of good research questions; relevance, originality, and rigour. Considering problems you have encountered as a learner or educator may be a useful way to generate relevant research topics. Alternatively, ask your chosen supervisor which topics they recommend. Read through recent issues of key journals in the field to see if there are any research topics that captivate your enthusiasm. Next make sure you are addressing an original question. Spend time looking at recent articles published on your topic of focus and see if there are any remaining gaps or tensions in the literature.

Write the background section of your proposal. Try to use the problem/gap/hook heuristic to clearly articulate the importance of the problem this study will address, the gap in the current literature (including what borders this gap), and a hook that justifies why this gap needs to be filled [2].

Time spent drafting, sharing, and redrafting here is time well spent as a well-crafted research question drives the project forward in a positive way with a clear sense of direction. Get the research question right and what follows becomes easier to accomplish.

Let the methods follow

As alluded to above, the third consideration for your research question is rigour. A rigorous study is philosophically aligned and internally coherent [3]. In order to achieve this, it is crucial that you choose a methodology aligned with your philosophical approach to the project and the research question (see Chapter 3). This ensures your project has maximal congruity and does not inadvertently design hidden points of failure into the project.

Consider the research onion model [4], it offers a good visual representation of how different research methods align to different research philosophies as a starting point for new researchers.

Seek feedback on your proposal

Ask for feedback on your proposal before finalising it. Your supervisor should be able to offer feedback, but it is also worth considering if there are any opportunities to get a fresh pair of eyes. For example, clinical education research group meetings and research design services. Hopefully, the feedback you receive is constructive, but regardless, any feedback can be useful if offering a new line of sight on your project, even if the feedback is negative.

Once you have got a first version of your project proposal, it is worth considering if there are any other resources you are going to need in order to successfully execute it. You may have picked your supervisor based on their topic interests, now consider whether they have the methodological expertise to support the project that has developed. If not, consider asking if you can have another informal supervisor to help guide you with the methodology, or again explore the possibility of formally introducing a second new co-supervisor to formalise the introduction of another person.

Depending on the methods you have chosen, you may have a significant amount of data collection and analysis to do. If the rules and regulations surrounding your project permit, think about collaborating with other researchers, new or experienced, you know to share the workload. If you have peers at a similar stage of their research development, you might be able to double or triple your individual experience of data analysis by being a second analyst on the projects of one or two peers as well as being lead analyst on your own project. This type of collaboration brings the added bonuses of increasing awareness of how other studies are being conducted, exposing you to subtle and sometimes not so subtle variations of analysis. You could extend the collaboration beyond the project to academic publication if the study merits it. This additional experience and any potential outputs all enhance your curriculum vitae!

However, please be aware that whilst some degree programmes or courses encourage this collegiate and collaborative approach, others do not. In particular, it is important to realise whilst project supervisors often contribute to data analysis in the wider research world, within degree programmes this is sometimes frowned upon or actively discouraged and can result in academic penalties being imposed on the student by their institution. Therefore, yet again, it is very important to be aware of any rules and regulations pertinent to your project before you start and that includes rules and regulations regarding supervisors.

Keeping it small, focused, and achievable

While it can be very tempting to design large projects with multiple data collection methods and large sample sizes, you have to balance this with feasibility. The potential size of a research project will depend on a wide range of factors including, but not limited to, the time available to commit to the project, the wider context in which the project sits (e.g. part of a degree programme or teaching fellowship), the funding available to support the project, and the very nature of the research question you are trying to answer.

Intercalated degree and master's projects, for example, are usually designed to be a first foray into research. Consequently, it is much better to construct a focused question, address it comprehensively, and finish your degree than it is to bite off more than it is realistic to chew. You can always conduct further studies afterwards, and even consider a doctorate in clinical education at a later date. Indeed, initial small projects can themselves provide the opportunity to gather pilot data that can then be used to apply for external funding for further research and can often lead to opportunities to gain research-orientated posts such as fellowships.

Plan for all eventualities

Formulate a well-planned, project management approach to your research, considering budgets, timeframes, and breaks (see Chapter 25). It is also good practice to be realistic with the planning of your own time – for example, everyone needs a break or a holiday and it would be wise to factor that into your project timetable.

A key part of planning research is thinking about what could go wrong as it progresses. For example, which parts are dependent on other people, what happens if you need to take a few weeks sick leave, and so on. Clearly, not all risks can be eliminated but most can be anticipated, and many can be mitigated by a prepreparedaction plan. Professional project managers typically document and manage such risks through risk registers, and these can also be helpful for small research projects to promote thinking about 'what happens if?'.

Good planning and organisation can certainly help identify and manage risks and promote timely intervention when things are not going quite according to plan. It will help you quickly identify if things are falling behind schedule so you are better able to meet your key research study milestones.

Go: conducting your research project

Write as you go

Whether you will simply need to write up a study report, a master's dissertation, a PhD thesis or a draft for publication submission – writing will always take longer than you anticipate (see Chapter 26). It is a good habit to start writing early and try to continue to write often throughout the project. Writing helps you to consolidate and interrogate your thoughts. Making field notes as your study progresses can greatly assist you in your subsequent write-up and in some forms of research is seen as a marker of rigour.

> 'Field notes are the researcher's documentation of events, conversations and behaviours observed in the field, and the researcher's reflections on them. Where and when field notes are documented will depend on the setting, the researcher and the participants being observed. [5]'

We recommend getting as much detail as possible written down in your first draft. However, be prepared for the possibility of revising much of your first draft and also subsequent early drafts. This is not a negative thing but is part of the natural evolution of your write-up. You start to connect the various strands of your analysis and thinking. This allows you to refine the alignment of the various sections of your write-up in order to reflect the coherent alignment of your entire research project.

Other recommendations that would help your write up include
- The use of good, clear tables. These can remove the need for whole paragraphs of your write-up whilst summarising your data beautifully.

- Learn to create good-quality diagrams. There are a number of online options that can help you do this that your institution may subscribe to (e.g. Canva).
- Try not to repeat what you say. If it is in a table, there is no need to tell the reader twice. When it comes to publication, space in scientific journals is limited!
- Sometimes research requires you to be balanced by being personally balanced too. Your burden of work, and your productivity will vary. However, being consistent, and utilising days where things are going well, and being relaxed on days where things are less good is also important.
- Diligence is key. You are only as good as the robustness, quality, and accuracy of your methods and your data. While it might not seem like it, every small or big project contributes to our understanding of this world and science only works when we can trust the data that we put out as a research community.

Later chapters in this part offer further guidance on writing dissertations (Chapter 26), writing for publication (Chapter 27), and disseminating your research findings (Chapter 28).

Keep on top of your references

First, check the reference style that you need for your writing. If you are writing a journal article check the instructions for authors in your first choice journal. If you are writing as part of a course of study, check the course handbook for regulations.

Keep track of the references you use as you go. Finding a reference retrospectively that you have used but not accurately recorded can be a real hassle. Recording them as you write is time and energy efficient and will avoid you missing any citations that you ought to be including. This may sound tedious, but it is one of the cornerstones of academic rigour and without it your research project will be weaker in its reporting. Additionally, if you submit to a journal, the peer reviewers and editors are likely to notice omissions, making it more difficult to publish.

If you do not already, we strongly urge you to consider using reference management software (e.g. Endnote, Mendeley, and Refworks). The time invested in learning to use a well-established reference management software package is never wasted and can be one of many useful learning experiences to be gained from your first research project. It will undoubtedly save you a lot of time later on in your project as it helps you to keep a good track of your references, which might be in lots of different sections of your write-up. The reference management software also offers you tremendous flexibility if you do decide to submit a research paper for journal publication. Different journals insist on different reference formats and being able to automatically and accurately switch from one to another can save you the many hours of work required to do this manually. If you are affiliated with a university, most will offer institutional subscriptions so it is worth checking if this is available. University libraries usually offer training too. If you do not have a university affiliation, then Mendeley is a good free option.

Accessing papers

All research projects will require the use of existing literature to inform the development of your research proposal, to underpin your research methodology, and support the discussion of your results. Accessing some papers may be easy as they are either open access or you may have an institutional subscription which provides you with free access to them. However, getting hold of others can prove more challenging. Having money available to support your work is usually a luxury that new researchers do not enjoy and we would strongly encourage you to think very carefully before personally paying for access to a specific paper or journal as papers can sometimes be genuinely accessed by other means.

The following is a nonexhaustive list of strategies to consider when thinking about those hard to access papers:

- Ask your supervisor – your supervisor may already have a copy they can share with you, especially if they are an expert in the subject or method to which the paper refers.
- Ask your librarian – librarians working in academic environments are usually experts in the various ways available to access papers, and this can include interlibrary-loan systems where libraries are able to borrow publications from one another.
- Ask your course director – your course may have access to specific publications if they are particularly pertinent to the course you are studying on, the research environment your study is being conducted in, or another student has made use of that same paper previously.
- Check online repositories – many authors will save accessible versions of their papers on websites such as ResearchGate or their institutional repositories.
- Email the corresponding author – if you cannot access it by any other means, it is perfectly acceptable to email the author to ask if they would

be prepared to share a copy with you. Often researchers are flattered that someone is taking an interest in their paper.

- If you are finding a particular paper especially hard to get, ask yourself if it is really that relevant or useful to your study, or whether a more easily accessible but similarly useful paper might be an alternative.

Use exemplars and reporting standards

No matter what format your write up is taking, we suggest looking through exemplars that can help you capture the required style and structure. There may even be different approaches illustrated by different examples in which case you could, in conjunction with your supervisor, carefully consider which approach might work best for you, your research project and your finished written work. If you are writing a journal article, check the journal's website for recent articles to use as exemplars. If you are writing a thesis or dissertation then check your university's library or ask your supervisor for examples. In the United Kingdom, the British Library stores digital versions of many doctoral theses that you can use to see different approaches to structure and writing (ethos.bl.uk).

In recent years, reporting standards have been published for almost all research designs [6]. The most common project designs include qualitative research [7], observational studies [8], and systematic reviews [9]. Find the standards aligned to your methods and review your evolving write-up against them. This will help you to identify gaps that you may need to address.

Make good use of your supervisor

One of the key ways to ensure that your project runs as smoothly as possible is to make good use of your supervisor. This may sound obvious but if you can establish a good working relationship with your supervisor then you will maximise the benefits of having them involved in your work and your development as a researcher.

We recommend you start at your first supervisory meeting by asking your supervisor to explain their expectations of you, their personal ground rules, and their preferred methods of communication and arrangement of meetings. It can be useful to explicitly consider each other's expectations of the supervisory relationship (see companion website for a resource that can be useful to facilitate this discussion). We recommend coming to an agreement regarding frequency of meetings, expected turnaround time for written feedback, research responsibilities, funding availability, support for professional development, publication and authorship [10]. After

that, do not be afraid to take the lead when it is appropriate to do so. For example, it can be helpful to send your supervisor(s) any work you want to discuss in advance of the meeting to give them the opportunity to read and digest it before you meet. If you have specific issues you want to discuss during your supervisory meetings, then sending a short agenda in advance can help to focus the discussion. Equally, sending over a summary of the discussion in the meeting, agreed actions, and timelines after the meeting can help to promote accountability. Supervisors generally enjoy supervising energetic and enthusiastic individuals who simply need guidance. Remember supervisors are not there to do your work for you, but to help you travel in the right direction without hitting too many bumps in the road. This is also easier to achieve if you have open and frank conversations with them. Supervisors can only provide clear guidance if they have all of the available information about your project and its progress. Keeping information from your supervisor because you are embarrassed about something that has gone wrong or are behind with the expected project progress will hinder the supervisor's ability to support you.

In contrast, if you are proactive and anticipatory in the information you provide to your supervisor this can help use any meeting time to give you the most support possible in the areas in which you most need it. Supervisors are usually busy people and even something as simple as pre-preparing most of the supervisory paperwork really helps free up their time for more educational and interesting aspects of your work. Finally, try to make the arrangements for your next meeting before leaving the current meeting, they can always be changed later on if necessary.

How to further capitalise on your hard work

By this point you will have put a lot of hard work into your research. Whilst completing your project is a significant achievement in itself, there are ample opportunities to further capitalise on this work that may be helpful to your research training and also for your career development. Submit abstracts to regional, national, and international clinical education conferences for posters, oral presentations, workshops, or round table discussions, whichever are most appropriate for the communication of your research findings (see Chapter 28). Consider submitting your work for prizes and awards too – and do not be put off doing this by the thought of competition. Fewer people apply for these things than you would think and you have to be in it to win it! Be sure to discuss with your supervisor the possibility of submitting your work for publication in a peer-reviewed journal (see Chapter 27). To keep up the momentum, try to complete these things as soon as possible after your research project has finished, otherwise day-to-day life will take over.

Summary

This chapter has offered tips on planning, progressing, writing up, and further benefitting from your research project. Tips about choosing your supervisor and developing the supervisory relationship have also been included. However, despite all this information and all that needs to be done to bring a research project to a successful conclusion, it must not be forgotten that to have the opportunity to explore an area of clinical education you are interested in, in a robust and methodical way is a joy and a privilege. So, the final piece of advice for this chapter to offer you has to be to encourage you to enjoy your research project and be proud of whatever it achieves for you personally and the academic community more generally.

Top tips

- Consider both the methodological and content expertise of potential supervisors.
- Discuss and agree expectations with your supervisor at the outset of your project.
- Capitalise on your work as soon as possible, by submitting conference abstracts, publications, or prize applications. Even if you are not successful on the first attempt, you may receive feedback that can strengthen your project and promote further learning and research.

Common pitfalls

- Trying to take on more than is feasible given your resources. First learn how to conduct a research project well and then you can build on it in further research.
- Bringing written work to discuss with your supervisor to the meeting. Sending it in advance will enable them to read it properly and give more meaningful feedback.
- Leaving the referencing until the end. Keep on top of these as you write to prevent you forgetting which to include or losing them.

Ethical issues

- Discuss and agree who will be included as authors of any research outputs from your project with your supervisor early on.
- Discuss with your supervisor which is the most appropriate ethics committee for your project.
- Make sure you get the appropriate permissions from supervisors, gatekeepers, and ethics committees.

References

1 Mattick, K., Johnston, J., and de la Croix, A. (2018). How to. . .write a good research question. *The Clinical Teacher* 15 (2): 104–108.

2 Lingard, L. (2015). Joining a conversation: the problem/gap/hook heuristic. *Perspectives on Medical Education* 4: 252–253.

3 Palermo, C., Reidlinger, D.P., and Rees, C.E. (2021). Internal coherence matters: Lessons for nutrition and dietetics research. *Nutrition and Dietetics* 78 (3): 252–267.

4 Saunders, M., Lewis, P., and Thornhill, A. (2012). *Research Methods for Business Students*, 6e. Pearson Education Limited.

5 University of Nottingham University (2021). Field notes. Understanding Qualitative Field Work. https://www.nottingham.ac.uk/helmopen/rlos/research-evidence-based-practice/designing-research/types-of-study/understanding-qualitative-field-work/section05.html#:~:text=Field%20notes%20are%20the%20researcher's,and%20the%20participants%20being%20observed (accessed 29 June 2022).

6 Equator-network.org. (2019). The EQUATOR Network. Enhancing the QUAlity and Transparency Of Health Research. https://www.equator-network.org/ (accessed 10 May 2023).

7 O'Brien, B.C., Harris, I.B., Beckman, T.J. et al. (2014). Standards for reporting qualitative research: a synthesis of recommendations. *Academic Medicine* 89 (9): 1245–1251.

8 von Elm, E., Altman, D.G., Egger, M. et al. (2007). Strengthening the Reporting of Observational Studies in Epidemiology (STROBE) statement: guidelines for reporting observational studies. *BMJ* 335 (7624): 806–808.

9 Gordon, M. and Gibbs, T. (2014). STORIES statement: publication standards for healthcare education evidence synthesis. *BMC Medicine* 12: 143.

10 McGill University (2023). Clarifying Expectations. Supervision – Graduate and Postdoctoral Support. https://www.mcgill.ca/gradsupervision/supervisors/expectations (accessed 07 February 2023).

25 Managing your project

Michelle D. Lazarus and Georgina C. Stephens

Learning objectives

By the end of this chapter, you should be able to:
- Define the term 'project' and communicate how this applies to clinical education research.
- Describe the stages involved in managing a clinical education research project.

- Identify, select, and describe resources which can support education research project management.
- Anticipate common pitfalls in education research project management and outline potential solutions.
- Apply practical project management techniques in clinical education research projects.

Introduction

A goal without a plan is just a wish.

Antoine de Saint-Exupéry,
writer and pioneering aviator

Many clinical education researchers have valuable ideas for projects. Without a clearly defined research plan, good ideas may languish, and worthy projects may fail prior to completion. A key challenge, even for experienced researchers, is effectively executing projects within their available time and resources. This chapter will draw upon the field of project management to help guide you in developing an effective project management plan to achieve your research goals. Importantly, project management is not about having everything 'go according to plan', but rather proactively anticipating setbacks and risks, and brainstorming ways around these.

Effective communication is key for successful project management – a theme that will be represented throughout this chapter by introducing different communication strategies and approaches. Communication should occur in a variety of ways throughout the lifecycle of the project, including meetings, emails, documents (such as project plans and task forms), and so on. Identifying preferred and successful communication methods between you and your supervisor or research team, as well as other project stakeholders, is an essential first step in project management.

Project management is a dedicated profession. Known as the 'discipline of discipline' [1], the focus of project management is supporting on-time delivery and necessary follow-through to achieve project success [2]. Project managers may draw on a range of different techniques and approaches relevant to their particular industry and projects [3].

The aim of this chapter is to explore some techniques which can be adapted and adopted from the project management profession to support clinical education research projects. Professional project managers typically have a bird's eye view of a project and are responsible for timely and successful delivery of project outcomes, whereas the day-to-day execution of project tasks often involves a team of workers. As a new clinical education researcher, you are likely to have roles in both managing and executing a project, alongside your supervisor and any other members of your research team. So, although you may have multiple roles within a research project, applying project management principles can help ensure you meet your project responsibilities, and that the project as a whole is successful.

What is a project?

The established characteristics of a project are that it is a well-defined, temporary endeavour, resulting in a unique output or goal. Although the magnitude and scope of clinical education research projects can

Starting Research in Clinical Education, First Edition. Edited by Eliot L. Rees, Alison Ledger, and Kim A. Walker.
© 2024 The Association for the Study of Medical Education (ASME). Published 2024 by John Wiley & Sons Ltd.
Companion website: www.wiley.com/go/clinicaleducation

vary widely from small, short projects with a couple of researchers to large multi-institutional or international projects lasting years, these project characteristics hold true.

As a new clinical education researcher, your project could be a contribution to a larger research programme, a student research project, or research undertaken alongside teaching activities. Outputs from these types of projects could be a degree thesis, conference presentation, or journal publication.

Project management focuses on the process undertaken to achieve the goal/outcome. In this way, a project has a lifecycle and is finite. Depending on the nature of the research, a single body of clinical education research may be best defined in terms of a series of successive yet related projects, where later projects depend on successful delivery of earlier outcomes. For example, early or interim outcomes which could be considered projects in their own right include completion of a literature review or securing grant funding, whereas later outcomes may include submission of a thesis or journal article. In this way, some research activities, especially dissemination of project outcomes, may continue well past the end point of an initial project. Such activities may even need to be defined as separate projects.

All clinical education research projects benefit from project management principles, but the approach and degree required will depend on the project context. We have developed a workbook based on Glassick's [4] criteria which can help you initiate and plan your research project (see project management workbook on the companion website).

Key to early stages of project management is the development of an effective and focused research question (see Chapter 2), and adequate preparation (see project management workbook on companion website). The project planning material and process are described in more detail in the following sections, with a focus on describing the stages of project management as if you were starting a research project from scratch. Practically, this may not always be the case (e.g. taking over management of a research project already in progress), however, the same overarching principles will apply.

Project management stages

There are five key stages to project management (Figure 25.1). Each stage is defined and described, with practical steps, in the following sections. Importantly, clinical education research projects, whilst finite, often feed forward and are linked to the next project.

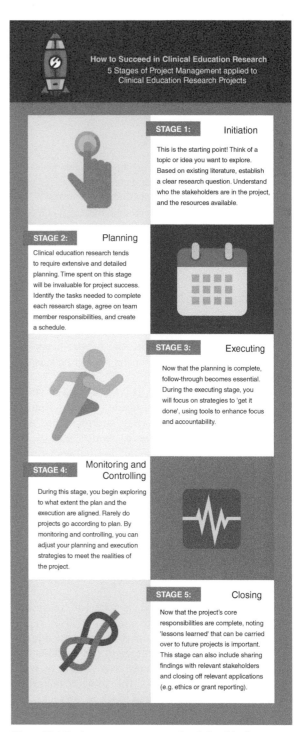

Figure 25.1 Project management can be defined in five stages, which may be applied to clinical education research.

Stage 1: initiation

Project initiation is the point at which a project begins. Herein the project is defined, stakeholders and resources are identified, and required approvals are sought. In clinical education research, the initiation stage will be informed by a literature review, establishing the research gap, and developed following refinement of a robust research question and/or hypothesis. Without a clearly defined research question, the project will be equally diffuse and unachievable, regardless of how effective the project management approach is.

By carefully considering project initiation, you will be able to understand both the need for the project, and its likelihood of successful completion. In this way, initiation allows you to make an informed decision whether to proceed with the project as intended, or terminate plans before significant time and resources are expended.

The first step is appointing a project manager who will be responsible for the day-to-day management of the project. As a new researcher, this is likely to be your role, although the person can differ depending on the nature of the project, the experience of research team members, and the extent of research funding. For example, the principal investigator, often alongside a research officer, may be best suited to manage large longitudinal projects, wherein less experienced researchers may participate in smaller components of the greater project. By contrast, master's students, PhD candidates, and teaching fellows may be expected to project manage their own research. In these cases, supervisors may provide relevant expertise and experience to guide you in your project management (e.g. by providing advice on appropriate timelines, stakeholder engagement, and/or research techniques).

If a project manager is taking over management of an existing project, they will still need to review all considerations laid out in this section to successfully manage the project across its remaining stages. Key considerations during the initiation stage are defining the project, understanding project stakeholders, and documenting an integrated project plan. Each of these stages is defined and described in more detail below.

Defining the project

Comprehensively defining the project is key to success across all stages. This aspect of project management hinges on knowledge of both the literature (i.e. general needs assessment) and your local research context (i.e. targeted needs assessment). For further details on conducting needs analyses, see resource on the companion website.

Importantly, defining the project is inseparable from identifying and engaging project stakeholders. For clarity, we discuss these elements of the project separately, but highlight that these will need to be considered in tandem to comprehensively attend to

initiation. As such, project initiation is likely to be highly iterative as these elements are increasingly drawn together.

Definitional aspects of your project ideally include a problem statement, research question(s), aim(s), objectives, approach, and anticipated outcome(s). The problem statement summarises the research challenge you are trying to address and should identify the relevant gap in existing literature and your own research context. The problem statement therefore informs the research question(s). The project aim then defines what you are setting out to achieve in the project. Project objectives are more specific than aims and will inform the scope and approach of your project. Objectives are most effective when they are specific, measurable, achievable, relevant, and timely (i.e. 'SMART').

'Measurable' within this context refers to how you judge and document the success (or failure) of the project, and how you will demonstrate the impact of your project. Measurable aspects will vary depending on the nature of your research, but may include the number of research participants (e.g. considering statistical significance or information power) [5], impact of publications resulting from the research (e.g. journal impact factor, Altmetric score, etc.), or an evaluation of how changes to educational practice impacts learners (e.g. student evaluation data).

To ensure project objectives are achievable, consider the resources you have available, such as funding, existing research infrastructure, and the expertise and availability of yourself and your research team. For the objective to be timely, consider how long you have to complete the project. This may be informed by factors such as the length of a degree programme, durations of grants or stipends, or other career and personal commitments. Project objectives, in turn, inform the approach of your project. Aligned with your research question, different research methods may be appropriate; however, these will need to fit within the objectives, feasibility, and risks that your project may have. For example, an initial pilot or feasibility study may be required, before embarking on a larger, resource-intensive project.

A project requires defined outcomes. These outcomes determine the project endpoint, also known as the project scope. Common clinical education research outcomes include dissemination (via journal article publication or conference presentations), submission of a thesis and/or degree conferral, or translation of research findings to educational practice. For larger projects, consider intermediate outcomes that are achievable (see 'planning' for more tips), such as research degree milestones and interim reports to grant funders. Intermediate outcomes are a great way of keeping larger projects on track for timely completion and preventing scope creep (described below).

Project stakeholders

Defining the project cannot be completed without understanding project stakeholders. Stakeholders are individuals or organisations who are involved in the project, or whose interests may be impacted by project execution or completion (see Chapter 5). Common clinical education research stakeholders are described in Table 25.1.

Team reflexive exercises can be helpful [6] to elucidate the research teams' prior experiences, relationship to the project, and worldviews, which may influence the project process and outcomes. Exploring how each stakeholder will contribute to the project, and which areas they will be responsible for is also important. Unpacking assumptions about supervisors and other research team member roles early can help identify the likely compatibility and success of the team, and whether the proposed team meets the project needs.

In addition to the research team, stakeholders may include research participants and a variety of institutions. Understanding your project stakeholders will help you anticipate the likelihood of successful data collection (Table 25.1). Consider, for example, your research participants. They may be able to provide advice on competing demands that may limit their capacity for participation, and thus whether the proposed methods are likely to be feasible. Also consider those who may not be directly involved in the project, but whose interests may need to be considered (e.g. healthcare consumers, other health care professionals, etc.)

By understanding project stakeholders, the principal investigator and project manager will also be able to determine any approvals that need to be obtained for the project, as well as project risks (see below). Depending on the project, multiple approvals may be required, including ethical approval from one or more institutions (e.g. university and/or health or social care service), and potential approval from training bodies (e.g. medical schools, postgraduate training programs). For more information on ethics in clinical education research, see Chapter 7. Approval processes can be lengthy, and thus may themselves require extensive planning and represent an important interim project outcome.

Risk register

Research does not always progress as planned. By defining the project and understanding stakeholders, you can proactively anticipate potential risks or setbacks, their likelihood of occurrence, and their consequences. These will be detailed in the project 'risk register' (see workbook on companion website) and include events that are likely to alter your timeline or projected outputs such as a low participation rate, unexpected results, failure to procure funding, change in research team members or supervisors, etc.

Understanding project risks will allow you to prioritise them and develop mitigation strategies ahead of their occurrence. Risks typically change throughout the course of a project, and thus the risk register is revisited during the 'monitoring and controlling' stage of the project to assess which risks are resolved, and which are ongoing (sometimes referred to as 'residual risks'). For example, a major early risk may be the recruitment of participants, which will be resolved by the point of data

Table 25.1 Common clinical education research stakeholder groups and key considerations for the project initiation phase

Stakeholder group	Examples	Key considerations
Research team	• Supervisor or lead/primary investigator • Co-investigators • Research assistants • Higher degree research students • Teaching fellows	• Roles and responsibilities • Relevant experience • Epistemology and reflexivity • Availability and competing demands • Motivations
Research participants	• Learners • Educators • Healthcare workers • Healthcare consumers/patients • Institutional leaders	• Relation between researcher and researched • Availability and competing demands • Risks and benefits of participation • Suitable methods
Institutions	• Educational institutions • Healthcare institutions • Regulatory bodies • Grant providers	• Approval processes • Reporting requirements

collection. Mitigation strategies could include multiple approaches to recruitment, or if appropriate, participant incentivisation. By contrast, inadequate provision of time for revisions of submitted manuscripts is a risk that may arise much later in the research timeline (e.g. uncertainty as to when the review process will be finalised could result in revisions being requested at a time when researchers are on leave, have already finished a secondment, etc.). It can be difficult to anticipate all risks, but developing a risk register in association with your supervisor will allow you to refine the project definition and better understand when and how risks may arise.

Integrating the project plan

Integrating the project plan draws together the results of your draft project definition, stakeholder assessments, and risk register. By this stage, you should be able to determine whether the project is achievable and can proceed beyond initiation, or whether the risks of the project are too great, and the resources too limited to progress.

If the project is to proceed, create a project plan document that includes the project definitions, and stakeholder roles and responsibilities. This document can then be distributed to all stakeholders for review and approval, with the finalised version forming a key reference throughout the project to ensure that project objectives and outcomes are met. A comprehensive research plan will then inform the more detailed project planning that follows.

Stage 2: planning

Research projects require extensive planning which tends to be 'front-loaded'. Whilst the initiation stage begins to provide an overview of the project and research team responsibilities, the planning stage should extensively detail specific project phases and tasks, and their scheduling.

The opportunity to revisit data collection sources is often prohibitively limited during clinical education research projects. Whilst data analysis may be flexible (in both timing and location), data collection is often far more inflexible. Study participation can be constrained by time (i.e. workload challenges) and availability (i.e. curricular timelines and participant timetables), and often cannot be re-engaged should further research be required.

Many clinical education research projects are context specific (e.g. how learners are impacted in a certain year or by a certain intervention), and thus revisiting participants is not only challenging, but could be irrelevant to the project and research question. For instance, if you are studying a particular clinical education assessment to evaluate its effectiveness, and the assessment only occurs once per year, you will have a finite window to collect data. For all of these reasons, extensive forward planning, to ensure relevant data is collected, is critical in clinical education research contexts.

Planning project phases

When planning your project, start by dividing it into broad research phases (Table 25.2). Within each phase, you will need to determine the roles and responsibilities of the research team members, identify the activities required to achieve each phase, and develop a timeline for completion.

Gantt charts are a form of bar chart commonly used in project management that can be valuable for providing an overview of research phases and timelines. Research phases and activities are listed on the vertical axis, and the timeline for completion on the horizontal axis. These are easily created in spreadsheet programs, many of which include Gantt chart templates.

Gantt charts may also highlight interdependent activities. For example, ethics applications are typically developed and submitted early in the project. They may be one of the first phases added to a Gantt chart, with the research phases that follow dependent on successful submission and approval. Assigning a team member responsible for the ethics application can help minimise the 'bystander effect' of assuming that 'someone else' is following through. Additional examples of activities and tasks that can be included on a Gantt chart are listed in Table 25.2, and a Gantt chart example and template is available on the companion website.

Working backwards from an endpoint can be an effective way to plan timelines. Endpoints are dependent on the given project, but may be thesis related, conference dates, or related to personal constraints. Sometimes the endpoints are narrower and include data collection completion, a report, archiving data, signoffs, etc.

Once the target endpoint is identified, review the Gantt chart phases to assign timelines (and leads) to each, working backwards from the target. For instance, data collection may only need a day, but ethics may need a few months. Next, you should break apart the phases into manageable tasks and subtasks.

Planning project tasks

Tasks are a series of activities with specific purposes related to the relevant research phase (Table 25.2). Tasks can be simple (e.g. uploading survey items into software) or complex (e.g. thematic analysis), and often include subtasks. For example, in the data collection phase of your research project, you are likely to identify a series of tasks including 'disseminate

Table 25.2 Common milestones included in clinical education research Gantt charts

Research phases	Tasks, roles and considerations	Estimated time involved
Ethical review	• Discuss application process with those experienced to gain insight into timelines and procedures relevant at your institution • Drafting application & associated documents (see data collection row below) • Editing • Submitting	A couple of weeks to a few months depending on the experience of the investigator(s) and the complexity of the study
Pilot data collection	• Consultations with experienced relevant researchers • Test run of data collection methods • Reviewing of areas for improvement • Development of improved data collection methods	One day to a few months. Typically, the pilot phase is shorter than the formal data collection, as the goal here is to test methods. For research studies with human participants, there can be miscommunication within the data collection process. This phase provides an opportunity to test your project before formal data collection starts
Data collection	• Drafting data collection protocols – (e.g. interview or survey questions) likely completed during the ethics application phase, and updated following pilot data collection • Consider who in the research team is best to collect data (e.g. power dynamics, confounding perspectives)	Cross-sectional studies with only a single data collection point may only need a single day, whilst longitudinal studies may span six months to a few years
Data analysis	• Qualitative research: transcription editing, initial coding • Quantitative research: data cleaning, statistical analysis • Synthesis and interpretation of data	Qualitative analysis typically takes six months to a year, depending on experience and approach Quantitative analysis tends to be more rapid (one to three months) Synthesis and interpretation of data can take another six months to a year.
Project feedback	• Advisory board	Meet a few times across the life of the project (variable)
Result dissemination	• Drafting abstracts • Developing talks/posters • Presenting • Manuscript development and editing • Manuscript submission	This can be ongoing, but tends to commence one to two years after the project starts

survey'. This dissemination task may have smaller subtasks including: developing a survey distribution list, sending the survey, and sending reminders. The further you can subdivide tasks, the more likely you can determine how to fit the research task into your existing workload. On a day your workload is heavy, you can still keep a research project moving along by focusing on the smaller task subdivisions. Whilst these smaller tasks may not feel like much at the time, collectively executed, they result in timely research project delivery.

There are several tools that can help you manage tasks and subtasks. Notebooks or bullet journals can help you maintain a task list as well as providing a space for capturing research notes and ideas [7, 8]. Apps such as Microsoft ToDo, Todoist, or any.do can be useful to keep track of whole

projects, set due dates for individual tasks, and allocate tasks or subtasks to other team members.

For each planning phase and/or task, assigning a lead to oversee and complete the task is critical for effective project planning. Without clear roles and responsibilities, the research project will likely languish. If you are leading a project, an approach would be to develop a draft of the project phases and tasks, and assign suggested leads that are then discussed and finalised at a team meeting. If you are conducting a student project, you may be the lead for most of the tasks, but it is worth highlighting when you will need input or feedback from your supervisor.

If you are leading a small project or part of a larger project, the project may appear narrow but you can still break it down into smaller phases and tasks.

Alternatively, consider a project where you are responsible for a certain aspect, for example, data collection. Phases may include: developing a recruitment strategy, designing an organisation and storage approach for the data, the data collection itself, and so on. Once you have developed your proposed phases, next you will discuss these with your research supervisor and team and make amendments. Once everyone agrees, consider sending out a summary to the team to ensure shared understanding. This document can then be used in the monitoring and controlling stage of your research project management and supplement the project plan with a more detailed description of specific project tasks and leads. Together these documents (project plan and task lead outline) can serve to enhance communication between the research team and provide a starting point for addressing challenges identified as the project continues.

Stage 3: Executing

The most challenging aspect of research project management is the follow-through of planned tasks (i.e. executing). This is because many researchers have considerable competing deadlines and often diverse expectations of times required for task completion, and relevant related subtasks.

Productivity

There are a few strategies that can help maximize productivity related to identified tasks [9]. The Pomodoro technique is a time management approach that supports brief periods of focussed work [10]. This technique includes both active working, and break times. Traditionally the working time is ~25 minutes, with five-minute breaks. However, the work: break ratio is flexible. Pomodoro techniques can be effective for executing tasks and subtasks identified in your project planning.

Another approach for successful research project execution is the use of writing retreats, either face-to-face or online. In writing retreats, expectations are set and action items are distributed across the team. This promotes accountability because participants have dedicated time (and to some extent, oversight) to achieve the pre-discussed goals.

Accountability

Execution and accountability are interwoven. Diarising your research tasks into your calendar can help. If you need external reinforcement to ensure follow-through, you can share this calendar invite with a collaborator. Additionally, shared online office applications (e.g. Microsoft Office 365, Google docs) can be valuable in team-based research projects. All team members can edit a single document, and the motivation of seeing others working can be helpful when struggling with your own productivity.

Key to success is minimising distraction and prioritising project work over competing activities. In the modern world email and social media can be distracting. Consider setting apps to 'do not disturb' when working, and 'batch checking' notifications at pre-determined times (e.g. 2–3 times a day).

It can be helpful to block out time on your calendar when writing. Ignoring distractions may be more feasible in short execution periods (e.g. Pomodoro), highlighting the value of these techniques in contemporary workplace contexts. Ultimately being accountable to yourself (or to others as needed), by having shared deadlines and engaging these strategies can enhance your project execution success.

Accountability also applies to the research team and supervisory meetings. Have an agenda prepared and sent out ahead of the meeting, and focus the meeting time on discussions that require group input for resolution and progression. Consider whether queries may be effectively addressed in an email. If so, you may be able to save precious meeting time for tasks that are ideally suited to collaborative discussion with your research team, such as resolving research challenges, and managing setbacks. Sending out a summary of the meeting is important to ensure effective communication and continued project execution.

Stage 4: Monitoring and controlling

The monitoring and controlling stage of the project encompasses evaluating to what extent the project is proceeding as planned, and how the project plan may need to be modified. Monitoring should occur frequently, and will compare the anticipated plan (i.e. task schedule, budget and risks) with the current reality.

Without prior experience, it may be difficult to anticipate the time each task will take. Keeping a research journal which includes the actual time spent on tasks, including start and finish times, is an ideal way of better understanding the time required for the project. This can then be used to more accurately plan the remaining project tasks, as well as future projects.

Controlling relates to dealing with changes in project scope. At times, project scope may need to be decreased, such as if time and resources become limited. Increase in project scope is commonly referred to as 'scope creep' and occurs often. Planned project objectives may change as initial data points are obtained, or further avenues for research identified as new literature is published.

For example, qualitative analysis of interview data may lead to development of unexpected themes worthy of further exploration (see illustrative case), or discussion of the project with potential stakeholders could expand data collection to other sites. In this way, increased scope can offer opportunities, but can also lead to challenges in planned project delivery timelines and/or outcomes. See Box 25.1 for a common type of scope creep.

To explore whether project scope creep is worth pursuing, first evaluate the need for changing objectives: Are the proposed additional objectives realistic and attainable? Even if the proposed changes are desirable to the project team, carefully consider how the project plan and schedule will need to change to accommodate changes in scope, and whether the scope now involves additional stakeholders or approval processes (e.g. ethics amendments). If there are insufficient resources (including researcher time), the proposed changes may be 'out of scope' of the present project, but could be undertaken at a later time when further resources become available. In this way, the 'out of scope' aspect may become a direction for future research. We recommend keeping a list of such ideas. Any changes to the project objectives should be discussed with all members of the research team and relevant stakeholders, with changes negotiated and documented in an update to the project plan.

Problems or setbacks frequently arise during projects, thus a key element of the project manager role is learning to anticipate problems (i.e. risks) before they arise, and addressing them when they do. Ideally, your risk register will have plans for risk mitigation, and timing for reviewing risks throughout the project. The reality is that unexpected risks and problems often arise. Start by understanding the source of the problem, and its actual or potential implications for the project outcomes and stakeholders. This will allow you to assess the importance of the problem, and prioritise addressing problems with the greatest potential to derail the project. Understanding the problem will also facilitate asking for targeted help from your research team, such as those who are best placed to assist based on their expertise and responsibility. Even experienced researchers encounter problems throughout projects, so whilst effective project management can't eliminate problems, it can help you identify problems early, and address them in a way that helps keep the project on track.

Stage 5: Closing

The closing stage of a project is frequently neglected, but helps ensure the success of the project, as well as future endeavours. Referring back to the project plan, closing includes assessing whether all outcomes of the project are complete and communicated to relevant stakeholders. Common examples of issues requiring attention include ending ethics applications, submitting grant reporting requirements, planning the long-term storage and/or destruction of data, sharing findings with participants and informing stakeholders about who will be the point of contact post-project (typically the principal investigator). A final team reflexive exercise is an ideal way of unpacking assumptions about what worked effectively for the project, and which areas could be improved for future projects [6]. Documenting lessons learned can then be used to inform the initiation stages of subsequent projects.

BOX 25.1   Illustrative case: identifying and controlling scope creep

Smita is a junior doctor seconded to a local medical school where she is teaching clinical anatomy. She is interested in gaining some research experience during the secondment, and becomes involved in a project already underway exploring medical students' experiences with professionalism during human donor dissection. The principal investigator (PI) completes an ethics amendment to add Smita as a co-investigator. Smita then begins to familiarise herself with the progress of the project so far. Smita's responsibilities as a co-investigator will be interviewing 10 students, analysing the collected data through a paired approach with the PI, and leading drafting of a research report (i.e., the main project outcome). Smita will return to clinical duties in four months, and plans to have all data collection, analysis and the first draft of the report complete by this time.

One month into the project, Smita meets with the PI to discuss progress. Smita has completed over half the interviews and has commenced data analysis. However, Smita is finding qualitative data analysis much more difficult and time consuming than she anticipated. Before she can raise her concerns with the PI, the PI is excited to tell Smita that following discussion with an anatomy education colleague at another institution, there may be an opportunity to expand the research to incorporate participants at that institution where students learn anatomy without dissection. The PI thinks it would be fascinating to compare and contrast the experiences of the two different cohorts of students.

- What does the research team need to consider to determine if the addition proposed by the PI is in or out of scope?

- If the proposed change in scope is made, what steps should be put in place to keep the updated project on track?

If the research team has completed a project plan, this can be used to help determine the extent to which the project scope has increased, and how this may impact team members' responsibilities and project resources. In this way, the project plan may help Smita, as a junior researcher, raise concerns about project scope with her supervisor in an objective manner. By first referring to the project plan that the team agreed upon, a potentially challenging conversation becomes a little easier to engage in. The research team will need to carefully evaluate whether the proposed change is realistic and achievable, as well as desirable in the view of the PI and other research team members. When considering what is realistic and achievable, all stakeholder needs should be considered. There are already signs that Smita may need to revise her project timeline, and require further assistance with data analysis. Thus, completing her existing responsibilities in a timely manner may already be difficult, without adding additional data collection and analysis related to the second institution. This proposed change in scope may therefore require significant additional resources, especially in relation to researcher time. The research team will need to assess if anyone has capacity for this (either those already in the team, or through the addition of further co-investigators), or whether this scope creep may be better considered a 'future direction' for when further time and resources become available.

Should sufficient resources be available, and the research team agree to pursue the change, comprehensive changes to the project plan, risk register and project plan will need to be made. Additional stakeholders may also necessitate updated approvals, and updated researcher roles and responsibilities will need to be negotiated and documented. In this case, Smita's involvement in the project is somewhat constrained by the duration of her secondment, so she will need to work with the PI to determine what aspects of the project she will now be responsible for, and, in particular, how the updated scope may impact the planned publication as the major project outcome.

Summary

Successful project management relies heavily on initiation and planning, with clinical education research projects often front-loaded through these early stages of project management. Key to success across all stages of research project management are effective communication strategies, including documentation (e.g. project plans, Gantt charts) and strategic use of meetings. Monitoring the project and adjusting your timelines as the project progresses, is valuable. Scope creep is common and may provide research opportunities, but should be evaluated and controlled to ensure that projects aren't derailed unnecessarily. Project management does not simply end when the project objectives are achieved, but continues through a closing stage wherein the research team reflects on what worked (or did not) to inform future project management. Whilst a project is a finite activity, successive and related projects may collectively contribute to a larger body or programme of research.

Top tips

- Clearly define your research question, project aims, and objectives.
- Identify a preferred communication strategy for your research team.
- Clarify and document roles and responsibilities of each research team member.
- Ask for feedback from experienced researchers about proposed research timelines and apply this to your project planning.
- Anticipate potential risks and setbacks and develop mitigation strategies, including contingencies if tasks take longer than anticipated.
- Identify effective strategies for holding yourself, and your research team, accountable.

Common pitfalls

- Trying to execute a research project that is too broad or nebulously defined.
- Getting distracted from the current project by the next project (or an expanded project scope), and not staying on task or on time.
- Failing to identify a method for effectively committing to deadlines.
- Poor communication leading to confusion about who is responsible for each task, and the deadlines associated with these tasks.
- Getting derailed by small setbacks, instead of planning for deviations.
- Not taking advantage to learn from those who have more experience.

Ethical issues

- Build time for review by a research ethics committee into your project timelines.
- Nominate a team member to oversee ethical processes before, during, and after the project.
- Ensure all research team members make reasonable contributions.
- Engage communication strategies (using agreed upon project plans, Gantt charts, etc.) to refer to when faced with challenging conversations due to power differentials in the team.

Further reading

Haniff, A. and Salama, M. (2016). *Project Management*. Oxford: Goodfellow Publishers Ltd.

Lientz, B. and Rea, K. (2007). *Project Management for the 21st Century*. Routledge.

Nicholls, J. (2020). *The Everyday Project Manager: Manager: A Primer for Learning the Principles of Successful Project Management*. London: Taylor and Francis.

References

1 Lientz, B. and Rea, K. (2007). *Project Management for the 21st Century*. Routledge.

2 Dinsmore, P.C. and Cabanis-Brewin, J. (2006). *The AMA Handbook of Project Management*. Amacom Books.

3 Haniff, A. and Salama, M. (2016). *Project management*. Goodfellow Publishers Ltd.

4 Glassick, C.E. (2000). Boyer's expanded definitions of scholarship, the standards for assessing scholarship, and the elusiveness of the scholarship of teaching. *Academic Medicine* 75 (9): 877–880.

5 Malterud, K., Siersma, V.D., and Guassora, A.D. (2016). Sample size in qualitative interview studies: guided by information power. *Qualitative Health Research* 26 (13): 1753–1760.

6 Barry, C.A., Britten, N., Barber, N. et al. (1999). Using reflexivity to optimize teamwork in qualitative research. *Qualitative Health Research* 9 (1): 26–44.

7 Tholander, J. and Normark, M. (2020). Crafting personal information-resistance, imperfection, and self-creation in bullet journaling. In: *CHI '20: Proceedings of the 2020 CHI Conference on Human Factors in Computing Systems*, 1–13. https://doi.org/10.1145/3313831.3376410.

8 Yiannouli, A. (2019). The point of a bullet journal. *The Veterinary Record* 185 (6): 180.

9 Bielczyk, N.Z., Ando, A., Badhwar, A. et al. (2020). Effective self-management for early career researchers in the natural and life sciences. *Neuron* 106 (2): 212–217.

10 Cirillo, F. (2018). *The Pomodoro Technique: The Life-Changing Time-Management System*. Random House.

26 Writing your dissertation

Frederick Speyer, Benjamin Davies, and Sarah Yardley

Learning objectives

By the end of this chapter, you should be able to:
- Apply a toolkit for planning the content and production of your dissertation.
- Pitch your narrative and voice appropriately for your research discipline or paradigm.
- Create a working environment that is designed for your individual needs.
- Recognise the dissertation has multiple purposes beyond simply communicating research findings.

Introduction

For many of you reading this chapter, the dissertation, (or thesis), may be the first time you will develop a substantial piece of writing. This chapter serves as an overview of the writing process applicable to both undergraduate and postgraduate study, and we will signpost you to further resources for deeper exploration throughout the chapter. Many of the principles can also apply more widely to presenting work in a written format (see Chapter 27).

Writing sits at a seminal point between the work conducted, and its communication to a wider audience. The field of clinical education spans a breadth of research settings, paradigms, and approaches; and as such, no one size fits all to the formula for dissertation writing. This chapter will provide advice on each component needed to successfully complete and submit work: understanding the purpose of the written product (i.e. the actual dissertation); planning structure; framing the narrative; time management and perseverance; and final touches to complete the work successfully. This is illustrated throughout the chapter using the story of Bailey (starting in Box 26.1)

The terms thesis and dissertation are used inconsistently and interchangeably by different academic institutions. Both terms cover a broadly similar concept, and so for simplicity, we shall use the term dissertation in this chapter.

Let me tell the world my story

BOX 26.1   Bailey tells the world her story

Bailey is an Emergency Medicine doctor with an interest in simulation training. As part of her master's in clinical education, she performed a qualitative study exploring how peer friendship groups impact upon performance within a simulated resuscitation setting. She approaches this from a constructivist perspective and uses in-depth qualitative interviewing to explore participants' experiences. She presented her findings at a departmental meeting. Her colleague, Mark, questioned the validity of Bailey's findings as there was no control group nor any statistical measure of performance. Bailey realised Mark was judging her work from a different paradigmatic stance, which led her to question how to present her work in her dissertation.

So, what is the purpose of a dissertation? You might say that it is to display a body of work achieved through a period of research as either a monograph or as a series of publications that will be examined by a panel of assessors for the conferment of an academic award. To an extent, this is true. However, a dissertation can go beyond simply reporting a work's outcome, and instead can be placed within an academic field to expand existing, or instigate new, academic conversations. Additionally, it offers

---

Starting Research in Clinical Education, First Edition. Edited by Eliot L. Rees, Alison Ledger, and Kim A. Walker.
© 2024 The Association for the Study of Medical Education (ASME). Published 2024 by John Wiley & Sons Ltd.
Companion website: www.wiley.com/go/clinicaleducation

the author scope to be reflexive and incorporate the story of their individual journey through a research programme towards becoming a more independent researcher.

Often the dissertation is seen as the final product, something that is written up as the end part of a linear process once the research has been conducted. However, the very act of writing can serve to clarify thoughts and becomes an integral part of the analytic research process in its own right. Therefore, it is best practice to conduct and write your research simultaneously, rather than leaving all the writing to the end.

You may enter the field of clinical education from a biomedical/clinical background that emphasises 'the scientific method', in which less emphasis is placed upon the concept of reflexivity and its influence upon the research process. Reflexivity is important in demonstrating rigour throughout your work, and for situating (contextualising) your work for your audience (see Chapter 3). If assessed through an incongruent paradigmatic lens, then your work can be misunderstood and therefore poorly received by your audience. By nailing your theoretical, conceptual, and methodological flags to the mast early in your dissertation, you signal to your audience your positionality in relation to your research, making explicit your paradigmatic stance, and encouraging your audience to read your work with, rather than against, your paradigm (worldview).

In summary, a dissertation ultimately enables the author to join an academic conversation, contribute to advancing a field, and demonstrate an ability to work to a credible standard. In doing so, it establishes the author within the wider academic community as an increasingly experienced researcher. Having established what a dissertation does, let us consider how to go about creating the dissertation (see Box 26.2).

No such thing as too much planning

BOX 26.2   Bailey contemplates her position in her research

Bailey's interaction with Mark has made her acutely aware of the need to communicate her positionality in relation to her research findings. However, she is struggling with where to start. On the one hand, she wants to outline her paradigmatic stance and explain this paradigm to readers who may not be familiar with this way of thinking; but on the other hand, she wants to entice the reader with the subject matter and worries that a deep exploration around the philosophy of science may put the reader off. As a result, she has become overwhelmed with possibilities and cannot see the big picture.

Start with the end goal in mind

It is never too early to start. This does not just mean putting pen to paper, or more likely now fingers to keyboards, but also relates to planning and structuring your dissertation. Constructing an output plan at the same time as designing the research will give your production an inherent structure aiding the fluency of presentation. Some of you may be reading this at a time when it needs to be applied retrospectively – do not panic but do read on!

Knowing your academic institution's requirements is essential. Some institutions have very rigid requirements around dissertation content and formatting, whilst others permit the author more freedom in construction. Previous dissertations may be available through your institution or national library, which may help guide your writing. Likewise, consider how your dissertation will be assessed. If it is part of a degree, there are usually criteria against which your dissertation will be marked and are known in advance.

It is very rare academic work appears from nowhere. More commonly, it is an extension of an existing baseline conversation within the academic literature. Lingard [1] offers the *Problem, Gap, Hook* heuristic as a mechanism for situating your work within the academic field, and this can be a useful springboard for deciding on where to begin your own storyline (see Chapter 27).

Overcoming blank canvas paralysis

Writing a dissertation is a creative process, and it is not uncommon for those within creative artforms to be crippled by indecision when starting. Imagine the artist standing motionless in front of a blank canvas, paralysed by its pristine luminosity, terrified that they will spoil its purity with a poorly placed brush mark. Likewise, the writer is tormented by the blinking cursor on the radiant blankness of the computer screen. Both situations can be overcome with a surprisingly similar approach.

The first step is the acceptance that what you create will not be perfect. Many intelligent people are driven by a desire for perfectionism, but as the quotation attributed to Voltaire states 'The best is the enemy of the good' [2]. What you write to begin with will not be perfect – it may not even be particularly good. What you submit as your final product may not have reached the elusive height of your own perfecting standards. Aim for success rather than focussing on perfection. A successful dissertation is a completed dissertation. You cannot complete what you have not started. With that in mind, write down anything, however ashamed you are of it, because once you take those first bold steps everything else will be easier.

Another strategy common to the artist and the writer is that of preliminary sketching. The first step to sketching is to establish the compositional form, ensuring the whole story fits into the predetermined space (canvas or word count) and the elements are harmonious (objects or storylines). Next is the selection of a communicative palette (paint colours or linguistic style). Then comes the dynamic range (placement of highlights or climaxes of story). All of this will be influenced by the contextual surroundings (placement in the gallery or relationship to academic field). The beauty of sketching out is the ability to experiment with your dissertation structure. Work out what works for you, your supervisor(s), your institution and ultimately your audience. It is not uncommon for a series of sketches to be created, and therefore the sketches should not be seen as fixed entities (for invariably adjustments will be made during the writing process), but more so as points of reference for when the author needs to take a step back from the details of writing to re-familiarise themselves with the overall landscape of their work.

Selecting your planning method

Without due consideration to planning, it can be easy to become constrained by the linearity conferred by the word processor. In English, written communicative information is organised in words that run from left-to-right, on lines that run from top-to-bottom. Other languages also commonly have linear structures. However, thoughts and ideas often inhabit our headspace as an energetic whirlwind and distilling this directly into prose can sometimes be problematic. There are many planning techniques, with a proliferation of apps and programmes available to execute these techniques. However, good old pen, paper, and a handful of sticky notes can be just as effective. The following are a few alternative strategies to the 'essay plan' for tackling the organisation of ideas:

1 Concept mapping helps group ideas into themes and ascertain hierarchy of importance.
2 Storyboarding helps visualise your main storyline(s) and branching subplots.
3 Gap filling helps assigning headings and filling in the gaps can help prevent going off at a tangent.

4 Photographing anything that is not a permanent record (e.g. using wipe clean boards and pens).
5 Moving into a more multidimensional space can liberate the mind and help find alternative routes past the stumbling blocks.

Compositional construction

A common conundrum that faces all writers is how to assimilate and construct their work into a dissertation. Many will be familiar with the *Introduction, Methods, Results and Discussion (IMRaD)* format. This can be a useful framework for reporting a single study, as might be the case in an academic journal. However, authors of research undertaken at master's or doctoral level might question how to apply a single overarching IMRaD structure to the whole of their dissertation; particularly if they have multiple components to their research, or perhaps wish to tell the story of both their research findings and their research journey.

Rather than focussing on what should go where, reconceptualise the decision making as how does placing specific information in a particular location influence the storytelling of your research? For example, in reporting the twists and turns of the research journey, how might the placement of this reporting affect the storyline if it were to be interwoven throughout the chapters versus consolidated into a single chapter.

Another approach is to zoom in and out, and plan along the three planes of the *macro, meso,* and *micro* levels.

- At a *macro* level ask yourself: What is the overall story I want to tell? What do I want this dissertation to achieve? How does my work relate to the existing academic field and what new knowledge does it contribute? Does my research lend itself to being presented as a single study or as multiple studies?
- At a *meso* level ask yourself: How do my chapters interrelate to tell my story? Should they start broadly and focus down? Should they start focussed and open up? Have I already published any of the work and should I include this in the dissertation? How will I signpost my audience within the work? Do I need any transitional chapters or linking sections?
- At a *micro* level ask yourself: How do I envisage the individual chapters? How will I segue into and out of chapters? How will I arrange my critical arguments? Do I want to use headings to organise my work? Would non-textual presentation be more appropriate? (e.g. tables, charts, infographics)

Ultimately, as Lingard [3] reminds us, 'Your research study – its methods and results – needs to be reported fully and accurately. Your research story, however, should be told as persuasively as possible.'

To facilitate a persuasive story, it can be useful to consider how you might like to *read* your work if you were to place yourself in the shoes of your audience. This will aid planning the form, structure, rhythm, and content of your dissertation. Consider the following: How would you set the scene? Who (or what) will be in your cast? How would you like to be guided through the story? Where would you envisage natural breaks? What will be the rhythm and tempo? Where will you place the climax(es)? How will you be kept engaged?

Having encouraged you to tell the story of your work and be creative in its construction, let us now turn to some stylistic elements of academic writing for conveying your message and framing your narrative. It is not just what you say, but how you say it (see Box 26.3).

Pitching your voice

BOX 26.3　Bailey's concerns about her pitch

Bailey's research centres around exploring people's experiences, and she is keen to write her dissertation in the first-person voice as she feels she is embedded within the research. However, she is concerned that this approach may be too colloquial and not appear academic.

Genre

What does the term *academic writing* mean? The answer, in part, depends upon the research paradigm and the outlet for communication. The concept of 'genre', as defined by Fairclough is 'the use of language associated with a particular social activity' [4]. If, 'Scientific research is a social activity centred on answering challenging questions' [5], then authors need to choose an appropriate and congruent language genre through which to communicate these answers. For example, whilst post-positivism (see Chapter 3) may favour writing that is formal, objective, and parsimonious, as one moves through the paradigmatic spectrum towards constructivism, academic writing can be thickly descriptive, exploratory, interpretative, and subjective. Both draw on evidence, albeit often of different varieties. Communicating through the outlet of an academic journal will use a different genre of language to, say, a national newspaper.

Tone and voice

Writers often believe they should adopt a neutral tone within academic writing. Watling [6] suggests that judicious use of tone can produce compelling research stories. Likewise, we all have our own idiosyncratic ways of speaking, and expressing this voice through your writing can make for a more personable narrative. Whilst the passive voice was historically favoured for academic writing (e.g. 'the literature was searched for. . .'), recent trends have seen a shift towards using a more active voice (e.g. 'I searched the literature for. . .'), which can be particularly useful in demonstrating your relationship with the research you have conducted, and your interpretation and presentation of results.

All language serves a purpose, and when communicating to your audience you should decide what you want language to do for you. For example, will it be narrative, informative, argumentative, aesthetic, or persuasive. As Varpio reminds us, 'our [research] solutions are accepted as truth until another, better proposition offers a more compelling explanation' [5]. She therefore encourages authors to communicate their findings using the three pillars of persuasive writing – ethos (the credibility of the writer), logos (the robustness of the logic), and pathos (the emotion stirred within the reader).

Historically, academic writing tended to be viewed as stuffy and inaccessible, as exemplified by Pinker in his pithy article 'Why academics stink at writing' [7]. In recent years, there has been a move towards creating more stylish and accessible academic prose. But, as Sword argues, whilst academics often aspire to create stylish writing, they rarely produce and publish it [8].

Fortunately, there are now many emerging resources to aid you with creating stylish writing in your dissertation. Many academic institutions provide courses and guides on academic writing. Some even employ dedicated academic support officers for one-on-one coaching. Much else is also freely available. As examples, Sword provides 10 tenets of stylish writing in her engaging and often humorous article [8], and for those who want more detail in her book 'The Writers' Diet [9]; and the journal *Perspectives in Medical Education* has an open-access series titled 'The Writer's Craft' [10].

Reading about writing and reading the work of others can provide a good foundation. However, there is nothing better to hone your craft than putting pen to paper (or more likely, pressing the keys on the keyboard) and then practising. Increasingly, digital technology is providing tools for real-time assessment of your writing to aid a more stylish output; whether already built into word processors (e.g. MS Word Editor) or as downloadable plug-ins (e.g. Grammarly [https://www.grammarly.com/office-addin], or The Writer's Diet [the author uses the same name for her app as the printed book] [https://appsource.microsoft.com/en-us/product/office/wa200002125?tab=overview]).

Last, remember that considerations of ethical issues are not confined to the process of gaining study approval, you may encounter ethical situations throughout your research (see Chapter 7). We also encourage you to be reflexive about these throughout your writing.

Time and place: setting yourself up for success

The time has come to start writing, which may seem like an almost insurmountable task at first. As described earlier, we have already provided strategies for getting started. This section provides practical advice on time management and perseverance to support your writing.

BOX 26.4   Bailey finds her space for writing

Having created a plan and covered some pages, Bailey is harnessing her motivational energy to crack on with writing the bulk of her dissertation. Writing her dissertation in the midst of a busy Emergency Department would not be suitable. She considered writing at home but opted for her local library as she wanted some distinction between home life and dissertation life. She also thought the library would offer a peaceful environment in which she could focus. However, she has become acutely irritated by the noises that punctuate the echoing silence, which she finds ironic given that her clinical work is situated within one of the nosiest areas of the hospital. What she has come to realise is that she thrives in places where there is a background hubbub providing a constant rhythm of energy that she can absorb, and that she finds the solitude of silence lonely and uninspiring.

Time and place

Making a timetable is an important first step to managing your time. This does not need to be detailed; it just needs to serve as a way of identifying windows of opportunity for you to write and for you to gain confidence by seeing progress. This timetable can extend as far into the future as your personal situation allows but creating an intention to write is an important starting point.

Next, you might want to think about how you structure those chunks of time. Time-management techniques, such as *Pomodoro* and *Timeboxing*, are great strategies for improving productivity.

Pomodoro strives to curb procrastination by earmarking chunks of time to undistracted output, whereas Timeboxing aims to prevent overcommitment to a task and creates pressure of a deadline to stimulate focus. If you are a chronic procrastinator, Pomodoro might be the technique for you. For the perfectionist who can lose track of time, Timeboxing might be worth a try.

Choosing your setting

Whilst some of you might flourish in a bustling social environment (see Box 26.4), the hubbub of café patrons' conversations providing the ambient soundtrack to your writing, others may prefer a quieter setting. Your university might have resources for you to use. You may already know what setting will work best, but experiment if you are unsure or if it is not working. It is also possible to manipulate an existing environment to suit your preferences, e.g. popping on a pair of headphones and listening to some relaxing or energetic music, or playing soundtracks that emulate the peaceful countryside. Varying settings can be reenergising, many of these can be found through freely available apps. Structured writing groups such as Shut Up and Write! or dedicated writing retreats [11] make the normally solitary exercise of writing more social (and accountable!).

Writing can be a tiring process and making your work area as ergonomic and comfortable as possible will help improve your productivity and limit distraction. Consider which chair you are going to use; what keyboard and mouse will be most comfortable; and whether a second monitor might help improve workflow. Remember to keep well hydrated with water, take regular screen breaks (e.g. every 20 minutes look 20 m into the distance for 20 seconds then blink 20 times), and savour your break times (perhaps with a treat or reward).

Making the most of digital tools

Whilst digital technology will not write your dissertation, automated tools can ease the process. For example, using the template and styles functions in your computer software allows you to adjust formatting quickly and consistently across a document, automatically generate tables of contents from your headings, and toggle between reference conventions at the click of a button. Reference management software will help keep track of your references and facilitate inserting references into your document. Some people find dictation software a faster way to get words onto the page. It is worth familiarising yourself with automated tools early on but always be open to considering such additions later in the writing process.

It is vital you are meticulous when it comes to saving and backing-up your work. Having your dissertation stored on a single device is a recipe for disaster. Backing up has become much simpler with the advent of synced cloud software, but whether it is the cloud, an external hard drive, or a prescribed university drive, make sure you back up your work. Make updated versions of your dissertation as it evolves and ensure each version is clearly labelled with the date; this will allow you to keep track of changes and enable you to revert to a previous version if required.

Running into a brick wall

Producing an individualised schedule and creating the perfect work environment cannot fully safeguard against the age-old nemesis of writer's block. It can occur at any time and without warning. You might start doubting the quality of your work or become so immersed in a section that you cannot see the way forward. Writing the next sentence seems like an overwhelming task but fretting over writer's block will not resolve the anguish. Writer's block often occurs because you have become stuck in a rut, and a change is required. Some questions you perhaps need to ask yourself are: would returning to your dissertation plan help regain overall direction; would speaking out loud help the words flow? Are you spending too much time self-editing? Sometimes, spending some time *free writing* with the sole purpose of getting thoughts down onto paper may help. Whatever is required, it is important to address it. Chatting things through with a critical friend or your supervisor may help sort out the stumbling block.

Practical considerations from first draft to finish line

Once the first complete draft is completed, the end is in sight. Nevertheless, there is still a little way to go before crossing that finishing line. This final section provides some strategies to support you to completion.

BOX 26.5   Bailey receives feedback

Bailey has been writing her dissertation tirelessly. She is relieved to send it to her supervisor for review, and even more excited when she sees a reply in her inbox. However, when she sees the flood of tracked changes in red across her work, she feels the bottom of her world fall beneath her.

Handing over the baton: working with your supervisor

Fostering a good relationship with your supervisor is key from the outset. They provide a much-needed source of information and guidance. They are not there to proofread, edit, or write your dissertation for you, but they will provide a much-needed source of information and guidance. A good supervisor will provide constructive criticism to help guide focus and boost your writing to higher standards. It can also be a good idea to make an informal contract with your supervisor at the outset so that you both know what to reasonably expect from the relationship. This could cover matters such as how often you will meet to discuss newly arising issues, how frequently your supervisor will review your work and how they would like it presented.

Receiving criticism can be challenging and having your hard work critiqued can feel very personal but be open minded (see Box 26.5). You may find yourself disagreeing with your supervisor's comments, but remember to maintain a good dialogue with them and not let it turn into a battle. A supervisor's feedback should not be followed blindly but rather seen as the beginning of a conversation to enhance your writing and as insight into how others interpret your work. Your dissertation will be all the better for it.

It's a marathon not a sprint: pace yourself and conserve energy

You will find the pace of your writing varies throughout the dissertation, some days the words will flow effortlessly, other days not so. There are some things which always take more time than you might imagine, e.g. organising tables, creating figures and diagrams, arranging appendices, checking reference lists, getting copyright clearance for reproduction. Some of this you could get done whilst writing, whereas others may be more appropriate to address after you have completed the bulk of your writing. Make sure you build in sufficient time because it nearly always takes longer than you anticipated.

No matter how organised you are sometimes life throws in unexpected events. These can range from a computer malfunction to a global pandemic. It is important to factor in some flexibility to your scheduling, liaise closely with, and talk to your supervisors. Be kind to yourself, and if necessary, explore the possibility to take a period of absence.

The home straight: final polishing

No matter how much you have done en-route to the finish, there will always be more to do before it is finally done and dusted. Editing and proofreading are essential to producing a good final product. Editing involves making changes to improve the clarity and overall package of your dissertation. Watling advises approaching editing by considering the story, structure, and style [12]. Proof-reading comprises identifying spelling mistakes, punctuation errors, and ensures consistency of formatting etc. At this stage, it is important to ensure your dissertation meets all your institution's formatting requirements. You should be aware and conform to these requirements from the outset, but double-checking is never a bad idea.

With guidance from your supervisor, you will be doing this throughout the writing process but it is also worth considering some outside help, where permitted (proofreading services need to be University approved). Getting someone unfamiliar with the immediate subject area to read your work can help ensure your messages and structure are clear and easy to follow. Ensure you allocate sufficient time to revise individual parts, but also to view the work as a whole. This allows for cohesion, signposting, and consideration of how the writing flows/makes sense as an entire work. However, make sure not to stray into the realms of receiving too much outside assistance. Someone else having significant input in your dissertation (whether a friend, relative, or essay-writing service) is universally prohibited by academic institutions.

The next race: writing for different formats to achieve impact

All good stories should have a beginning, a middle, and an end, but we also know that many have a sequel. As well as being the culmination of a body of work, for many of you the dissertation will be part of a longer career trajectory. Whilst it is important to finish the job in hand and get the dissertation written, it is also worth being mindful of how the dissertation might fit with any future career or research plans. Who knows what cliff-hanger you might want your dissertation to end on!

You may wish to influence policy, practice, or praxis [13]. This may require you to publish in academic journals or communicate with stakeholders through other media (see Chapters 27 and 28). We caution that trying to simply edit your dissertation into a journal article or policy document will not be successful. Instead think of your dissertation as an encyclopaedia or other reference source. If writing for another format, particularly one much shorter, then start afresh and repeat the principles we have suggested to create a draft narrative for the new work before going back to select material from the dissertation to flesh it out.

Summary

This chapter has offered advice for starting, keeping up, and completing your dissertation writing. Key principles include careful planning, deciding on appropriate pitch, finding time and space for writing, responding to feedback, and polishing your dissertation. Many of these principles will be transferable to other forms of research dissemination. We hope our advice will encourage you to share your work more widely than your academic institutions' archives.

Tops tips

- Begin with the endgame in mind and accept that what you create will not be perfect.
- Start writing early, by planning and structuring your dissertation.
- Organise your writing using appropriate tools and ensure you know any institutional requirements.
- Set up a work environment that suits your preferences and be open to changing this if it is not working for particular tasks or phases of writing.
- Employ time management strategies to keep your dissertation moving forward.

Common pitfalls

- Starting writing too late. Dissertation writing always takes longer than you think.
- Expecting to only write each chapter once. Dissertation work is iterative, and you will need to revise in response to feedback.
- Becoming disheartened in response to supervisor feedback. Remember supervisors are offering feedback that will improve the quality of your final submission, but final decisions are ultimately yours.
- Storing your dissertation work on a single device. Always back up your work to avoid disaster.

Ethical issues

- Confidentiality and anonymity when reporting data. Take care not to identify your participants unless they have consented to being identified.
- Attribute others' work to avoid plagiarism. When building on your own work, cite your previous submissions or publications.
- Avoid gaining too much assistance from others. Academic institutions prohibit significant input from supervisors, friends and relatives, and proofreading services.

References

1 Lingard, L. and Watling, C. (2021). Problem/gap/hook introductions. In: *Story, Not Study: 30 Brief Lessons to Inspire Health Researchers as Writers*, 7–14. Cham: Springer.

2 Knowles, E. (ed.) *Oxford Dictionary of Quotations*, 8e. Oxford University Press. p. 804.

3 Lingard, L. (2017). Does your discussion realize its potential? *Perspectives on Medical Education* 6 (5): 344–346.

4 Fairclough, N. (1993). Critical discourse analysis and the marketization of public discourse: the universities. *Discourse & Society* 4 (2): 133–168.

5 Varpio, L. (2018). Using rhetorical appeals to credibility, logic, and emotions to increase your persuasiveness. *Perspectives on Medical Education* 7 (3): 207–210.

6 Watling, C. (2017). Tuning your writing. *Perspectives on Medical Education* 6 (3): 189–191.

7 Pinker, S. (2014). Why academics stink at writing. *The Chronicle of Higher Education* 61 (5): 2–9.

8 Sword, H. (2009). Writing higher education differently: a manifesto on style. *Studies in Higher Education* 34 (3): 319–336.

9 Sword, H. (2015). *The Writer's Diet*. Auckland University Press.

10 Lingard, L. (2015). The writer's craft. *Perspectives on Medical Education* 4 (2): 79–80.

11 Bell, M. and Murray, R. (2021). Structured academic writing retreats in healthcare professional practice. *The Clinical Teacher* 18 (3): 243–246.

12 Watling, C. (2016). The three 'S's of editing: story, structure, and style. *Perspectives on Medical Education* 5 (5): 300–302.

13 Ng, S.L. and Wright, S.R. (2017). When I say. . . praxis. *Medical Education* 51 (8): 784–786.

27 Writing for publication

Amaya Ellawala and Aileen Barrett

Learning objectives

By the end of this chapter, you should be able to:
- Recognise the nuances of publication in a journal.
- Determine the 'fit' of your work for a journal.
- Position your work for publication and choose the appropriate article type.
- Manage reviewer and editor comments and respond to feedback.
- Create a writing strategy.

Introduction

Many new clinical education researchers aspire to publish their work, usually in a peer-reviewed journal. However, getting a project to the publication stage requires more than a good idea. It also requires skills in academic writing, an understanding of the conversation you are joining [1] and a willingness to challenge and be challenged [2]. For those attempting to publish educational research for the first time, it may also require an epistemological shift, embracing new ideas on not just how research is conducted, but how we ask the critical questions informing that work.

The aim of this chapter is to provide you with a framework to make your publication decisions and choices, in particular, which journal may be the most appropriate for your research which is usually a first step for new clinical education researchers. Once your decision has been made, the chapter provides further information on the publishing process, how to deal with rejection, and improve your writing.

Getting started

> "Where shall I begin, please your Majesty?" he asked. "Begin at the beginning," the King said gravely, "and go on till you come to the end: then stop."
> Lewis Carroll, Alice in Wonderland

In this context, 'the beginning' means the design phase of your project. Attempting to 'write up' a project without the necessary background work (and without ethical approval) may become an insurmountable challenge.

Guided by previous chapters in this book, you should now be aware that the success of any research study is dependent on a good research question (see Chapter 2), an aligned methodological approach (see Chapter 3), and the relevant ethical approval (see Chapter 7). As you start to shape your research, also consider how you might share it in the future (see Chapter 28). The factors that are likely to enhance the chances of successfully publishing your work, including the various components of rigorous approaches to research, are already discussed throughout this book.

Once you have shaped your project, it may be useful to identify the health professions education journals and platforms (which may include preprints and social media platforms) currently publishing similar-style work. This will require some searching (mostly online) and discussions potentially with other experienced professionals, for example, librarians, other researchers, your supervisor. This is particularly important in pointing you towards journals with which you are not familiar [3].

Where to publish

When deciding which journal to publish in, there are several key questions to consider:
- Which journals are publishing similar work to you where you can add to the evidence base?
- Where are authors in your field publishing their work?
- Do you have options to publish an 'open access' paper and what are the cost implications?

Starting Research in Clinical Education, First Edition. Edited by Eliot L. Rees, Alison Ledger, and Kim A. Walker.
© 2024 The Association for the Study of Medical Education (ASME). Published 2024 by John Wiley & Sons Ltd.
Companion website: www.wiley.com/go/clinicaleducation

- Is impact factor an important consideration for you?
- Are you targeting a national or international audience?
- Is your audience predominantly educators, researchers, or clinical teachers?

Rees et al. [4] identified six factors clinical education authors prioritise when making choices about which journal to submit their manuscript: fit, impact, editorial reputation, speed of dissemination, breadth of dissemination, and guidance from others. They found that prioritising 'fit' and deciding on a target journal early in the research process were associated with greater likelihood of being accepted for publication in the authors' first-choice journal. They recommend authors determine where their manuscript might 'fit' by familiarising themselves with the breadth of journals in the field through reading recent articles, editorials, author instructions, and discussing with supervisors and experienced colleagues [4]. Attending 'writing for publication' workshops at conferences can also be an opportunity to meet editors and gain an insight into the priorities for their journals.

When determining where your research may best 'fit', we suggest you first consider the scope of the journal. For example, a research study exploring undergraduates' perspectives on clinical placements to a journal specifically focused on graduate medical education is likely to be met with a desk rejection (i.e., rejected without being sent out for peer review). Next, you should consider the audience you want to reach with your research. This may help you decide whether you want to submit to a clinical journal, a clinical education journal, or a general education journal. Each of these groups will

also have generalist and specialist journals. Maggio et al. [3] describe a list of 24 medical education journals that serve as a useful starting point.

When you have identified a journal to which you might like to submit, pay close attention to the journal's scope and its mission or vision statement. What is the aim of the journal? Do you know its likely readership profile or demographics? This information is usually available on the journal's webpage, but you will also find guidance by reading editorials, commentaries, and other articles to better understand the conversations and debates taking place within its pages.

Article type

Another key consideration is what type of article to write. Clinical educational research, as you will have recognised by now, comes in many different guises. So do article types. Journals have different article types which are designed to provide platforms and structures relevant to their specific readership, mission, and approaches. Although research articles are often the first thought for a publication, there are other types that may be more relevant.

Many journals now provide space for descriptions of innovations or curriculum development initiatives. Quality improvement (QI) projects, using recognised models and frameworks developed for healthcare, may also be published using a QI-appropriate structure. Research studies in health professions education may also be structured in different ways, and some journals may have separate sections for review articles versus empirical research. Table 27.1 provides an overview of some common article types seen in the clinical education literature.

Table 27.1 Examples of article types

Article types	Description
Original research	A research article that has the traditional IMRaD format: Introduction, Methods, Results, and Discussion
Innovation	A report of a novel intervention or new way of combining theory and evidence
Specific sections, e.g. good ideas, How to. . ., toolbox	A section specific to the journal. These tend to be shorter than research reports and can highlight key developments
Commentary, Insight, Perspective, Editorial	A scholarly commentary on a topic or article, often commissioned by an editor. Sometimes one can be submitted without an invite or by pitching an idea to an editor
Letters to the Editor	A letter about an article you wish to expand on (provide more information or reference your own project) or contradict (more controversial). These can be a good way to get started in publishing
Special issue – specific article topics/content	A response to an open call for articles for a special issue on a specific topic. If your work fits into this, then this can be a good way to highlight your work alongside other articles in a similar area
Reviews	A section where an individual reviews or comments on the research articles in the journal. This is a way of writing without using your own research
Methodological papers	A paper that provides detail and guidance on aspects of research design, methodology, or methods

When deciding which type of article to write for your work, there are a number of things to consider. First and foremost, it is critical to define your work so that you can position it within the relevant article type. Pay close attention to the *author guidelines* for each article type within the journal. You should never assume that each article requires a 'introduction-methods-results-discussion' format. Indeed, this is generally only used for research studies. Some journals will have specific criteria for research papers, including, for example, the integration of conceptual or theoretical frameworks [5]. Curriculum developments or teaching approaches, on the other hand, are usually now positioned as descriptive pieces, underpinned by educational theory, and supported by an evaluation strategy.

Awareness of these requirements will help, as you consider the 'why' and 'how' of your work and what it is likely to contribute to the field. As you develop your project and consider your publication options, seek out the publisher resources that are usually freely available on their websites. Academic writing guides, frameworks for ethical approval, and other useful hints and tips (also available from publishers) can also help to improve the quality of your initial submission.

Ethical issues

As a guide, any data collected with the intention to publish must be approved by a research ethics committee. Editors will check for this approval on any submission and where ethical approval has not been sought, even the highest quality papers may be rejected solely on those grounds (see Chapter 7). Each journal will detail the ethical approval assurances required for submissions. Data protection and management, informed consent, and details of any exemptions from full ethical review are usually sought. Evaluations of teaching innovations and quality increasingly, but not always, require some type of ethical review.

Authorship is often a contested and contentious area [6]. For guidance see the International Committee of Medical Journal Editors (https://www.icmje.org/) for specific criteria on authorship entitlement. Having early discussions around authorship (though uncomfortable, particularly for you as a new researcher) will help to guide the writing process and determine a strategy that works for the team. It is good practice to agree on the order of authors prior to any writing [7] and expect all authors to give final approval of the paper.

Writing the story of your work

Now you have chosen your journal and the type of publication, it is important to work on the detail. Clinical education authors do not always use the traditional IMRaD format (see Table 27.1), and instead use creative writing strategies, such as storytelling and the 'problem/gap/hook' heuristic [1]. While a rigorously designed and conducted piece of work is essential, this alone is not always enough. You need to be able to draw your reader in, convince the reader (or editors and reviewers in the first instance) your work is important and worth publishing. Taking the typical structure of a research article as an example, we will now offer guidance for each part.

Title

Constructing a catchy title is vital [8, 9]. A title performs the same function as perhaps a billboard or advert – it catches the eye, conveys information, and most importantly creates interest – making it a key part of any paper. However, while being eye-catching, the title must also maintain a scholarly tone and accurately reflect the scope of the work, so as not to mislead the reader [9].

Titles are extremely important for indexing in databases such as Scopus, PubMed and others. Keywords in titles are used by databases and search engines to pull up relevant search results. If the title does not contain important key words, it might never be found by an interested reader. A useful way of identifying keywords is to think what terms readers would use when searching for your article. For example, if a paper on role modelling does not contain the term 'role model' in the title, it may not appear in any search on the topic. Another strategy is to use sub-titles – thereby the main title could be the catchy element, while the sub-title conveys the main essence of the paper.

In other words, a title needs to include both key search terms and attract readers' interest. To illustrate these points further, consider these two options for a study on doctor–patient communication skills: 'The tapestry of doctor–patient communication skills: unravelling the threads' and 'A study exploring doctor–patient communication skills'. Which one grabs your attention?

Abstract

Like the title, an abstract attracts the reader and determines whether they read on or not. The vast majority of readers never proceed beyond the abstract. Therefore, it is vital it captures attention and succinctly conveys the most important messages of the article, giving the reader adequate motivation to continue reading [10]. The abstract should not only highlight the key findings of the study but also convince the reader of the robustness of the work. It is not a murder mystery and there are no spoiler alerts. You need to clearly articulate the 'so what' of your work in this abstract, i.e. why is this *relevant* and *important* to the reader?

Introduction

The title and abstract may have caught the interest of the reader, but how do you ensure they stay riveted beyond the initial lines? The first few paragraphs of your introduction play a key role in this regard and should be used to position your research within the body of related literature and showcase the importance of your work. Several approaches can be used to this end, one of which is the 'problem-gap-hook' method [1]. Here, the first couple of paragraphs provide a snapshot of a problem related to the area of research, and then highlight a gap in knowledge surrounding this problem. Finally, the reader is 'hooked' in by highlighting why this gap is of significance, thereby establishing the importance of the work described in the paper. This method aims to convince the reader of the paper's importance at the outset, establishing key messages early on, and ensuring that interest does not wane.

Methods

Although this may seem one of the easiest parts of the manuscript to write, the methods section must provide sufficient detail and explanation to allow the work to be reproduced and/or understood. It is easy to miss out key items such as characteristics of participants, and the processes or interventions employed, as you are so familiar with the research. It is equally important not to overcomplicate by providing too much detail about your methods. If the methods have previously been used, then a reference will suffice. If a questionnaire has been used, this is often provided as supplementary material. The methods section should state how the objective was achieved, think of it as a roadmap from the beginning to the destination. Journals will generally ask reviewers to comment on whether the methods have been described well, can be replicated, and to judge whether the study is valid or credible.

Results

This section must clearly articulate the key findings and is perhaps the most important part of your article since your research is probably aiming to fill a gap in previous research on your topic. It is probably the hardest one to make interesting for the reader. It is a good idea to include figures or tables to provide some visual stimulation to the article, even though key points will also be included in the text. It is sometimes useful to put the results in chronological order or systematic order, e.g. characteristics of participants, inclusion, and exclusion criteria and your key statistical outcomes if used. It should also report all the findings, positive and negative as these are equally important to be stated. Connections between the findings or comparisons are better left for the discussion. A well-written research section is capable of generating interest in your research.

Discussion

'How does this impact me and my work?' This is the question every reader asks, possibly subconsciously, when reading a journal article. It is essential, therefore, you tell the reader exactly what the findings of your work mean and how they can be used in varying contexts. Making the study aims and the positionality of researchers explicit can help the reader make sense of your work. Particularly in the case of journals that have a multiprofessional readership and a global presence, your findings must have some level of relevance outside your specific context, as readers will want to glean some 'lessons learned' they may apply in their own setting. Within your discussion, you need to clearly articulate how your findings influence educational practice and policy. You should draw on existing research and describe how your study adds to this literature, but also highlight where gaps remain that could be addressed in future research. This may be included as part of the discussion section, or as a conclusion. Use previously published papers from your chosen journal as a guide to the best location for this information.

It is also necessary to describe both the strengths and limitations of your research. For the limitations, it is helpful to consider how these may affect how your findings are interpreted.

Style, language, and structure

How do you make the read interesting? How do you steer your paper away from the label of 'tedious' or 'dull'? Writing style, language, and structure have a crucial role to play, in particular in drafting your 'results/findings' section. This skill is learned, practised, and enhanced over time.

It is important to familiarise yourself with your chosen journal's writing style. Careful scrutiny of articles within a journal can reveal similarities in writing style and structure. Aligning your work with these can bolster chances of your work being considered a good fit for the journal. The prescribed word count is also an important consideration in determining the structure and content of the paper. Many journals have curated collections of academic writing resources, which are valuable tools in polishing your written work.

We recommend you review any relevant reporting guidelines or standards for the type of study you are conducting. Doing this early within the research process can help to ensure you have considered all of the appropriate domains. The Equator Network (http://www.equator-network.org) [11] provides a comprehensive guide to reporting standards for different types of research. Make sure you choose standards that are appropriate for your chosen research paradigm (see Chapter 3).

Writing a paper is rarely a solo effort; collaborative and team writing bring their own challenges in attempting to ensure a seamless 'flow' and consistent style across the article. Working on a single voice from the start of the project will ensure this is evident within the paper, but this requires effort and shared visions of the final product [12, 13]. It is usual for the first author to determine the voice, but understandably everyone must contribute.

Graphics

If a picture tells a thousand words, then a graph or figure, cleverly positioned, can help you articulate your results, and take-home messages while remaining within the word count [14]. As an author, you want to tell the entire story of your work and each detail is, at that point, critical to its telling! However, as a reader, there is a balance between having enough detail to gauge the trustworthiness and meaning of the work and concisely getting to the point.

Figures, boxes, and tables can allow you to achieve this balance. For example, information that can be provided in a series of bullet points might neatly tell the reader what content was included in a module development. Figures such as photos or pictures can eliminate the need for a description of a simulation scenario set-up.

Some journals with online platforms also offer the option to include supplementary files or appendices that readers can access alongside the article. This may allow you to share your research instruments such as surveys, interview schedules, or topic guides.

Writing strategy

We have outlined many of the decisions you have to make before you even start typing on the keyboard. Having a writing strategy is as important as your

research protocol. This will help guide you through the process especially if you are working with a larger team. First and foremost, set aside time, preferably in blocks to help you get started. Developing a timeline will help focus your mind and ensure you write regularly. Too much time in between, often means progress can be slow as you will have to reconnect with the data and outputs. Writing retreats, which offer uninterrupted time away from work to write with some support from experienced researchers may be beneficial, especially at the beginning. It will take time to get to a finished product, but setting down thoughts on paper, what story you want to tell and determining the key message will benefit you in the longer term.

It can be lonely working on your own and collaborative work and writing can be beneficial as it will allow you to share ideas and receive feedback.

Submitting your paper; from manuscript to accepted article

The process of submitting a manuscript is relatively straightforward (albeit often long!) once you have ensured your work conforms to the scope, remit, intent, and structure of your chosen journal and article type (see Figure 27.1).

As part of the process, you may also need to submit a cover letter, although many editors choose not to read it and let the paper stand on its own. You do not need to explain why this paper fits within the journal, this should be evident from reading the manuscript. However, where it is required, this initial contact with the editor will allow you to start a conversation with them, so use their name and title, not just 'Dear Editor'! If writing a cover letter, ensure you clearly and concisely (one short paragraph) outline why your paper is relevant and of potential value to the journal's readership.

Peer review

The role and value of peer review in the evaluation of research remains unparalleled. As an author, it allows you to become part of a conversation and also part of a community engaged in your field or topic. It is also a very useful exercise in developing your writing skills [15]. However, receiving feedback from peers and experts is not without its challenges including how to respond to reviewers' comments, a subject we will address later.

Reviewers are invited to provide overall comments on the paper, along with specific queries, comments, suggestions, and a recommendation on the paper's readiness or suitability for publication.

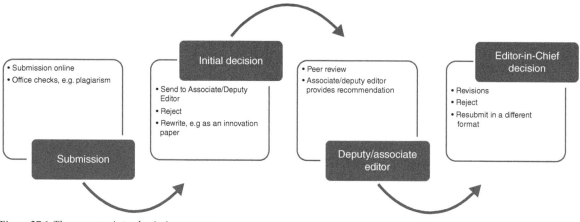

Figure 27.1 The manuscript submission process.

They are guided by the author guidelines for the journal, but also by a collective approach to determining the 'what, how and why' of the individual paper [16]. Once all peer reviews have been completed, the associate or deputy editor will collate this feedback, and along with the Editor-in-Chief, make a decision on the paper. This decision is also informed by critical choices around current hot topics, and what this submission adds to the journal's ethos and priorities.

Decoding the decision; from major to minor

Manuscripts are rarely accepted without some requested revisions. These may range from minor structural changes to major methodological concerns that need to be addressed. Importantly, a 'major revisions' decision does not guarantee that your paper will be published even if you address all the requested revisions. Rather, it means that the editors and reviewers generally like the paper, or feel it has potential, but have some serious concerns about an aspect(s) of the research and need more information to determine whether the paper is likely to be suitable for publication. This is another conversation point in your publication journey which often results in a better paper. You may not agree with all of the reviewer comments/suggestions, and this process allows you to discuss such areas with the editors [17, 18]. For example, you may address a specific suggestion by saying 'while we note the reviewer's suggestion with interest, the focus of this statement was to ensure that the process we used was transparently described and would rather not amend this section'.

Each journal will detail its process for accepting revised manuscripts, but you will generally be required to submit two copies, one with the changes highlighted (or 'tracked') and another 'clean' copy of the revised version. However, it is also very useful to the editors if you can detail the changes using a revisions template (please see companion website for example response template), explaining what change was suggested, your reply to the editor/reviewer, and a signpost to the change within the manuscript.

Individual journals and publishers often also have specific guidance, and it is worth reading around some editorials and guides to managing revisions specifically in the context of clinical education.

The publication journey: rejection is not failure

The road to publication is long and arduous. Rejection is an inevitability for all researchers at some point in their journey. Acceptance rates for papers can be lower than 10% for some journals. Therefore, you are more likely to have a manuscript rejected than accepted. Bitter though it may be, rejection should not be viewed as failure. Feedback provided by editors and reviewers can be invaluable in uplifting the standard of the paper and bolstering chances of publication in the future. They may also provide useful advice on where to consider publishing next. Addressing suggested revisions before resubmitting elsewhere could improve chances of a favourable outcome. Take heart in the fact that each time a paper is reviewed, it only serves to make it stronger.

Recognising the potential duplication of efforts taken to review papers that go through relentless cycles of rejection, some journals provide a 'fast-track' option. This is a means by which a manuscript rejected by one journal is submitted to another, along with previous records of peer review and author responses. Based on these, the handling editor can decide if the manuscript can be accepted immediately or if further peer review is needed, thereby shortening processing time and use of resources [15]. Making use of such options can significantly reduce the time taken to publish your work.

When you finally manage to savour the sweet success of publication, first be sure to celebrate! Remember though, this is not the end of the journey. Rather, it is the closing of one chapter and the beginning of another. As Lingard [1] observes, publishing serves to promote scholarly discourse. Therefore, publication of your paper may serve as the starting point for a conversation or signal a turn in an ongoing discussion. It is important to remember therefore that contributions to this discourse from the academic community may arrive in various forms, for example as a letter to the editor critiquing your work. It is obligatory to respond to such critique to ensure that scholarly dialogue flourishes.

It is equally important to remember it is in the best interests of the authors and the journal to increase the visibility of your research. Successfully publishing your work is only half the battle, ensuring that the academic community actually reads your work is the other. There are many methods and channels that can be harnessed to promote visibility. Web-based research communities are ideal platforms on which to disseminate your work. Linking publications to your social media profiles in a timely manner can ensure that you garner a wider readership, thereby enhancing your reach within the world of research [19] (see Chapter 28).

Social media (SoMe) is steadily growing in popularity as a medium for scholarly dissemination. Social media platforms are powerful tools for sharing your work far and wide and can reach diverse communities of readers instantaneously. To this end, many journals allow authors to include their social media handles on their papers, thereby allowing readers to engage with the authors in a more informal setting and develop virtual communities of scholarly discussion [20]. See Chapter 28 for further ideas for dissemination outside of the traditional manuscript.

Depending on the copyright clauses of the publisher, you may be allowed to share abstracts or full papers on these various platforms. A straightforward route to this is sharing a link to an electronic format of your work. Another, possibly more effective method, is creating a visual abstract. Visual abstracts are graphical summaries of the key points of a paper. They are more likely to capture attention than written text, by conveying the most significant messages to the reader at a glance. The toolbox on graphic design developed by Asif and Burton [14] can serve as an invaluable resource when developing visual abstracts.

Summary

Publishing your work is a significant professional achievement; optimise every opportunity to do so by preparing well, putting the groundwork into your study design and by surrounding yourself with peers and colleagues who can support you. This chapter has provided guidance for developing a publishable submission. At every step of the publication journey, we recommend keeping clear, concise, and captivating notes. Do not be disheartened if your submission is not accepted first time around; reviewer feedback will help you to continue refining your writing.

Top tips

- Start thinking about publication as you begin to plan your project.
- Choose which journal you intend to submit to and familiarise yourself with the journal's mission, submission guidelines, and academic writing resources.
- Write a compelling story.
- Apply a range of methods for presenting information. Create figures and tables which convey your findings with an economy of words.
- Consider reviewer feedback carefully, identifying where improvement is needed and where you can push back.

Common pitfalls

- Attempting to write up a good idea or project after it has been implemented. It is important to do the background work and get relevant ethical approval.
- Not allowing enough time to write and publish. Be realistic about the time frames not only for the writing but also for the publication journey.
- Not agreeing authorship at the beginning. Agree order and contributions before starting writing.

Ethical issues

- Ethical approval cannot be retrospective. This needs to be in place before starting work.
- Make sure you are accurate and honest in reporting your findings. Report all relevant findings, whether positive, neutral, or negative.

Further reading

Lingard, L. and Watling, C. *Story Not Study: 30 Brief Lessons to Inspire Health Researchers as Writers*. Springer. ISBN: 978-3-030-71362-1.

Academic Medicine Blog: Writing effectively and navigating the publication process: advice from the editors of academic medicine. https://academicmedicineblog.org/?s=writing+effectively

References

1 Lingard, L. (2015). Joining a conversation: the problem/gap/hook heuristic. *Perspectives on Medical Education* 4: 252–253.

2 Han, J.J., Soegaard Ballester, J.M., and Aarons, C.B. (2021). Finding alignment between numbers and values in medical education. *Medical Education* 55: 553–555.

3 Maggio, L.A., Ninkov, A., Frank, J.R. et al. (2022). Delineating the field of medical education: bibliometric research approach(es). *Medical Education* 56 (4): 387–394.

4 Rees, E.L., Burton, O., Asif, A. et al. (2022). A method for the madness: an international survey of health professions education authors' journal choice. *Perspectives on Medical Education* 11 (3): 165–172.

5 Bordage, G. (2009). Conceptual frameworks to illuminate and magnify. *Medical Education* 43 (4): 312–319.

6 Konopasky, A., O'Brien, B.C., Artino, A.R. et al. (2022). I, we and they: a linguistic and narrative exploration of the authorship process. *Medical Education* 56 (4): 456–464.

7 Maggio, L.A., Artino, A.R. Jr., Watling, C.J. et al. (2019). Exploring researchers' perspectives on authorship decision making. *Medical Education* 53 (12): 1253–1262.

8 Lingard, L. (2016). Bonfire red titles. Perspect. *Medical Education* 5 (3): 179–181.

9 AMRounds. (2018). Why titles are important. https://academicmedicineblog.org/why-titles-are-important (accessed 11 May 2023).

10 Cook, D.A. and Bordage, G. (2016). Twelve tips on writing abstracts and titles: how to get people to use and cite your work. *Medical Teacher* 38 (11): 1100–1104.

11 The Equator Network. (2022). Reporting guidelines. https://www.equator-network.org/reporting-guidelines (accessed 11 May 2023).

12 Ramani, S., McKimm, J., Forrest, K. et al. (2022). Co-creating scholarship through collaborative writing in health professions education: AMEE Guide No. 143. *Medical Teacher* (4): 44, 342–352.

13 Findyartini, A., Ramani, S., McKimm, J., and Fornari, A. (2021). Collaborative writing for clinical educators: recommendations from a community of scholars. *The Clinical Teacher* 18: 330–335.

14 Asif, A. and Burton, O. (2021). Comic sans or common sense? Graphic design for clinical teachers. *The Clinical Teacher* 18: 583–589.

15 Ellaway, R., Tolsgaard, M., and Norman, G. (2020). Peer review is not a lottery: AHSE's fast track. *Advances in Health Sciences Education* 25 (3): 519–521.

16 Jauregui, J., Artino, A.R. Jr., Ilgen, J.S. et al. (2022). Publishing your scholarship: a survey of pearls from top reviewers. *Medical Education Online* 27: 1.

17 Sullivan, G.M., Simpson, D., Yarris, L.M., and Artino, A.R. Jr. (2019). Writing author response letters that get editors to "yes.". *Journal of Graduate Medical Education* 11 (2): 119–123.

18 Meyer, H.S., Carline, J., and Durning, S.J. (2016). Ten tips to move from 'revisions needed' to resubmission. *Academic Medicine* 91 (12): e15.

19 Gallo, T. (2016). Congratulations! Your article has been accepted. Now what? Media, social media, and other outlets for promoting your work. *Academic Medicine* 91 (12): e9.

20 Yarris, L.M., Chan, T.M., Gottlieb, M., and Juve, A.M. (2019). Finding your people in the digital age: virtual communities of practice to promote education scholarship. *Journal of Graduate Medical Education* 11 (1): 1–5.

28 Disseminating your findings

Jonathan Guckian and Teresa Chan

Learning objectives

By the end of this chapter, you should be able to:
- Identify a range of approaches to disseminating your clinical education research.
- Formulate a basic dissemination strategy for your research projects, centred around understanding of relevant audiences.
- Describe the opportunities, limitations, and risks of dissemination via journal publication, meeting presentation, social media, and multimedia.

Introduction

Now that you have completed your project, you might be thinking that you are done. That is not the case. Simply generating new evidence is insufficient in today's noisy world. As researchers in an applied field, we must engage in methods to close the gap between knowing and doing. Remember: it is never too early to plan a dissemination strategy. In this chapter, we will shed light on how you can connect with your intended audience to raise awareness and possibly affect change.

There are numerous ways in which you can engage in knowledge dissemination, translation, and implementation of your findings. These will enable you to affect change in your clinical or educational environments.

What is knowledge dissemination?
Knowledge dissemination is a component of both *knowledge translation* and *implementation science*. Knowledge translation is a dynamic and iterative process involving the application of knowledge to improve health and healthcare systems [1]. Implementation science focuses on the implementation of research into reality, seeking to test if and how interventions might work in real-life settings [2].

Knowledge dissemination focuses on the initial parts of the knowledge translation and implementation science processes, for example, raising awareness of your scientific work. Its purpose is to 'create a positive impact on the acquisition of knowledge, attitudes, and practice' [3].

Planning your dissemination strategy

As a new researcher doing your first project, your job will be to engage in knowledge dissemination and plan your strategy. This will enable you to recruit others to support you in engaging in knowledge translation or implementation later on. Often new researchers will forget to plan for this step in advance.

Planning is important with a focus on the end-user and readers of your research as well as your stakeholders (see Chapter 5). It may also change the way you think about various aspects of the research. If you have written a grant proposal, there are usually sections where you write in your dissemination plan. This may vary depending on the stage of the research (see Table 28.1).

Key questions for designing your dissemination strategy
It may seem intimidating at first to design a dissemination strategy. Answering a few key questions can help you plan the way forward.

What are your dissemination aims?

Sharing your work should not simply be done for the sake of it. Clarifying your aims will guide your dissemination strategy. If you wish to influence educational policy, this should lead you to specific meetings and influence the language of your dissemination. If your desire is to support educational practice 'on the ground', then you may find podcasts, YouTube videos or meetings supporting practical learning points most beneficial to communicate your message.

Starting Research in Clinical Education, First Edition. Edited by Eliot L. Rees, Alison Ledger, and Kim A. Walker.
© 2024 The Association for the Study of Medical Education (ASME). Published 2024 by John Wiley & Sons Ltd.
Companion website: www.wiley.com/go/clinicaleducation

Table 28.1 Dissemination considerations at different project stages

Project stage	Dissemination considerations
Grant writing	Budgeting for knowledge dissemination (e.g. travel to conferences, printing posters)
Abstract writing	Submitting to key conferences
Manuscript writing	Preparing your manuscript for a key audience
Figure generation	Ensuring that your figures are easily read and digested Some authors will prepublish their figures in the public domain (e.g. WikiCommons) and then cite their open access figure within the paper to ensure others can use their figures freely
Post-publication	Planning to share the paper post-publication via various sources (e.g. tweeting about your publication; writing a blog post about your findings; being invited to be part of a podcast)

Who is your audience and what are their needs?

If your audience is a homogenous group with similar interests and behaviours, it may be sensible to focus on one dissemination format, i.e. presenting at a specific academic meeting or targeting one social media platform. However, if your audience is more diverse, this may necessitate a 'multi-pronged' approach, with careful curation of message for different stakeholders across various formats.

What modality best fits your findings?

At first, the conclusions of your research may seem to naturally fit one specific dissemination modality. Research featuring numerous graphs and tables may suit academic journal publication, rather than contributing to busy presentation slides or posters. However, creative approaches such as Social Media Tweetorials may challenge you to break down complex research into brief, digestible chunks and inspire you to find new ways to get the word out.

What is your timeline?

Depending on your findings you may find there are faster and slower dissemination processes. Abstracts can usually be presented within months, whereas some journals may take closer to a year (or more) to go from a submitted manuscript to a full paper.

What might be the financial cost of dissemination?

It is important to bear in mind certain methods for dissemination can cost more than others. Presenting at a conference will entail registration fees, travel, and subsistence costs and possibly the price of printing a poster. Various types of publication may also require publication fees (see Chapter 27). Financial support in the form of grants, or being aware of available institutional support, may help you map out what is practically feasible in terms of dissemination, and this can favour certain modalities, such as social media rather than meeting attendance.

What skills or resources are available to you?

At certain institutions, you may have access to technologies, printing, or individual collaborators which can drive dissemination through specific modalities. Subscription to graphic software or design support may favour poster development. Your institution or collaborators may have links to social media or multimedia platforms such as podcasts which can amplify your message.

Ways to disseminate

Academic journal publication

Most researchers will see publication as the main target for their work. When seeking to engage your audience via publication, it is important to know there are a wide range and types of publications. Consider the article types that can be found in various journals as to which is the most appropriate (see Chapter 27).

There can be a lot of pressure on new researchers to publish, especially in institutions where supervisors are being pressured to 'publish or perish' themselves [4, 5]. Traditionally, scholarly outputs have been measured through citations or the h-index, which is a quantitative means of calculating publication impact [6]. While this may be slowly changing, with the advent of other types of alternative metrics [7] and new forms of scholarship [8], academia has never been known to change quickly. However, publishing can have the advantage of adding to one's curriculum vitae (CV), which can be an important part of career development.

There are some key points to think about when publishing. Consider your audience. All journals have unique target audiences. Therefore, take some time to read the articles within a journal to ascertain if it is a right fit for you and whether they have published similar articles to yours.

Conferences

He who attends meetings regularly, even if he does not impart his experience to others, must leave a better man, better by the knowledge he has absorbed while listening to others.

Dr. M Feingold, 1925 [9]

Almost 100 years ago, Dr. Marcus Feingold wrote of the key role of the medical meeting in sharing ideas and values beyond our own circles, for the betterment of those entrusted to our care. Despite advances in technology and accessibility (not to mention gendered language), the inherent emotions and values depicted remain true for the 'ideal' meeting. A meeting or conference should provoke emotions of determination, admiration, and desire for imitation.

Conferences can be as diverse as their participants, ranging from mass congresses of thousands to smaller local gatherings. It is not necessary to address vast crowds to share clinical education research. Instead, you should carefully consider the audience size, career stages, and specialist interest in selecting the best means of spreading your message as detailed in Table 28.2.

Oral presentation

At the heart of the meeting is the presentation. The most common meeting myth is that the presenter is the most essential figure in the room. This is a misconception. The audience is far more important. Every successful orator has one core role, telling a story [10], which is driven by the audience present. Consider career stages, specialty interests, demographics, and accessibility when crafting your story [11]. Start by writing down the potential needs of your audience, as well as the potential challenges they face. A general audience may necessitate removal of jargon and inclusion of metaphor or broader imagery [12], whilst specialists may hunger for depth or academic challenge.

Table 28.2 Categories of meeting presentations

Presentation type	Description
Oral presentation	Opportunity to share key messages regarding research undertaken or relevant concepts to meeting audience. Usually supported by slide deck/PowerPoint presentation and may be delivered to large or small audiences. Usually didactic and followed by questions
Poster	Historically, a printed summation of research findings displayed amongst similar works, whereby event delegates may browse between presentations or during breaks. More recently, these have been supplemented by 'e-posters' of varying formats, including graphical abstracts displayed on screens
Workshops	Small to medium size group sessions led by a session chair which are designed to be more interactive than didactic presentations. May involve collaborative activities and often longer than research presentations. Usually focus on sharing skills rather than disseminating research findings

Once you better understand your audience, you are ready to craft your story. The popular P-cubed approach [13] advocates for a stepwise approach, structuring groups of ideas, organising an overarching narrative, and featuring key objectives with memorable moments. Supportive materials should only be considered after this. Variable guidance exists on composing effective PowerPoint presentation slides, but the overarching principle is less is more [14]. Reading verbatim from busy slides is a common pitfall of the presenter [15], so you must remember the audience should be captivated by your story, not your slides. Avoid distracting fonts and animations. Instead, consider fonts which are accessible to those with visual impairment. If graphs or similar figures require more than a few seconds to understand, remove them. Slides featuring long references are usually ignored and instead these should be considered for a handout or QR code. Delivery is the final and often most challenging step in oral presentations. Get to know your nerves and avoid avoidance behaviours. Practice breeds familiarity and can help settle anxiety as well as helping you look again and critique any weak areas of your talk. Belief in your story, simplification of supporting materials, and understanding of your audience will provide the best foundation to any presentation.

Posters

The historic four foot, self-printed 'poster' has begun to evolve, giving way recently to a diverse array of formats including video pitches, visual abstracts, and QR-code-driven 'e-posters' [16]. Posters represent a less intimidating opportunity for new researchers to dip their toes into the academic world and disseminate projects which may not quite reach the threshold of publication [17].

Posters require as much strategy as presentations. Know not only your audience but also their behaviours and limitations. A key tenet of any poster should be brevity and focus on key messages. Too many people make the mistake of oversaturating their poster with swathes of text, complex figures, and copious references in minuscule font. Delegates usually spend little more than a few moments casting their eyes over your poster (in person or online) and retain very little during meetings dominated by high cognitive load [18]. The challenge is first to draw the delegate in with a concise, clear, and interesting title. Once ensnared, the reader must be able to ingest your story quickly and easily. Therefore, portray no more than a handful of core messages, using creative but simple graphics. Such simplicity should facilitate clarity of message, which must surprise, entertain, or challenge.

Practical preparation for your poster is required. Study the meeting programme to determine exactly when poster viewing will occur, whether they must be accompanied by pitches, and where they will be hosted [19]. Stand by your poster at key moments and prepare complementary materials such as pre-prints, copies of data, or further reading. One study even claims that colour coordination between attire and posters may be a driver for increased visitation [20].

There are numerous guides with conflicting advice for the arrangement, font, and colour of posters [18, 21]. Consider visual accessibility with a light background stationed behind a single, large, clear, sans serif, dark-coloured font for contrast [22]. Remember the basics, nothing is more jarring than a poster printed on a paper size or orientation which is not recommended by the organiser. Whilst expensive or complex software does not guarantee successful dissemination, consideration of production platforms should be seen as an opportunity rather than a cause for anxiety. Microsoft PowerPoint may be a staple of traditional posters but new platforms have been developed which facilitate inexpensive, innovative approaches even for the novice, e.g. Canva [23] or Figma [24]. Those experienced in graphic design may consider Adobe Illustrator or Photoshop [25], and guidance or support may be available from your local medical illustration department.

As mentioned earlier, many conferences are now moving to online posters, sometimes known as e-posters or accessible short communications. Many of the principles and key requirements are the same as for the printed version. However, the ability to engage your audience and promote your work is even more difficult and new, innovative approaches may be required.

As a researcher, you may not have a wide range of niche technical skills, such as graphic design. However, consideration of dissemination strategies early in your project may help you consider assistance from colleagues with relevant expertise.

Several studies highlight the limitation of posters as a dissemination tool, citing limited delegate visitation [26] and lack of discussion [27] as factors for a disconnect between those authors and potential audiences. Longer term utility is also questionable, with a Cochrane Review highlighting only 63% of results from posters was later published in full and were vulnerable to publication bias [28]. Care must be taken that posters remain an educational experience, so they do not become little more than a means for conferences to attract registrations and act as 'CV fodder'.

Workshops

Workshops may be utilised in clinical education to share research with educators, to allow educators to collectively consider how their teaching practice can be enhanced, or for educators to learn more about research methodology or methods. Therefore, it can be an opportunity to present and disseminate findings without that being the primary reason for the workshop. Whatever is being presented, many of the principles outlined previously apply. It is essential to know and engage your audience, provide a clear message, and minimise over stimulation with lots of busy slides and information. Workshops can be highly variable and allow for greater creative freedom in terms of presentation. This may facilitate more interaction and activities, which can provide a break from the uniformity which can contribute to conference fatigue. As with other presentation mediums, it is important to avoid overcomplicating your message. Activities with low cognitive load can still provide some of the more memorable meeting experiences.

Networking

Despite the chaotic and often opportunistic nature of the conference experience, a strategy for networking can be as helpful as a presentation or poster, opening up opportunities for mentorship [29], leadership development [30], and support for promotions or grants [31], as well as disseminating your work. A simple first step should be to carefully construct and rehearse a concise elevator pitch for a project. Conference mobile apps or online spaces often allow early visibility of delegate profiles, therefore curation of your profile with interests and external links to professional works should be complemented by an understanding of the interests of other delegates. Clear identification of potential collaborators or mentors in advance may calm the perceived pandemonium of a meeting. Prepare business cards with up-to-date contact details in advance to allow follow-up from networking.

Meetings should not be considered a panacea for dissemination in clinical education. Conferences are unquestionably an industry in themselves, with most faculty familiar with correspondence from 'predatory' conferences [32]. Cost of training is a rising problem amongst early career educators and sources of funding since the COVID-19 pandemic is increasingly challenging to source. It is reasonable to question the utility of attendance at expensive meetings, with evidence suggesting that cheaper student or trainee events may provide comparable or even superior learning value at a fraction of the cost [33]. This cost is not always purely financial, with growing concerns regarding the environmental impact of meetings. Organisers have been encouraged to host meetings at major population centres, close to attendee locality, so as to offset the significant carbon footprint associated with air travel [34]. With a surge in technology-enhanced learning since the pandemic, virtual meetings have been proposed as a major solution to this problem. Virtual platforms may eliminate geographical barriers preventing early career educator attendance, in addition to supporting input from those in low- to middle-income nations [35]. Moreover, such platforms have been demonstrated to increase attendance from under-represented communities. However, virtual meetings do carry major diversity implications, with anecdotal evidence suggesting that women are more likely to be spoken over or interrupted by men during virtual meetings compared to face-to-face conferences [36].

Social media

In the 21st century landscape, social media (SoMe) dominates as a means to network, translate knowledge, and share narratives. Loosely defined as online platforms designed for multidirectional content creation and curation or community collaboration [37], SoMe is increasingly used by scientists, researchers, and journals to further clinical education conversation. SoMe's legitimacy as a tool for knowledge translation lies in the emerging power of online communities [38]. Such networks enable immediacy of message and sustainable approaches. Academics have adapted their research behaviours to suit SoMe, harnessing its multi-directional functionality to listen and then translate research into practice [39]. The impact of SoMe can be underscored by the creation of a host of social media editors, who engage with authors and participate in innovative ways to advance scholarship [40].

In terms of sheer reach, evidence suggests sharing research via Twitter may facilitate engagement with new audiences [41]. Said reach has a democratising effect, where users with limited resources or social capital can engage directly with world experts and negotiate knowledge. Such engagement can be instantaneous, with live discussion occurring during in-person or virtual events, across continents and hierarchies. Such disruption is driven by the largely free or low-cost nature of SoMe, in addition to a culture where open access is celebrated [42]. The inherently conversational nature of most SoMe ensures the author not only disseminates but also receives direct feedback.

This can benefit author and scientific practice alike, such as with the public outcry and subsequent retraction of a vascular surgery article where male surgeons criticised what they perceived to be inappropriate attire of female colleagues [43]. This '#medbikini' response typified the power of SoMe to challenge gender stereotypes and systemic inequalities within academia. With marginalised populations as strong consumers of SoMe, it is perhaps the responsibility of academics to engage with such open-access approaches.

The most prominent, traditional measure of scientific article impact is via citations. With the rise of SoMe as a dissemination tool, the Altmetric Attention Score has been developed to conceptualise how an article may have been shared or interacted with on SoMe [7]. One study has demonstrated positive correlation between Altmetric and 5-year citations, particularly related to Twitter [44]. However, within clinical education, a study found that Twitter metrics (mention counts and potential exposure in terms of followers) had weak correlations with access or citation counts, limiting its utility as a measure of scholarly impact [45]. Whilst Altmetric itself has not been demonstrated to directly influence journal *Impact Factor*, such data may complement traditional approaches to measuring impact and inform wider dissemination strategy. Examples of social media dissemination approaches are detailed in Table 28.3.

Experience with SoMe, in conjunction with a keen attention to metrics, will provide you with an understanding of audience behaviours. This may include intuition for the days and time followers are most likely to engage, preferred hashtags, appropriate tone, and relevant platforms for the type of article being promoted. Such comprehension can facilitate scheduling content in advance, which significantly decreases the workload but still maintains visibility and impact. Collaboration with other accounts may also increase impact and reach, therefore contacting popular accounts in advance of publication of materials may generate more interaction, in addition to proactive tagging of such accounts. Keeping messages concise and complemented by striking graphics can prove impactful, with visual tweets gathering significantly more attention and retention [48]. Quick wins may be achieved via the inclusion of polls to encourage basic interaction, whilst keeping threads brief and including summary posts should help with clarity of message. The user journey is fundamentally helped by fewer clicks, therefore a simple step for video materials is to directly embed media into a

Table 28.3 Social Media dissemination approaches and their advantages and disadvantages

Approach	Description	Advantages	Disadvantages
Tweetorials/threads	Linked consecutive Tweets, often breaking down complex information into short bursts	• Ability to pre-prepare • Share information through narrative • Simple to monitor metrics	• Tweets may be viewed out of context • Threads require manual expansion • Peer review is organic but inconsistent
Tweeting the meeting	Real-time conversation, reaction, and critical appraisal during events by delegates and those unable to attend	• Broadens reach of meeting and included works beyond physical space of meeting • Equalising effect of reaching those who cannot afford to attend conference • Opportunity to improve professional 'brand' in presence of relevant peers and institutions	• May be highly dependent on 'clinical education influencers' • Associated with significant cognitive load • Challenges presented include risk to intellectual property and lack of real-world context lost in translation
Visual abstracts/ infographics	Visual reproduction of study background, aims, and conclusions through graphic design approach	• Engagement with Instagram audience • Visual appeal, ease of navigation, clear take-home messages • Significant increase in Altmetric score [46]	• Requires significant resource for creation • Variation in quality creator dependent • Does not appear to increase full-text readership
Journal clubs	Virtual communities of practice discussing and debating single or multiple research papers, often on regular basis	• Can develop regular audience and reinforce community experience • May increase Altmetric scores and access to journal web pages [47] • Can facilitate more detailed and nuanced discussion through structure and moderation compared to live-tweeting meetings	• Require significant preparation • Quality of discussion highly dependent on moderator activity • Brief time window limits accessibility across all time zones

Tweet, rather than provide an external Youtube link. SoMe 'influencers' are held in variable regard within academic circles, there are few surer ways to guarantee widespread interest in a research post on SoMe than via sharing by a popular account. Such accounts may be individuals or institutions, therefore consider contacting your journal's social media editor when planning dissemination.

Despite strong links to successful academic communication, SoMe is often met with mistrust and scepticism. This is not without merit, as the medium is deeply complex, intimidating, and even dangerous in the wrong hands. A recent study demonstrated that on SoMe, false stories were 70% more likely to be retweeted and were spread 10 times faster than true stories [49]. SoMe misinformation has been demonstrated across a variety of academic medical fields, unsurprisingly contributing to mistrust and the need for criticality [50]. This phenomenon, in addition to the need to navigate self-promotion and pre-existing biases contributes to the cognitive load which can limit the efficacy of SoMe as a dissemination tool. Careful curation of your timeline, including following only reliable sources, as well as

encouraging a culture of challenging inaccurate information and taking breaks from SoMe are examples of 'healthier' SoMe practices. Deliberate trolling, bullying, or antagonisation is unfortunately common and also unpredictable and challenging to plan for. Whilst common advice is 'do not feed the troll,' this approach has been criticised as silencing victims and is situated as part of a victim-blaming narrative, particularly when considering such online violence against women [51]. Responsibility lies with SoMe corporations and leaders in academic communities, to call for systemic and cultural intolerance of such harassment, to provide a safer environment for research dissemination.

Multimedia

If you are creative and bold, take advantage of new multimedia technologies beyond social media to capitalise on your research. Prominent amongst such approaches are podcasts and YouTubing.

Podcasts are mainly audio-based, unilateral, and feature conversations between hosts and guests or follow a narrative thread. They have been demonstrated within clinical education to provide entertainment whilst also allowing listeners to keep up with relevant literature and improve knowledge [52]. Already having reached mainstream popularity, they have surged within clinical communities as a means of maintaining creative communications during the COVID-19 pandemic. Whilst it is difficult to directly measure the impact of podcasts upon learning, their popularity has been well documented, with one study of 356 United States residents finding that 88% reported listening to medical education podcasts at least once a month [53]. Key to podcast popularity appears to be convenience, authority of source, and relative brevity, with the ideal podcast length in one study suggested to be 10–20 minutes [54]. Journals have capitalised on this, including within medical education and the format is ideal for transposition of the educational journal club into audio format, for example with the KeyLime podcast [55].

YouTube features a number of the dissemination advantages of social media, including immense popularity and support for communities. Indeed, much of the evidence related to the efficacy of SoMe for research dissemination includes YouTube. However, the platform stands apart from most others as an opportunity for depth, with its video approach facilitating a diverse range of potential dissemination approaches. Its global reach ensures a broad audience, and its comment section provides potential for immediate feedback so that creators can become more familiar with the needs of subscribers. Robust evaluative studies of YouTube as an educational tool are surprisingly lacking, though a scoping review highlighted technical quality, comprehensiveness, perceived accuracy, credibility of authorship, and teaching quality as important factors linked to 'quality' YouTube resources in clinical education [56]. Of interest, one study reported no correlation between learner engagement and quality of YouTube videos amongst United States residents and fellows [57].

Most podcast and YouTube content creators within the clinical education community actively seek new guests and welcome those passionate about their research and prepared to discuss what it may mean for practice. Consider contacting your favourite shows, with a brief pitch selling the relevance of your work. Podcasters and YouTube hosts are less likely to provide harsh rejection than academic journals! In such a communication, include two or three keywords early on to catch attention, ensure brevity, and avoid exaggeration. Once you have secured time on a show, you should prepare with a similar strategy to a presentation or networking. Formulate an 'elevator pitch', which should be brief and speak to the relevance of the study. Rehearse this repeatedly, and strip this down to a single-line introduction, which should sound natural to the listener. Conversations with hosts can be daunting, as many worry their words may later haunt them. General principles to follow include avoiding any issues you would not wish to make public, particularly anything identifiable. You should share your story and express your humanity through emotion and honesty. Detail the importance and timeliness of your work and explain why your research is meaningful [58]. Clarify in advance if you have the right to request removal of any content you are not happy with after recording, and do not be afraid to exercise this right if you have any concerns whatsoever. If video is involved, avoid cluttered environments.

Appropriate lighting and audio are more important than the quality of technical recording equipment. In particular, learners will tolerate lower quality video, but not low-quality audio. Consider purchasing a simple USB microphone, which can improve sound quality immeasurably compared to standard smartphone or laptop audio feeds. It may be worth investing in a higher quality USB microphone, particularly if you are considering regular virtual presentations or distance teaching. Sound quality can be aided by dampening; however, this can prove complex and expensive. Simple steps can involve closing curtains, covering gaps under doors and identifying all the noise within your room. Concerning lighting, alongside choosing a well-lit room for recording, further lighting support can be provided by a ring light.

Whilst engaging with multimedia can prove a bold and rewarding choice for research dissemination, such approaches can be intimidating for the uninitiated. They require a high level of effort and commitment and not insignificant associated costs if high-quality delivery is desired. Much like SoMe, reliability of platforms may be called into question, with misinformation particularly rife on YouTube [59]. It is therefore key to undertake your own research on shows before joining them to speak, as association with an unreliable platform can damage academic credibility. Unlike SoMe, podcasts do not facilitate effective or immediate opportunities for feedback or response, which can limit the criticism so central to rigorous academic debate. An example of how this may work is explained in the illustrated case study (Box 28.1)

BOX 28.1   Illustrated case study

Clodagh listens to a podcast which cites a study on well-being and burnout amongst medical graduates. Reading the study, she decides to undertake a research project on the financial cost of training in her specialty. She undertakes this research, with rich and surprising data collected.

Clodagh decides to start by writing the study up for publication, with a target audience including both her peers and leaders with influence in postgraduate medical education. She realised it will take some time to reach publication, so decides to write a brief abstract and submits it to a national conference, gaining acceptance as a poster. Her visual abstract has stark, clear messaging regarding the financial cost of training. A delegate at the conference views the poster and invites her to speak at a regional meeting of educators. Clodagh tailors her talk to the audience, discussing ways training could be better funded. Her paper is then accepted by a journal. To increase the impact and further disseminate the findings, she breaks down the text into the most important pieces. A tweetorial is developed, tagging in key national figures in clinical education and influential staff, using the hashtag #CostofResidency and creating a poll asking her audience how much they spend on training costs and saves the analytics for this. She asks to feature on the journal podcast, where she discusses the cost of training more widely and key lessons from her study.

Octavian, another new researcher listens to her podcast and decides to undertake a study on the emotional burden of residency training. Through effective dissemination, a future generation of research has been inspired.

Summary

Dissemination should not be an afterthought in undertaking clinical education research. Instead, dissemination strategies should be woven into the overall approach to your project, with consideration of creative, efficient means of sharing your messages. Dissemination is your opportunity to share the work that has such meaning to you. Therefore, crafting a story that is concise, practical, and captures the imagination of your audience is essential. No single medium is perfect, but the most impactful posters, presentations, articles, and Tweets all share common themes: careful preparation, audience consideration, and minimisation of cognitive load. Consideration of dissemination at each stage of your research will make this sometimes intimidating step much more manageable.

Common pitfalls

- No strategic thinking to dissemination. Use the guiding questions in this chapter to maximise research impact.
- Overcomplication of message. Craft a clear and accessible story.
- Producing presentation slides and posters which are overwhelmingly busy with text or media content. Aim to minimise cognitive load.
- Sharing your research on platforms with reputations for misinformation or lack of academic rigour, i.e. YouTube channels or predatory journals. Instead, reach out to reputable hosts or create your own multimedia presentations.

Ethical issues

- Social media ethics can be challenging to navigate, with availability of research disseminated varying across platforms and misinformation rife. Consult local guidance or research ethics staff for advice on navigating this complex medium.
- Intellectual property is an important consideration when publishing multimedia content online. Explore whether you retain ownership to your research work when publishing online.
- Ensure that you have relevant permissions for posting in social media and that messages are not exaggerated when sharing your research. Check you can edit media if you are not happy with the content.

Top tips

- Plan dissemination from the outset of research (and budget for it).
- Think carefully who your audience is and tailor to them. Only use humour when appropriate.
- Work smartly and efficiently – make things count twice. For example, export your slides to JPG file and then use it as the visuals within a tweetorial.
- Creativity and patience may be rewarded with increased reach of your message.

References

1 Government of Canada (2005). Canadian Institutes of Health Research. About us – CIHR. https://cihr-irsc.gc.ca/e/29418.html (accessed 11 May 2023).

2 Khalil, H. (2016). Knowledge translation and implementation science: what is the difference? *JBI Evidence Implementation* 14 (2): 39–40.

3 Lafrenière, D., Menuz, V., Hurlimann, T., and Godard, B. (2013). Knowledge dissemination interventions: a literature review. *SAGE Open* 3 (3).

4 Relman, A.S. (1977). Publish or perish – or both. *The New England Journal of Medicine* 297: 724–725. Massachusetts Medical Society.

5 McGrail, M.R., Rickard, C.M., and Jones, R. (2006). Publish or perish: a systematic review of interventions to increase academic publication rates. *Higher Education Research and Development* 25 (1): 19–35.

6 Murphy, L.S., Kraus, C.K., Lotfipour, S. et al. (2018). Measuring scholarly productivity: a primer for junior faculty. Part III: understanding publication metrics. *The Western Journal of Emergency Medicine* 19 (6): 1003–1011.

7 Bornmann, L. (2014). Do altmetrics point to the broader impact of research? An overview of benefits and disadvantages of altmetrics. *Journal of Informetrics* 8 (4): 895–903.

8 Chan, T.M. and Kuehl, D.R. (2019). On lampposts, sneetches, and stars: a call to go beyond bibliometrics for determining academic value. *Academic Emergency Medicine* 26 (6): 688–694.

9 Feingold, M. (1925). The habit of attending medical meetings. *Journal of the American Medical Association* 85 (2): 83.

10 Mai, C.L., Minehart, R.D., and Pian-Smith, M.C. (2019). Seven tips for giving an engaging and memorable presentation. *BJA Education* 19 (9): 274–275.

11 Kavanagh, J. (2006). Giving presentations without palpitations. *BMJ* 332 (7555): s242–s243.

12 Gewin, V. (2019). Top tips for giving an engaging talk. *Nature* 568 (7750): 133–135.

13 ffolliet (2014). How to 'do' a presentation #htdap. pcubedpresentations.http://ffolliet.com/2014/10/05/how-to-do-a-presentation (accessed 11 May 2023).

14 Harolds, J.A. (2012). Tips for giving a memorable presentation, part IV: using and composing PowerPoint slides. *Clinical Nuclear Medicine* 37 (10): 977–980.

15 Schmaltz, R.M. and Enström, R. (2014). Death to weak PowerPoint: strategies to create effective visual presentations. *Frontiers in Psychology* 5. Article 1138.

16 Naseem, S., Rafi, S., Qazi, M.A. et al. (2021). Conventional to virtual poster presentation in scholars' day during coronavirus disease-19 lock down: medical students' performance and perspective. *International Journal of Health Sciences* 15 (6): 23–27.

17 Ahlers-Schmidt, C.R., Chesser, A., Maher, J., and Vernon, S. (2009). Dissemination of student and resident research: publication rates after poster presentation. *Medical Teacher* 31 (3): 315–315.

18 Saperstein, A., Lennon, R., Olsen, C. et al. (2016). Information retention among attendees at a traditional poster presentation session. *Acta Medica Academica* 1 (45): 180–181.

19 Ramsewak, A. (2012). Create a poster presentation. *Education for Primary Care* 23 (5): 360–361, 1.

20 Keegan, D.A. and Bannister, S.L. (2003). Effect of colour coordination of attire with poster presentation on poster popularity. *CMAJ* 169 (12): 1291–1292.

21 Kaimal, S. and Thappa, D. (2010). The art and science of medical poster presentation. *Indian Journal of Dermatology, Venereology and Leprology* 76 (6): 718–720.

22 Papanas, N., Georgiadis, G.S., Demetriou, M. et al. (2019). Creating a successful poster: "beauty is truth, truth beauty". *The International Journal of Lower Extremity Wounds* 18 (1): 6–9.

23 Canva. Canva. https://www.canva.com.

24 Figma. Figma. https://figma.com.

25 Adobe. Adobe Products. https://www.adobe.com/au/products.html.

26 Salzl, G., Gölder, S., Timmer, A. et al. (2008). Poster exhibitions at National Conferences: education or farce? *Deutsches Ärzteblatt International* 105 (5): 78–83.

27 Goodhand, J., Giles, C., Wahed, M. et al. (2011). Poster presentations at medical conferences: an effective way of disseminating research? *Clinical Medicine* 11 (2): 138–141.

28 Scherer, R.W., Langenberg, P., and von Elm, E. (2007). Full publication of results initially presented in abstracts. *Cochrane Database of Systematic Reviews* 18 (2): MR000005.

29 Jackson, V.A., Palepu, A., Szalacha, L. et al. (2003). 'Having the right chemistry': a qualitative study of mentoring in academic medicine. *Academic Medicine: Journal of the Association of American Medical Colleges* 78 (3): 328–334.

30 Warren, O.J. and Carnall, R. (2011). Medical leadership: why it's important, what is required, and how we develop it. *Postgraduate Medical Journal* 87 (1023): 27–32.

31 Streeter, J. (2014). Networking in academia. *EMBO Reports* 15 (11): 1109–1112.

32 Lang, R., Mintz, M., Krentz, H.B., and Gill, M.J. (2019). An approach to conference selection and evaluation: advice to avoid "predatory" conferences. *Scientometrics* 118 (2): 687–698.

33 Sharp, E.W., Curlewis, K., and Clarke, T.H.S. (2019). Stop paying through the nose: student and trainee medical conferences offer better value for money than professional alternatives. *Postgraduate Medical Journal* 95 (1129): 577–582.

34 Leddin, D., Galts, C., McRobert, E. et al. (2022). The carbon cost of travel to a medical conference: modelling the annual meeting of the Canadian Association of Gastroenterology. *Journal of the Canadian Association of Gastroenterology* 5 (2): 52–58.

35 Wu, J., Rajesh, A., Huang, Y.N. et al. (2022). Virtual meetings promise to eliminate geographical and administrative barriers and increase accessibility, diversity and inclusivity. *Nature Biotechnology* 40 (1): 133–137.

36 Gupta, A. (2022). It's not just you: in online meetings, many women can't get a word in – The New York Times. https://www.nytimes.com/2020/04/14/us/zoom-meetings-gender.html (accessed 11 May 2023).

37 Guckian, J., Utukuri, M., Asif, A. et al. (2021). Social media in undergraduate medical education: a systematic review. *Medical Education* 55 (11): 1227–1241.

38 Chan, T.M., Dzara, K., Dimeo, S.P. et al. (2020). Social media in knowledge translation and education for physicians and trainees: a scoping review. *Perspectives on Medical Education* 9 (1): 20–30.

39 Chan, T., Trueger, N.S., Roland, D., and Thoma, B. (2018). Evidence-based medicine in the era of social media: scholarly engagement through participation and online interaction. *Canadian Journal of Emergency Medicine* 20 (1): 3–8.

40 Lopez, M., Chan, T.M., Thoma, B. et al. (2019). The social media editor at medical journals: responsibilities, goals, barriers, and facilitators. *Academic Medicine: Journal of the Association of American Medical Colleges* 94 (5): 701–707.

41 Buckarma, E.H., Thiels, C.A., Gas, B.L. et al. (2017). Influence of social media on the dissemination of a traditional surgical research article. *Journal of Surgical Education* 74 (1): 79–83.

42 Chan, T.M., Stehman, C., Gottlieb, M., and Thoma, B. A short history of free open access medical education. The past, present, and future. *ATS Scholar* 1 (2): 87–100.

43 Hardouin, S., Cheng, T.W., Mitchell, E.L. et al. (2020). RETRACTED: prevalence of unprofessional social media content among young vascular surgeons. *Journal of Vascular Surgery* 72 (2): 667–671.

44 Ayoub, F., Ouni, A., Case, R. et al. (2021). Dissemination of gastroenterology and hepatology research on social media platforms is associated with increased citation count. *The American Journal of Gastroenterology* 116 (10): 2137–2139.

45 Amath, A., Ambacher, K., Leddy, J.J. et al. (2017). Comparing alternative and traditional dissemination metrics in medical education. *Medical Education* 51 (9): 935–941.

46 Huang, S., Martin, L.J., Yeh, C.H. et al. (2018). The effect of an infographic promotion on research dissemination and readership: a randomized controlled trial. *Canadian Journal of Emergency Medicine* 20 (6): 826–833.

47 Wray, C.M., Auerbach, A.D., and Arora, V.M. (2018). The adoption of an online journal Club to improve research dissemination and social media engagement among hospitalists. *Journal of Hospital Medicine* 13 (11): 764–769.

48 Ibrahim, A.M., Lillemoe, K.D., Klingensmith, M.E., and Dimick, J.B. (2017). Visual abstracts to disseminate research on social media: a prospective, Case-control crossover study. *Annals of Surgery* 266 (6): e46.

49 Vosoughi, S., Roy, D., and Aral, S. (2018). The spread of true and false news online. *Science* 359 (6380): 1146–1151.

50 Suarez-Lledo, V. and Alvarez-Galvez, J. (2021). Prevalence of health misinformation on social media: systematic review. *Journal of Medical Internet Research* 23 (1): e17187.

51 Lumsden, K. and Morgan, H. (2017). Media framing of trolling and online abuse: silencing strategies, symbolic violence, and victim blaming. *Feminist Media Studies* 17 (6): 926–940.

52 Malecki, S.L., Quinn, K.L., Zilbert, N. et al. (2019). Understanding the use and perceived impact of a medical podcast: qualitative study. *JMIR Medical Education* 5 (2): e12901.

53 Riddell, J., Swaminathan, A., Lee, M. et al. (2017). A survey of emergency medicine Residents' use of educational podcasts. *The Western Journal of Emergency Medicine* 18 (2): 229–234.

54 Cosimini, M.J., Cho, D., Liley, F., and Espinoza, J. (2017). Podcasting in medical education: how long should an educational podcast be? *Journal of Graduate Medical Education* 9 (3): 388–389.

55 KeyLIME (2023). KeyLIME Podcasts: Key Literature in Medical Education https://keylimepodcast.libsyn.com (accessed 29 May 2023).

56 Curran, V., Simmons, K., Matthews, L. et al. (2020). YouTube as an educational resource in medical education: a scoping review. *Medical Science Education* 30 (4): 1775–1782.

57 Desai, T., Sanghani, V., Fang, X. et al. (2013). Assessing a nephrology-focused YouTube channel's potential to educate health care providers. *Journal of Nephrology* 26 (1): 81–85.

58 Bigham, B.L. and Chan, T.M. (2018). Going viral and interacting with the press. *Journal of the American College of Radiology* 15 (1): 153–154.

59 Li, H.O.Y., Pastukhova, E., Brandts-Longtin, O. et al. (2022). YouTube as a source of misinformation on COVID-19 vaccination: a systematic analysis. *BMJ Global Health* 7 (3): e008334.

29 Developing your career

Gillian Vance, Sarah Simpson, Sue Jackson, and Richard Conn

Learning objectives

By the end of this chapter, you should be able to:
- Appreciate the breadth of careers in clinical education.

- Recognise opportunities to build skills and experience in clinical education research.
- Construct an effective plan for a career path.

Introduction

The rapidly changing landscape of healthcare presents many opportunities for clinical education research to inform the evidence base for education and training. This requires a steady pipeline of researchers who get started in research activities, develop relevant skills and qualifications, and successfully establish a career in the discipline. Yet evidence suggests that the pipeline of researchers is broken. For example, only a very small proportion of clinicians who reach senior academic positions in medical schools in the United Kingdom (UK) are listed in medical education [1]. Further, as this national data does not distinguish between researchers and those with programme delivery and leadership roles, it means the number of academics who are working predominantly in a research capacity is likely to be much lower. This situation is likely to be, at least, equally as challenging in other healthcare professions. Among the factors contributing to this historical lack of clinical education researchers is the poor specification of career paths and development opportunities, and a lack of guidance on how to navigate these. Addressing these issues may support many talented professionals to achieve success in research and rise to the much wider challenge of establishing clinical education research as a recognised, well-funded, and credible career option [2].

In this chapter, we set out to simplify the varied and often confusing routes [3, 4] to developing a research profile in clinical education. We will provide you with clear practical guidance on how to identify and take actionable steps towards a successful career in clinical education research. We have supplemented our advice with examples and illustrations. We also provide case studies of five professionals with varying career journeys in clinical education, which are available on the companion website. We hope this chapter will benefit everyone with the drive and intellectual curiosity to explore and address the important questions affecting clinical education and training, whether you are wishing to develop research within a wider educational role or have an aspiration to develop a dedicated career in clinical education research.

Careers in clinical education

We begin by exploring career options in clinical education in more depth. This task is complicated because those working in clinical education often balance multiple activities – teaching, leadership, research, and, for many, clinical practice. Moreover, as the discipline of clinical education has evolved, the number and types of educational roles have expanded and diversified. Terminology and job titles, which vary significantly between professions, institutions, settings, and geographical locations, confound what exactly a 'career in clinical education' looks like. Most clinicians are involved in clinical education to some degree, with teaching a long-established duty of healthcare professionals [5, 6]. Formal educational roles may include commitments to research, teaching or educational leadership, or a combination of these. Roles may be in healthcare organisations, universities, or with training bodies that have oversight of postgraduate training. Clinicians may combine these roles with clinical practice (sometimes referred to as 'clinical academics'). Professionals from other scientific backgrounds (e.g. psychology, sociology) also contribute, as do, increasingly, patients and patient representatives.

Starting Research in Clinical Education, First Edition. Edited by Eliot L. Rees, Alison Ledger, and Kim A. Walker.
© 2024 The Association for the Study of Medical Education (ASME). Published 2024 by John Wiley & Sons Ltd.
Companion website: www.wiley.com/go/clinicaleducation

Clinical education roles: A framework

Given this landscape, it is unsurprising that those who have clinical education aspirations find career progression unclear, difficult to navigate, and even 'serendipitous' [4]. This is especially true for those interested in research. Whilst many roles involve research activity, it is often conducted alongside other educational or clinical commitments. Dedicated clinical education research roles (whilst existing in some institutions and countries) are less well established than in other academic fields, e.g. biomedical research, as are the relevant training pathways.

To help guide career choices, and drawing on other work in this area [7, 8], we aim to clarify clinical education roles by proposing a framework with four overarching roles: leader, educator, teacher, and researcher (Table 29.1). These roles overlap and are interrelated, meaning that the framework encompasses both those who are primarily leaders, teachers etc., and those who practise multiple educational activities in combination. Clinical practice is not included within this framework (to ensure the framework is inclusive of professionals who do not practise clinically) but given the ultimate goal of clinical education is to benefit patients, clinical practice should directly or indirectly inform and energise all roles within it.

The framework avoids the term 'scholar' (which has been previously been used as a byword for clinical education researcher [7]) because all roles should be underpinned by scholarship, as reflected in Boyer's expanded definition of scholarship [10]. This framework makes clear that there is parity between roles, whilst also creating space for dedicated clinical education researchers who can contribute alongside those who conduct research in other capacities. We believe providing such roles, and training pathways towards such roles, to be a key step as clinical education evolves and develops. Those considering these careers can use this framework to support them in reflecting on their own skills, interests, and priorities, in evaluating the possibilities offered by a particular clinical or educational role and in planning the next steps for their career development.

The remainder of this chapter explores, in practical terms, how you can develop interests and build your career, paying particular attention to the role of research. Aligning with the framework above, we detail key steps in this process: developing foundational skills, seeking further qualifications and training, and establishing research independence and output.

Developing foundational skills

Having a set of core research skills will benefit all roles in clinical education. This section starts by examining the essential skills needed and how you might develop these. We also offer advice on how to build supportive relationships with colleagues and peers. The section will help you review your research needs and lay the foundations for your ongoing research involvement.

Developing essential research skills

If you are a new researcher, you will benefit from training in research methods. Generic skills, such as literature searching, critical appraisal, and academic writing, are essential for all educational practitioners. An introduction to quantitative and qualitative research approaches, as well as the practicalities of study design, delivery, and dissemination of findings will give you a valuable knowledge base to get started. You can find introductions to these in the respective chapters within this book. There is also a wealth of different training options, from one-off workshops to more formal graduate-level programmes, including those leading to degree qualifications. Explore what is available in your area, and what best meets your needs. Do seek out opportunities to become involved in research projects as this will allow you to apply your learning, deepen your understanding of research concepts, and develop your skills through practice. Contributing to projects is a great way to get a 'foot in the door' and get to know and work with experienced research teams.

Key activities that support development of these essential research skills are summarised in Table 29.2.

Mentorship and collaboration

Given the wide range of roles in clinical education, it is beneficial to find mentors who can help you navigate the local landscape, whilst also opening your eyes to the wider national and international picture. They can support you in setting your career goals, guide different parts of your development and help foster useful professional relationships and connections [12]. Good mentors can be difficult to find, but they do not necessarily need to be within the same specialty or profession, nor be geographically nearby, given the advent of videoconferencing [12]. In selecting a mentor, reflect on your mentorship needs and career goals. Schedule a time to meet and discuss your thoughts, plans, and expectations of them as a mentor, should they agree to consider your request.

Table 29.1 Framework of overlapping roles within clinical education and associated activities, skills, qualifications, and research involvement

	Researcher	Leader	Educator	Teacher
Definition	Conducts and leads research into educational issues	Leads educational programmes or departments and oversees teams of teachers and educators [9]	Designs, develops and evaluates educational modules, programmes, and curricula	Teaches health professionals and student health professionals, playing critical roles in their professional development [7]
Foundational skills	Expertise in educational theory and methodology appropriate to research area	Broad understanding of educational theory and evidence base for educational practice	Expertise in educational theory and evidence base in relation to area of educational practice; may also have research training and experience	Experienced in teaching methods, practical pedagogy, and giving and seeking feedback
Further qualifications[a]	Usually doctoral	Often master's or above	Usually, a formal qualification, often master's or above	Variable – no formal training through to recognised courses/certificates/diplomas/master's
Research independence and output	Leading research programmes; seeking grant funding; research supervision; national/international collaboration. Publications and evidence of impact are key and used in assessing performance	Variable – not primary to role but may act as collaborators/work with researchers, particularly to address curricular problems. Publications possible, but leadership goals are the priority	May collaborate in/lead research, which may include rigorous evaluation and implementation of educational initiatives. May be involved in research supervision. Publications form part of overall educational portfolio	Variable – from no involvement to conducting research relating to teaching activities and presenting teaching initiatives at conferences, etc. Publications possible but not essential to the teaching role

[a] Higher qualifications include certificate, diploma, and master's degree courses and doctorates/PhD.

Table 29.2 Activities to build foundational skills in clinical education research

Professional activity	Research skill/outcome
Reading	• Become familiar with the language and structure of research publications • Gain an understanding of the existing evidence base – what is already known in the literature about a particular topic and what is still missing
Participation in journal clubs	• Develop skills in critical appraisal of study design, recruitment strategies, and statistical and qualitative analysis
Mentorship	• Locate mentors to help you navigate your career goals and open your eyes to local, national, and international perspectives
Collaboration	• Seek collaboration with other researchers to support the development of skills and build your professional reputation
Peer reviewing	• Gain experience in peer-reviewing research articles. Reviewing others' work offers insights into a wider range of methodology and broader contemporary issues in clinical education [11]
Membership of professional society	• Build a professional network of useful contacts and like-minded peers • Identify opportunities for collaboration, small pots of funding, prizes, conferences, and presentation • Become a member of an accredited scheme promoting teaching excellence, e.g. Advance HE (UK), TEQSA (Australia)
Attendance at workshops and conferences	• Develop awareness of emerging research and 'hot topics'. • Build a professional network • Identify opportunities to get involved or collaborate in research studies • Present your early study findings and receive feedback as you progress
Teaching	• Gain experience of teaching in a variety of formats and settings • Gain experience in assessment of learning and evaluation of teaching • Develop an awareness of learner needs, preferences, professional development, and how to support these • Scope ideas for clinical education research
Involvement in research	• Become familiar with research planning: attend or contribute to patient and public involvement, proposal writing, ethical review or other research governance activities • Gain experience of steps in the research process: literature review, study design, study delivery (e.g. recruiting participants, gaining consent, facilitating an educational 'intervention', interviewing participants, entering data, undertaking qualitative and quantitative analyses) • Gain experience of dissemination: prepare abstracts, poster and oral presentations, prepare and submit manuscripts for publication

Forming networks and collaborating with other researchers is also very valuable. By engaging with the wider research community, you will continue to develop your skills, access further research opportunities, and build your professional reputation. Explore joining a professional society. In Box 29.1, see an example of a national networking initiative that creates a forum for professionals with interest in developing clinical education research careers.

Peer review

Although you may be experienced in having your work peer-reviewed as a researcher, acting as a peer reviewer can also be beneficial for developing your career. This may sound daunting, but it may be helpful to start by volunteering to review draft manuscripts ahead of submission to a journal. This will not only promote insight into a variety of research approaches but also develop your research communication skills if you ask for feedback on your reviews. You could also consider participating in peer review for academic journals as part of a group or 'peer review club'. This is an excellent way to proactively learn how others respond to the same submission [11] and is promoted by some journals. Journal websites contain helpful guidance on how to conduct a peer review but also look out for workshops, short courses, and mentored peer reviewer schemes. Good peer reviewing takes practice, so the more you do, the more confident you will become. It will also help you refine your ideas and develop research practices.

Accessing small pots of funding

Research takes resource which is often difficult to find. Funding to support your research is always beneficial. Education research tends to be less expensive than clinical research and small funding pots can go a long way in supporting costs such as transcribing recorded data and dissemination activities. Applications for funding provide important early experience, even when you are not successful the first time around. You will almost always gain helpful feedback and develop useful contacts to inform the next application. Through applying for funding, you also establish your interest in a particular area of education research.

Funding is available from a range of sources, more than you may realise, and often targeted at early career researchers. Internal funding opportunities may be offered by your university or healthcare organisation, while external funding is awarded by many professional bodies, societies, and charities (e.g. the Association for the Study of Medical Education). Membership of a professional society offering funding may be a prerequisite for eligibility, but this will also give you access to all the opportunities within that community, including advanced notice of grant deadlines. Funders may also have online resources around aspects of research process and useful guidance on their assessment criteria. Read these carefully! If you are successfully funded, they will expect updates on progress, but this helps to maintain the research momentum.

Seeking further qualifications and training

As you progress as a researcher, it will be crucial for you to develop further research expertise, broaden your connections within the research community,

and produce peer-reviewed academic outputs. Achieving these goals requires additional training, support, and time.

To help you navigate this stage, we outline some of the main structured training opportunities available to you as a new researcher.

Choosing to do a further qualification

If you are aiming to pursue a career involving clinical education research, a higher degree will support your professional development and is an essential requirement for many academic roles. Undertaking further postgraduate education can be transformative in terms of career progression. As there are many different programmes of study available, you need to consider the options in relation to your personal circumstances and career goals. Look at Table 29.1 to help you reflect on your current position as leader, educator, researcher, or teacher. What are your plans for development?

Two distinct forms of postgraduate education are master's and doctoral degrees. The key difference is the level of independent research. A master's degree is an intense but short period of study encompassing both taught elements and supervised research training. A doctorate, however, is the result of a longer period of study and is awarded on the production of a significant piece of independent research that makes a unique contribution to the clinical education field. To be a dedicated clinical education researcher you should consider a doctorate. However, undertaking a master's first can provide the necessary grounding in educational theory and research methodology before commencing your doctorate.

Table 29.3 provides a general overview of master's and doctoral study processes. Doctorate options include Doctor of Philosophy (PhD) as well as other doctoral-level qualifications, e.g. Doctor of Education (EdD), Doctor of Medicine (MD). There may be some geographical variations but the essence of further degrees is the same.

Specific considerations

There are several specific considerations that you should factor in your planning, as the decision to undertake a postgraduate degree is an important one.

Setting

Irrespective of your choice of master's or doctoral study, your degree will be awarded by a university, so you should explore what different universities offer. If there are taught elements, do these modules interest you? Who are the experts who might teach you? Who might you approach for supervision? What topics do most students seem to investigate?

Table 29.3 Outline and comparison of master's and doctoral study

	Master's degree	Doctorate
Goal	To gain a solid foundation in education theory and research methodology	To gain expert knowledge and experience in a particular area To make a contribution to the evidence base To support long-term career aspirations (especially when pursuing positions that require a doctorate)
Duration	Usually one-year full time, or two years part-time	Usually three years full-time or five years upwards for part-time
Cost	Less expensive than a doctorate Cost may vary slightly between institutions	Generally more expensive than master's as a result of the time taken to complete Scholarships may be available to provide funding while studying (sometimes matched to a clinician's salary) Part-time students will be able to continue some employment if they wish
Method of study	Series of core lectures and taught modules, exams, and assignments	Independent research supported by a supervisory team
Dissertation/Thesis	Supervised research dissertation	A novel body of work in the form of a thesis or, depending on your institution a doctorate-by-publication might be possible. This involves the submission of high-quality published papers (typically 3–4) and a linking narrative

Does the university offer flexible or part-time options for those wanting to work clinically while studying?

Subject

This is key – not only because your outputs need to build on existing knowledge for a master's, or be an original contribution for doctoral study, but it should be a subject that you feel passionately about, or a problem that you think needs further examination. Just to note, master's candidates may not always have an option to choose their research topic, whereas doctoral students are expected to choose, or at least significantly shape, their own area of research. Revisit Chapters 1 and 2 for related advice on developing a research topic and questions.

Supervisors

Having chosen your research subject, the next important consideration is your supervisory team, since this is critical for success [13]. Reflect on *your* methodological preferences when considering supervision. Most doctoral students have one primary supervisor and one or two secondary (or subsidiary) supervisors. Within your supervisory team you should aim to ensure you have at least one person with expertise in the topic and at least one with expertise in the proposed methods. They will also need to meet the particular eligibility criteria of the university.

It is worth sounding out possible supervisors from within your wider networks, including from different healthcare disciplines, to expand thought processes and methodological approaches. Make contact with people who you believe you will work well with – good communication and rapport are essential elements of effective supervision [13].

Funding

Undertaking further qualifications can be expensive and self-funding can be difficult. However, there may be part and full funding options available. The most straightforward way is to apply for an advertised university studentship or submit a proposal for a doctoral fellowship [14]. Many universities now offer scholarship funding for applicants with limited financial support, or who require part-time study options, have caring responsibilities, or come from groups which are historically under-represented in academia.

Healthcare professionals often wish to continue in clinical training or practice alongside their research study. This is possible within some fellowship schemes (e.g. NIHR [15]). Other clinicians wishing to maintain paid employment may be able to do so in part-time or through flexible programmes of study [16]. You may be able to negotiate with your employer about funding and study time since there are recognised benefits for you and your organisation's research culture if you undertake research that relates to issues in your workplace.

Making your study experience a great one

The path to a clinical education degree can be challenging, especially for those undertaking research alongside clinical or teaching commitments. Be careful to ring-fence time for study and keep track of milestones for project delivery and university review processes. If appropriate, identify and negotiate blocks of research time to immerse yourself into the project (see Chapter 25).

While the primary management of a doctoral dissertation project will lie with you, the supervisory team can help facilitate your progress and maintain motivation, so do take advantage of all their support. Make sure supervision meetings are scheduled regularly and planned around your work commitments. Be prepared to produce work in preparation for supervision meetings and be open to receiving both positive and negative feedback [13]. The original time plan submitted with your proposal might slip slightly, but make sure you are on top of your progression milestones, as these are important for both funder and university requirements.

Most doctoral candidates find their studies challenging at one time or another, making it difficult to maintain momentum and enthusiasm [13]. Loss of motivation, lack of confidence, and 'imposter syndrome' are well recognised [17]. Your supervisory team, and the postgraduate office within the educational institution, are there to support you. There are also resources available that can help you make your study a very positive experience. For example, Vitae, an online community for researcher development has sections dedicated to supporting doctoral students (www.vitae.ac.uk). Remember a higher degree can be a highly rewarding and transformative experience, both personally and professionally.

Career paths in research

So far, our focus has been on practical ways to develop your research skills, form supportive connections, and obtaining higher qualifications. We now need to consider routes to building your career, which will enable ongoing professional development and research productivity.

Generally, pathways in clinical education have been informal and heavily reliant on individuals 'finding their own way'. However, this can lead to many talented individuals being discouraged from pursuing an academic career that they may have otherwise considered [18]. Hence, we will share examples of formal, funded positions that could support your progress along an academic track.

Research fellowships

Earlier, we considered the value of undertaking a period of doctoral study, acknowledging the practical requirements and demands. A funded doctoral research fellowship offers the ideal way to have protected time for customised training and to carry out the research project. If you are a health care practitioner, some funders also match clinical salaries and allow a proportion of the programme to be spent undertaking clinical activities in order to maintain competence and skills.

However, these fellowships are highly competitive, and you will need to make an excellent application. You will need to set out a clear picture of why the research matters and how it will be carried out. In addition, you may need to make the case for your suitability and that of the environment you will be working in. Tips on how to approach these elements are shown in Table 29.4.

Table 29.4 The essentials of a good research proposal (adapted from Frost et al. [19])

Domain	Guidance
Clarity of writing	Write clearly, using language pitched to an informed non-expert
Proposal	Demonstrate why this study is important. The research should be applicable at a national or international level
Person	Demonstrate your passion for becoming an academic. Highlight previous study (e.g. at undergraduate or master's level) and any publications. Show how a PhD will develop your career
Place	Reflect on your research knowledge limitations and show how you will develop these within your institution and training environment. Align yourself with a high-quality research institution (often measured by published indexes of an institution's research success). Make sure you have a suitable supervisor(s) with the expertise you need to succeed
Project	Provide an excellent, clearly written research plan. Ensure the research will be deliverable
Stakeholder involvement	Your plan must demonstrate how you will work in partnership with patients, members of the public and other relevant stakeholders (for example, healthcare students and staff). There should be a defined stakeholder involvement plan at the start of your application which is threaded throughout your project
Timescales	Be organised. Allow enough time to write your application, secure sign-off from institution leadership and finance personnel, and gain rounds of feedback from others, enabling you to pre-empt issues and make it stand out

Other fellowships

There are other funded posts that allow healthcare professionals to take 'time out' of formal training or practice, which can facilitate development of research skills and activities.

One of the most common options is a teaching/education fellow post. Whilst the main function of these posts is delivery of teaching activities, the experience provides a rich source of research questions, which, in turn, may drive the evidence base for improvements.

Another option is to consider a fellowship in leadership and management. There are a number of schemes open to clinicians in medicine, dentistry, nursing and pharmacy (e.g. in the UK, from the Faculty of Medical Leadership and Management [20]). The discipline of leadership and management seeks to positively change issues affecting healthcare delivery. These might relate to policy, organisational ('system') processes or workforce practice, and often therefore encompass educational issues. Fellowships tend to provide opportunities for research experience. These schemes offer another great start point to becoming a skilled researcher with expertise in a particular subject area relevant to clinical education.

Establishing research independence

The transition from early career to independent researcher often presents competing priorities which may be clinical, professional, and personal [21, 22]. Commonly reported challenges are funding, insecurities with career progression, and access to appropriate support [21–23]. To maintain momentum, start to think about how to progress your research and career. What should come next? Coaching conversations with mentors and supervisors can help you gain focus and set a direction for moving your research forward [22].

You have invested considerable time in your career already, possibly attaining a higher qualification, so be sure to capitalise on every professional opportunity this offers. Consider possibilities to convert your work into publications and conference presentations. Set yourself time and milestones to produce relevant manuscripts whilst the work is fresh in your mind. Getting your findings 'out there' and engaging with the wider research community will help to build your professional profile, support ongoing career progression, and even attract employment opportunities (see Chapter 28).

Sharing your work at conferences is an opportunity to gain constructive feedback from like-minded peers that challenges your thinking and promotes generation of new ideas. In clinical education, work can often be presented at both education-specific and clinical discipline-specific meetings, maximising possibilities to have impact and to meet other interested colleagues. Collaborating with other research teams can have multiple benefits. It is an opportunity to learn new skills, which may be outwith your comfort zone, or gain understanding of new theories that stimulate thinking, and so enrich your work. Furthermore, multi-centre research affords larger scale studies and sharing of resources [24].

Maintaining your profile

Peer recognition of your research outputs helps your academic reputation and professional profile. One of the biggest challenges is maintaining an adequate publication output. Start studies with research outputs in mind to ensure you undertake and focus your work in such a way that it is likely to be accepted for conference presentations and journal submissions. Your output also needs to be visible to the wider research community. Publishing your work in the peer reviewed journals most appropriate to your subject area and having your work cited by other authors will enhance your reputation over time. An additional way to increase your visibility is to use research repositories (e.g. ResearchGate) and maintain a professional social media profile. Here you can share publications, updates about your research activity, and engage in discussion with others in the academic community.

Funding

As stated earlier, funding is a great resource. Gaining it is both one of the greatest achievements and greatest challenges in research [21, 23]. If you are unsuccessful the first time, try to focus on the positives of new connections, experience of funding processes, and feedback to strengthen the case for your research the next time around. Whether 'small pot' funding or larger awards (e.g. post-doctoral level fellowships), any funding you do receive should be used to its maximum potential to develop yourself. Consider using small pot funding to support pilot studies to underpin applications for larger pot funding and fellowships.

Becoming independent

It can be difficult to emerge from the shadow of your research supervisors/mentors and to gain recognition in your own right. Some advocate using this transition period in your career to move institutions.

Of course, personally, and indeed professionally, this move may not be desirable or possible.

A good supervisor will have supported development of the skills you need to lead research projects yourself and (co-)supervise your own research students. Look for opportunities to get involved with master's and/or doctoral supervision. This process, as well as being an enjoyable chance to 'pay it forward', will help you establish your own research portfolio, support 'getting your name known', and promote the transition to independent researcher.

Summary

Research forms one aspect of the many and varied roles of those working within clinical education. In this chapter, we have also acknowledged clinical education research as a distinct career destination, on par with clinical research, with major potential to benefit patient care through transformation of the healthcare workforce [25].

Interest in clinical education research is growing [26, 27]. Issues that are clearly within the scope of clinical education research, such as crises in workforce and retention, staff wellbeing, and burnout [28–30] are receiving attention within mainstream media. Funding bodies are now explicitly making clinical education research a strategic priority. Nevertheless, challenges continue to exist for those developing a career in clinical education research. These include a lack of initial awareness about career opportunities, the variety and complexity of career pathways, the differing perception of clinical education research in relation to other research disciplines, and difficulties in obtaining funding [31]. These challenges are greater for some professional groups than others, and there is much work still to be done to make academic career paths accessible, visible, and attractive [32, 33].

Despite these challenges, we believe that opportunities in clinical education research are greater than ever before and that the discipline may be reaching a tipping point. This chapter has endeavoured to demystify the routes into a career involving clinical education research, offering a framework to make sense of the complementary roles that clinical education involves. It has signposted development opportunities at various career stages, as well as structured training programmes that may provide smoother pathways to progress in the discipline. We hope this chapter will provide both inspiration and practical guidance for aspiring clinical education researchers.

Top tips

- Consider what you see as your primary educational role: researcher, educator, leader, or teacher. When considering whether to undertake further qualifications or apply for an educational position, consider which of these roles are foregrounded and how this fits with your career goals.
- Seek out opportunities to contribute to ongoing research to start to develop your foundational research skills. This could include peer review activities.
- In discussion with a mentor or supervisor, think about and develop a clear professional development plan detailing the skills and training you need to progress your research.
- Weigh up the merits and limitations of master's and doctoral study and decide on what is the right programme for you and when further study would be best for you personally and professionally.
- Secure small pots of funding to undertake pilot work that could inform a larger grant proposal.

Common pitfalls

- Not applying for opportunities as you think there will be better applicants. You have got to be in it to win it.
- Relying only on your own profession and institution for opportunities, rather than looking beyond your immediate environment. Join national and international organisations and online communities to understand hot topics and upcoming funding opportunities.
- Becoming disheartened if your first application for funding is unsuccessful. This is common and should be seen as an opportunity to gain feedback and refine your proposal for next time.
- Taking on too much and not being able to deliver on everything. It is better to do less, but do it well.

Ethical issues

- Make sure you have the time and resources to finish projects you start. It is unethical to collect data that you will not go on to use or share the findings from.

References

1 Medical Schools Council (2018). Survey of medical clinical academic staffing levels 2018. www.med-schools.ac.uk/media/2491/msc-clinical-academic-survey-report-2018.pdf (accessed October 2022).

2 Archer, J., McManus, C., Woolf, K. et al. (2015). Without proper research funding, how can medical education be evidence based? *BMJ* 350: h3445.

3 Sabel, E. and Archer, J. (2014). "Medical education is the ugly duckling of the medical world" and other challenges to medical educators' identity construction: a qualitative study. *Academic Medicine* 89 (11): 1474–1480.

4 Hu, W.C.Y., Thistlethwaite, J.E., Weller, J. et al. (2015). "It was serendipity": a qualitative study of academic careers in medical education. *Medical Education* 49 (11): 1124–1136.

5 General Medical Council (2013). Good medical practice. https://www.gmc-uk.org/-/media/documents/good-medical-practice—english-20200128_pdf-51527435.pdf (accessed October 2022).

6 Nursing and Midwifery Council (2018). The code. Professional standards of practice and behaviour for nurses, midwives and nursing associates. www.nmc.org.uk/standards/code (accessed October 2022).

7 Ramani, S., McKimm, J., Thampy, H. et al. (2020). From clinical educators to educational scholars and leaders: strategies for developing and advancing a career in health professions education. *The Clinical Teacher* 17 (5): 477–482.

8 Health Education England (2022). Capital nurse career framework. https://www.hee.nhs.uk/our-work/capitalnurse/workstreams/career-framework (accessed October 2022).

9 McKimm, J. and O'Sullivan, H. (2016). When I say . . . leadership. *Medical Education* 50 (9): 896–897.

10 Boyer, E. (1990). *Scholarship Reconsidered: Priorities of the Professoriate*. New York: Wiley.

11 Eva, K.W. (2021). Altruism as enlightened self-interest: how helping others through peer review helps you. *Medical Education* 55 (8): 880–882.

12 Sherbino, J. (2018). You don't need a mentor; you need a board of directors. *Canadian Journal of Emergency Medicine* 20 (6): 816–817.

13 Phillips, E. and Pugh, D. (2015). *How to Get a PhD: A Handbook for Students and their Supervisors*, 6e. Oxford: Oxford University Press.

14 Williams, K., Bethall, E., Lawton, J. et al. (2010). *Planning your PhD*. London: Bloomsbury Publishing.

15 National Institute for Health Research. NIHR fellowship programme. www.nihr.ac.uk/explore-nihr/academy-programmes/fellowship-programme.htm (accessed October 2022).

16 Logan, P., Gallimore, D., and Jordan, S. (2016). Transition from clinician to academic: an interview study of the experiences of UK and Australian registered nurses. *Journal of Advanced Nursing* 72 (3): 593–604.

17 Vitae (2022). Staying positive during your doctorate. www.vitae.ac.uk/doing-research/doing-a-doctorate/during-your-doctorate-the-middle-phase/staying-positive-during-your-doctorate (accessed October 2022).

18 Moderning Medical Careers and the UK Clinical Research Collaboration (2005). Medically- and dentally-qualified academic staff: Recommendations for training the researchers and educators of the future. https://www.ukcrc.org/wp-content/uploads/2014/03/Medically_and_Dentally-qualified_Academic_Staff_Report.pdf (accessed October 2022).

19 Frost, G. (2019). What makes an application excellent? NIHR Research Blog. www.nihr.ac.uk/blog/what-makes-an-application-excellent/10987 (accessed October 2022).

20 Faculty of Medical Leadership and Management. FMLM fellowship. www.fmlm.ac.uk/fmlm-fellowship (accessed October 2022).

21 Deane, J.A. and Clunie, G. (2021). Healthcare professionals in research (HPiR) Facebook community: a survey of U.K. doctoral and postdoctoral healthcare professionals outside of medicine. *BMC Medical Education* 21 (1): 1–9.

22 de Lange, W., Kars, M.C., Poslawsky, I.E. et al. (2019). Postdoctoral Nurses' experiences with leadership and career development: a qualitative study. *Journal of Nursing Scholarship* 51 (6): 689–698.

23 Ranieri, V., Barratt, H., Fulop, N., and Rees, G. (2016). Factors that influence career progression among postdoctoral clinical academics: a scoping review of the literature. *BMJ Open* 6 (10): 1–7.

24 Cheng, A., Kessler, D., Mackinnon, R. et al. (2017). Conducting multicenter research in healthcare simulation: lessons learned from the INSPIRE network. *Advances in Simulation* 2: 6.

25 Academy of Medical Sciences (2020). Transforming health through innovation: Integrating the NHS and academia. https://acmedsci.ac.uk/file-download/23932583 (accessed October 2022).

26 van der Vleuten, C.P.M. (2014). Medical education research: a vibrant community of research and education practice. *Medical Education* 48 (8): 761–767.

27 Jaarsma, D., Scherpbier, A., Van Der Vleuten, C., and Ten Cate, O. (2013). Stimulating medical education research in the Netherlands. *Medical Teacher* 35 (4): 277–281.

28 Carrieri, D., Briscoe, S., Jackson, M. et al. (2018). BMJ open 'care under pressure': a realist review of interventions to tackle doctors' mental ill-health and its impacts on the clinical workforce and patient care. *BMJ Open* 8 (2): 1–8. https://doi.org/10.1136/bmjopen-2017-021273.

29 Turale, S. and Nantsupawat, A. (2021). Clinician mental health, nursing shortages and the COVID-19 pandemic: crises within crises. *International Nursing Review* 68 (1): 12–14.

30 Scheffler, R.M. and Arnold, D.R. (2019). Projecting shortages and surpluses of doctors and nurses in the OECD: what looms ahead. *Health Economics, Policy, and Law* 14 (2): 274–290.

31 Todres, M., Stephenson, A., and Jones, R. (2007). Medical education research remains the poor relation. *BMJ* 335 (7615): 333–335.

32 Trusson, D., Rowley, E., and Bramley, L. (2019). A mixed-methods study of challenges and benefits of clinical academic careers for nurses, midwives and allied health professionals. *BMJ Open* 9 (10): e030595.

33 Gibson, J.M.E. (2019). Shouldn't we all be clinical academics? *Journal of Advanced Nursing* 75 (9): 1817–1818.

Conclusion

Starting research in clinical education can be an exciting but challenging adventure. As with anything, with help and support, you are more likely to succeed in your journey. This book has had a two-year gestation, but we hope you think it has been worthwhile. It is aimed at new clinical education researchers, to enable you to successfully conduct research and begin the initial steps on your career. It has purposely been divided into five parts covering different areas but also emphasising the voyage of discovery from initial thoughts, through the methodology, to writing up and dissemination.

While no book can be comprehensive, we have highlighted what we think are the key elements of a successful research project. These include traditional types of research and more novel methods now being used in clinical education. The balance is tipped towards qualitative methods as new clinical education researchers are often less familiar with these. This text will act as a window through which you can learn and develop your skills and knowledge. As with any book, the text is in an order, but it is not anticipated that everyone will read the book from start to finish. However, we do recommend that it is worth looking at chapters you might not initially be interested in, to step outside of your comfort zone and explore. You never know what you might learn or discover.

There are common threads across the *Top tips*, *Common pitfalls*, and *Ethical issues*, which perhaps you would expect. We are sure you are familiar with team working, possibly in a clinical situation. Research is almost always a collaborative effort, and you can learn a great deal from working not only from others in your team but also liaising with experts and stakeholders in their fields. It is important at the beginning to ensure everyone knows their role, what is expected of them, and their contribution from start to finish including dissemination of results. Most researchers, even the most experienced, usually want to talk about their work and are keen to support others. We encourage you to be curious, open-minded, and persistent in your pursuit of advice. Others can, and often will, help.

Another key theme is time and project management. Research always takes longer than you expect. Arriving at a research topic is only the first step. You need to then carefully consider the design and the feasibility of your project within the time and resources available. A good research protocol and project plan will reap dividends – this is as important as the actual research itself.

We have emphasised the need to engage in critical thinking and ongoing reflection. We hope this book serves as an invaluable resource as you move forward in your academic and professional career.

Eliot L. Rees
Alison Ledger
Kim A. Walker

Starting Research in Clinical Education, First Edition. Edited by Eliot L. Rees, Alison Ledger, and Kim A. Walker.
© 2024 The Association for the Study of Medical Education (ASME). Published 2024 by John Wiley & Sons Ltd.
Companion website: www.wiley.com/go/clinicaleducation

Index

A

AAA Code of Ethics *see* American Anthropological Association (AAA) Code of Ethics
abstract, 233, 255–256, 262
  visual, 259
academic databases, searching, 5
academic journal publication, 262
accountability, 233, 241
ACPs *see* advanced clinical practitioners (ACPs)
action research, 107, 110
  Carr and Kemmis's model, 108
  critical, 107
  by educators, 108
  feature of, 107
  practical, 107–109
    critical and self-critical evaluation, 110
    cycle 2 planning, 110
    desired outcomes, achieving, 108–109
    dissemination of action research, 110
    implementing and monitoring change, 109–110
    planning change, 109
    stakeholders, recruiting, 109
    stakeholders in preliminary discussions of problems, 109
  practitioner, 107, 108, 111
    act, 111
    observe, 111
    plan, 111
    reflect, 111
  principles of, 107
  technical, 107
  types of, 107–108
Adobe Illustrator, 264

advanced clinical practitioners (ACPs), 133
alpha value, 205
Altmetric Explorer, 119
Altmetric scores, 118, 265
American Anthropological Association (AAA) Code of Ethics, 150
ANalysis Of VAriance (ANOVA) test, 205–206, 210
Annual Review of Competence Progression (ARCP), 129, 217
ANOVA test *see* ANalysis Of VAriance (ANOVA) test
application programming interfaces (APIs), 119
ARCP *see* Annual Review of Competence Progression (ARCP)
artefact elicitation, 137
article types, 254–255
asymmetric distribution, 202
audio/video recording, of interview, 131
audio/visual materials, using, 149
authenticity, 28
author guidelines, 255, 258
authorship, 63, 255
  cultural perspectives on, 63
  ghost, 63
  honorary/gift, 63
authorship order, 63
auto-ethnography, 159
axiology, 25, 27, 28

B

bar chart, 203, 239
behaviourism, 32

Best Evidence in Medical Education (BEME)
  collaboration, 69, 80
betas, 208
Big Data, 213
  accessing, 216–218
  in clinical education, 213–215
  multiple datasets, linking, 218
    data cleaning and exploration, 218–220
    missing data, 220
    software and coding, 218
    statistical analysis, 220
  and other data sources in clinical education, 215
  preparation and planning, 215–216
  reporting and dissemination, 220–221
big datasets, 213–215, 218–220
  gaining access to, 217
  working with, 215–220
Big Q qualitative research, 165, 167, 170
binary logistic regression, 209
block randomisation, 194
Bonferroni correction, 206
Boolean operators, 82
bootstrapping, defined, 214
box plots, 201, 203, 204
business cards, 264

C

Canva, 264
capacity building, stakeholder involvement facilitating, 40
career, 271
  in clinical education, 271–272
  foundational skills, developing, 272

career (*cont'd*)
  essential research skills,
    developing, 272
  mentorship and collaboration,
    272–274
  peer review, 274
  small pots of funding,
    accessing, 274–275
  research independence,
    establishing, 278
  funding, 278
  independent, becoming,
    278–279
  profile, maintaining, 278
  seeking further qualifications
    and training, 275
  funding, 276
  setting, 275–276
  subject, 276
career paths in research, 277
  other fellowships, 278
  research fellowships, 277
Carr and Kemmis's action research
    model, 107, 108
categorical data, 202, 203
categorisation, 32
causal inference, 24, 206, 214
cause-and-effect relationship, 25
central tendency, 202–203
CHAT *see* Cultural Historical
    Activity Theory (CHAT)
Chi-square test, 204, 205, 210
CI *see* confidence intervals (CI)
citation management software, 6
clinical academics, 271
clinical education research, 4
closed-ended questions, 186–187
closed question, 131
close-ended items, 186
cluster sampling, 49
CMOC *see* context-mechanism-
    outcome configuration
    (CMOC)
Cochrane Risk of Bias tool, 83
Cochrane's Six-Step Stakeholder
    Engagement Framework, 41
codebook thematic analysis,
    169, 170
codes, 168–169
code saturation, 51

code/syntax, defined, 214
coding reliability thematic analysis,
    168–169
coercion, 60, 62
cognitive-behavioural theories,
    33, 34
cognitive interviewing, 188
cognitive testing *see* cognitive
    interviewing
coherence, achieving, 22
cohort studies, 214
collaboration, 274
committee chair, 229
communication, 233, 235,
    243, 267
  of roles, goals, and expectations,
    43–44
communication skills, 35, 36,
    206, 208
communication skills variable, 208
Communities of Practice, 35
community–academic
    partnerships, 42
compensation, 44
competence, 183, 277
  and confidence, 17–18
composite narratives, 161
compositional construction,
    247–248
concept mapping, 247
conceptual framework, 5, 91, 104
conceptual generalisability/
    transferability, 49
conferences, 262
  networking, 264–265
  oral presentation, 263
  posters, 263–264
  workshops, 263, 264
confidence, 128, 134, 175, 176
  and competence, 17–18
  and trust, 148
confidence intervals (CI), 208, 209
confounding by indication, 193
confounding variables, 209
consolidated criteria for reporting
    qualitative research
    (COREQ), 73
CONSORT guidelines, 197
constructivism, 21, 28, 32, 99, 101
  markers of rigour in, 28

constructivist epistemology, 26, 28
  defined, 22
constructivist ontology, defined, 22
constructivist paradigm, 22, 26, 28,
    62, 133
constructivist research, 27
constructivist research design
  data collection and analysis,
    27–28
  dimensions of problem/
    phenomenon, 25–26
  'good' research, conducting, 28
  knowledge, 26–27
  methodology, 27
content experts, 80, 82, 118
context, 33, 74
  defined, 90
  in realist reviews, 74
context-mechanism-outcome
    configuration (CMOC), 74,
    90, 93, 95
contextualisation, 26
continuous data, 202
convenience sampling, 49
convergent design, 102
correlation, 206
  negative, 206
  positive, 206, 265
  scatter plots of, 207
  squared, 208
counterbalancing, 197
credibility, 28, 42, 109, 178, 185, 267
critical action research, 107
critical appraisal, 6, 83, 272
criticality, in education research,
    4, 266
critical reflection, 107, 109
cross-over design, 101, 109
c-statistic, 209
Cultural Historical Activity Theory
    (CHAT), 32, 33, 36
cultural-historical category, 33
curriculum developments, 255
curriculum vitae (CV), 231, 262

D

data *see also* Big Data; online data
    collection
  categorical, 202, 203
  continuous, 202

de-identifying, 60–61
discrete, 201
extract, 84
interactive, 118–119
missing, 220
nominal, 202
normally distributed, 202
observational, 117–118
online, 117–119
ordinal, 202
pseudonymised, 218
qualitative, 24
quantitative, 201–202
semi-structured, 213
structured, 213, 214
unstructured, 213
data analysis, 17, 23, 28, 97, 105,
    120, 139, 209, 218, 230, 231,
    239, 240
data cleaning and exploration,
    218–220
data collection, 8, 25, 27, 40, 51, 60,
    91, 99, 103, 104, 119, 128–129,
    131, 147, 150, 239–241
  face-to-face methods of, 129
  observational, 118
  online, 61, 116
  pilot, 240
  qualitative, 96, 125, 149
data dictionary, 216
  defined, 214
data extraction, 80, 84, 119
data extraction form, 84
data holders, 215, 216–220
data linkage, 218
data management, 61, 83
Data Management Plan, 61
data mining approaches, 120
Data Protection Impact
    Assessment, 61
data quality and integrity, 119–120
data saturation, 51
datasets, 166–169, 202–203, 216
    see also big datasets; multiple
    datasets, linking
de-anonymisation, 218
  defined, 214
defining clinical education
    research, 3–5
de-identifying data, 60–61

demi-regularity, 90, 91
density histogram, 203–204
dependability, 133, 178
dependent relationships, 60
descriptive statistics, 120, 201
  central tendency, 202
  data, types of, 201–202
  dispersion, 202–203
  frequency distribution, 202
  graphic presentations, 203–204
dichotomous options, 186
'difficult to access' groups, 48
digital recording, of interview, 131
digital scholarship, 118
digital tools, 249–250
discrete data, 201
discussion section, 256
dispersion, 202–203
dissemination strategy, 261, 262
  academic journal publication,
    262
  conferences, 262
    networking, 264–265
    oral presentation, 263
    posters, 263–264
    workshops, 263, 264
  key questions for designing,
    261–262
  knowledge dissemination, 261
  multimedia, 266–267
  planning, 261–262
  social media, 265–266
dissemination task, 240
dissertation, writing, 245
  compositional construction,
    247–248
    different formats, writing
      for, 251
    editing and proofreading, 251
    pace of writing, 250–251
    supervisor, working with, 250
  planning method, selecting, 247
  starting with the end goal in
    mind, 246
  time-management techniques,
    249
    choosing the setting, 249
    digital tools, making the most
      of, 249–250
    writer's block, 250

diverse supervision team, working
    with, 175, 179
Doctorate, 275, 276
documents, collecting, 149
double screening, 83
duplicate screening, 79, 83
dust-bowl empiricism, 215

E
editing, 251
educational phenomena, 18
educational surveys, 189
education research, 3–4
effective communication, 235,
    241, 243
epistemology, 24, 26, 28
  constructivist, 22, 26, 28
  defined, 22
  post-positivist, 22
e-posters, 263–264
The Equator Network, 80, 257
essential research skills,
    developing, 272
ethical considerations, 63, 120–121,
    150, 171
ethical principles in research, 57
  clinical education, research
    in, 58
  historical perspective, 58
ethical research, conducting, 57
  exiting ethics, 63
    dissemination, ethics
      surrounding, 63–64
    exiting responsibilities, 63
  procedural ethics, 58
    compliance with ethical
      principles, 61
    data management, 61
    de-identifying data, 60–61
    documentation required,
      59–60
    online data collection, 61
  relational ethics, 62
    external stakeholders, 62–63
    situational ethics, 62
    insider research, 62
ethical review, 240
ethics and informed consent, 150
ethics committee, 59–60
ethics committee chairs, 229

ethnographic fieldwork, 145–147
  analysing and writing up
      ethnographic research, 149
  audio/visual materials,
      using, 149
  basis of, 146
  documents, collecting, 149
  fieldnotes, recording, 149
  long-term, 146, 147
  methods, 146
      participant observation versus
          observation, 147
  recording fieldnotes, 149
ethnographic research, 148–151
  analysing and writing up, 149
  types of, 148
ethnographic study, planning, 147
  field site, choosing, 147–148
  study participants, 148–149
  types of ethnography, choosing
      from, 147
ethnography, 145
  auto, 159
  challenges of, 150–151
  of clinical education, 146
  ethics and informed consent, 150
  focused, 148
  history and value of, 145–146
  informed case study, 148
  meta, 82
  micro, 148
  mini, 148
  participant burden, 150
  quick, 148
  rapid, 148
  reflexivity as an ethnographer,
      150
  short-term, 148
  visual, 149
evidence-based education, 4
evidence syntheses, 69, 72
  choosing the appropriate
      evidence synthesis
      approach, 75
  in clinical education, 69–70
  comparison of, 71
  narrative reviews, 74–75
  realist reviews, 74
  scoping review, 73–74
  systematic reviews, 70

mixed methods systematic
    reviews, 73
  qualitative systematic
      reviews, 73
  quantitative systematic
      reviews, 72
  umbrella reviews, 75
evidence synthesis project, 79
  key steps in, 81
    analysing and synthesising,
        84–85
    data extraction, 84
    defining the scope, 81–82
    dissemination, 85
    screening and selecting
        documents, 83–84
    searching for evidence, 82–83
  planning, 80–81
  project team, assembling, 79–80
evocative dissemination
    methods, 141
exiting ethics, 57, 63
  ethics surrounding
      dissemination, 63–64
  exiting responsibilities, 63
experiment, 191–192
  controlled, 72
  defined, 191
  seven steps to designing, 192
    compare, 197–198
    control groups, 193
    hypothesis, 192
    manipulating participants,
        195–196
    measurement process, 196–197
    randomisation, 193–194
    sampling and power, 194–195
expert practitioners, 216
expert researchers, 73, 176, 216
expert validation, 187
explanatory sequential design, 102
exploratory sequential design, 102
external stakeholders, 62–63

F
Facebook, 118, 119, 213
face-to-face interview, 129
factorial relationship, 192
familiarity between participants,
    128

fieldnotes, recording, 149
Figma, 264
'final' programme theory, 93
FINER research questions, 15, 16
first steps in clinical education
    research, 9, 10
flexibility, 52, 73, 82, 85, 92, 105,
    129, 141, 171, 172
focused ethnography, 148
focused research questions, 13,
    14, 169
focus groups *see* interviews and
    focus groups
foundational skills, developing, 272
  essential research skills,
      developing, 272
  funding, 274–275
  mentorship and collaboration,
      272–274
  peer review, 274
framework analysis, 169
frequency distribution, 202, 219
functional analysis, 160
funding, 42–43, 274–275, 278

G
Gantt chart, 217, 239, 240
gap filling, 247
gatekeeper, 8, 52–53, 229
General Data Protection Regulation
    (GDPR), 59, 217
  defined, 214
generalisability, 99, 108, 119.
    194. 205
  sampling decisions and their
      effects on, 49–50
General Medical Council's (GMC)
    List of Registered Medical
    Practitioners, 217
General Practitioners (GPs),
    166–167
genre, 248
ggplot2, 220
ghost authorship, 63
good clinical education research,
    4–5
Good Reporting of A Mixed
    Methods Study
    (GRAMMS), 104
Google, 5

Google Analytics, 118–120
Google Scholar, 6, 82
GPs *see* General Practitioners (GPs)
grand theories, 32
graphic presentations, 203–204
graphics, 257
guided walks, 137

H
haven function, 218
Hawthorne effect, 195
health data warehouses, 214
Health Research Authority (HRA)
 approval process, 59
help, getting, 8
 finding someone to help, 8
 meeting, expectations from, 9
 meeting, preparation for, 9
heterogenous groups, 128
hierarchy of responsibility, 150
histograms, 203–204, 220
historical control groups, 193
homogenous groups, 128
honorary/gift authorship, 63
HRA approval process *see* Health
 Research Authority (HRA)
 approval process
humility, 26
hypothesis-driven study
 designs, 17

I
Ibry chart, 216, 217
 defined, 214
ICMJE *see* International Committee
 of Medical Journal Editors
 (ICMJE)
I-enquiry, 111
iKT *see* integrated knowledge
 translation (iKT)
illusion of causality, 193
IMRaD format *see* Introduction,
 Methods, Results and
 Discussion (IMRaD) format
independent and dependent
 variables, 204
independent researcher, 278–279
indexing services, 5–6
inferential statistical tests,
 choosing, 205

inferential statistics, 201, 204
 correlation, 206
 determining statistical
  significance, 204–205
 independent and dependent
  variables, 204
 inferential statistical tests,
  choosing, 205
 multiple comparisons, 205–206
 regression analysis, 206–208
  logistic regression, 209
 relationships, identifying, 206
information power, 51
information privacy, 121
information technology (IT)
 team, 117
informed consent process, 121
innovation, 69, 254
insider research, 62
'in situ' interview, 130
Institutional Review Boards
 (IRBs), 59
intangible incentives, 62
integrated knowledge translation
 (iKT), 39, 40
'intention-to-treat' analysis, 197
interactive data, 118–119
International Committee of Medical
 Journal Editors (ICMJE),
 63, 255
intervention, 90
 complex, 92, 93
 educational, 97, 109
 social media (SoMe), 115
interviewees, 131
 interviews *see also* visual
  elicitation
 cognitive interviewing,
  employing, 188
 face-to-face, 129
 formats of, 130
 'in situ' interview, 130
 narrative, 130
 online, 129
 phone, 133
 semi-structured, 129, 130
 structured, 130
 traditional seated one-on-one
  interview, 130
 types of, 130

 unstructured, 129, 130
 walking, 130
interviews and focus groups,
 127–128
 case example, 133–134
 choosing, 129–130
 conducting, 130–133
 ensuring rigour in, 133
 recording, 131
  ending the interview or focus
   group, 132
  getting started, 131
  promoting participation, 132
 researcher reflexivity and
  positionality, 132–133
 sampling in, 128–129
 strengths and considerations, 128
 topic guide, 130–131
 transcribing, 132
interview to the double, 130
Introduction, Methods, Results and
 Discussion (IMRaD) format,
 178, 247, 255
introduction, of research article, 256
involved stakeholders, similarity
 of, 43
involvement in research, 274
IRBs *see* Institutional Review
 Boards (IRBs)
item-specific response options,
 186–187

J
journal clubs, 266
 participation in, 274

K
knowledge dissemination, 261

L
learner reactions, focusing on, 17
learning-as-acquisition, 32–33
learning-as-participation, 32
Likert items, 186
Likert scale, 24, 186, 202
linear regression, 208–210
linguistic interpretation, 160
link analysis, 120
literature search, 5–6
logistic regression, 206, 209, 210

logistics, 42
longitudinal studies, 214, 222

M
manuscript submission
      process, 258
markers of rigour, 25, 28
Master's degree, 275–276
meaning saturation, 51
measurable aspects, 237
mechanism
      defined, 90
      in realist reviews, 74
medical education, 82
Medical Education Research Study
      Quality Instrument
      (MERSQI), 72
meeting, 233, 264
      expectations from, 9
      'ideal', 263
      online, 141
      preparation for, 9
      presentations, 263
      supervision, 178
      video, 132
      virtual, 265
Mendeley, 118, 119
mentorship, 274
      and collaboration, 272–274
meta-data, 216
      defined, 214
meta-ethnography, 82
methodological choices, 27
      case studies, 34–36
methodological papers, 254
methodology
      choosing, 27
      defined, 22
      post-positivist, 24
methods, 256
      defined, 22
      versus subject expertise, 228
micro-ethnography, 148
middle-range theories, 32
mini-ethnographic case study, 148
missing data, 215, 220
missing data imputation,
      defined, 214
mixed methods research, 99, 100
      benefits and challenges, 104–105

choosing, 100–101
considerations when planning,
      101
design options, 102–103
planning and designing mixed
      methods project, 101
      design, choosing, 101–103
      integration, 103–104
      purpose of using, 100
      quality criteria for, 104
      reporting, 104
mixed methods systematic
      reviews, 73
Moodle, 120
multimedia technologies,
      266–267
multiple comparisons, 205–206
multiple datasets, linking, 218
      data cleaning and exploration,
            218–220
      missing data, 220
      software and coding, 218
      statistical analysis, 220
multiple imputation, 220
multiple regression analysis, 208
multiple sociological dimensions,
      160
multivariate analysis, 204

N
narrative data, 157, 159
      theorizing from, 161
narrative interview, 51, 130
narrative research, 155
      countering critiques of, 157
      and decision-making, 159
      different about, 157
      narrative and, 155
      need to choose, 156–157
      philosophy of, 156
      quality criteria, 161
      strengths of, 158
narrative reviews, 70, 74–75
narratives, 157
      analysing, 159
            functional analysis, 160
            linguistic interpretation, 160
            plot-based analyses, 160
            sociological dimensions, 160
      gathering, 158–159

presenting, 160–161
      selecting, 159
National Institute for Health
      Research, 275
negative correlation, 206
negative experiences, 167, 168
Netherlands Code of Conduct for
      Research Integrity, 58
networking, 264–265
new researchers' struggles,
      learning from, 175
      diverse supervision team,
            working with, 179
      getting from data to themes,
            175–177
      possibility of making changes
            along the way, 178–179
      subjectivity and interpretation,
            dealing with, 177–178
nominal data, 202
nominal questions, 186
nonobtrusive data *see*
      observational data
non-participant observation, 147
non-positivist Big Q paradigm, 169
non-randomised sample
      approach, 50
normally distributed data, 202

O
Objective Structured Clinical
      Examinations (OSCEs),
      34–36, 90
objectivity, 26, 168, 169, 177
observational data, 109, 117–118,
      121, 192
obtrusive data *see* interactive data
odds ratio (OR), 72, 209
online data, 115–117
      interactive data, 118–119
      observational data, 117–118
online data collection, 6, 115
      data analysis, 120
      data collection, 119
      data quality and integrity,
            119–120
      ethical considerations, 120–121
      online platforms, types of, 117
      study considerations, 116–117
      types of online data, 117

interactive data, 118–119
observational data, 117–118
online focus groups, 128
online interviews, 116, 129
online meeting, 141
online platform, 115–117, 119–121
online surveys, 189
online versus face-to-face interviews and focus groups, 129
ontology, 23
  constructivist, 22
  defined, 22
  post-positivist, 22, 23
open-ended questions, 130, 187
open question, 131
opportunistic sampling, 52
oral presentation. 220, 233, 263
ordinal data, 202
ordinal items, 186
original research, 4, 254
OR *see* odds ratio (OR)
OSCEs *see* Objective Structured Clinical Examinations (OSCEs)
outcome, in realist reviews, 73–74, 90
outcome variables, 204, 205, 208–209

P
papers, accessing, 232–233
paradigm
  constructivist, 22, 26, 28, 62, 133
  defined, 22
  non-positivist Big Q paradigm, 169
  post-positivist, 22, 49, 62, 168
  qualitative, 165
participant burden, 150
Participant Information Sheet, 53, 60
participant observation, 147
participants, 48, 60, 116, 121, 128, 137
  burden for, 150
  choosing, 148–149
  information, 53–54
  observation, 147
  potential, 52–53, 60

Participants, Interventions, Comparisons, Outcomes (PICO) format, 72, 82
participatory research, 39
patient and public involvement (PPI), 39
patient engagement, 39
patterned meaning, 166
P-cubed approach, 263
peer review, 257–258, 274
perfectionism, 246
Personal and Public Involvement (PPI) groups, 84
personal narrative, 155
person-centredness, 80, 82
perspective, 7
  distanced, 32
  'fact finding', 16
  theoretical, 31, 32
phone interviews, 133
photographs, 137, 139–141
Photoshop, 264
photo-elicitation, 137, 139, 140
  how to use, 141
  key considerations when using, 141
pie chart, 203
pilot data collection, 240
pilot testing, 186–187
pirate plots, 220
placement, 13
plagiarism, 63–64
planning method, selecting, 247
plot-based analyses, 160
podcasts, 116, 266–267
point of view video elicitation, 141
  how to use, 142
  key considerations when using, 142
point-of-view elicitation, 137
Pomodoro technique, 241, 249
porting, defined, 214
positionality, 132–133, 178
  case studies, 33–36
  and reflexivity, 36
  researcher reflexivity and, 132–133
positionality, identifying, 132–133
positive correlation, 206, 265
positive experiences, 27, 167, 277

posters, 263–264
post-positivism, 21, 24–25, 70, 165
post-positivist epistemology, defined, 22, 24
post-positivist framing, 168
post-positivist ontology, 23
  defined, 22
post-positivist paradigm, 22, 49, 62, 168
post-positivist research design, 178, 179
  data collection and analysis, 24–25
  dimensions of problem/ phenomenon, 23–24
  'good' research, conducting, 25
  kind of knowledge hoping to produce with research, 24
  methodology, choosing, 24
potential participants, 52–53, 60, 196
potential stakeholders, 40, 109, 242
power, 50, 194
power differentials and tokenism, 43
PowerPoint, 263, 264
PPEET *see* Public and Patient Engagement Evaluation Tool (PPEET)
PPI *see* patient and public involvement (PPI)
practical action research, 107–109
  act, 111
  critical and self-critical evaluation, 110
  cycle 2 planning, 110
  desired outcomes, achieving, 108–109
  dissemination of action research, 110
  in education, 108
  implementing and monitoring change, 109–110
  observe, 111
  plan, 111
  planning change, 109
  reflect, 111
  stakeholders, recruiting, 109
  stakeholders in preliminary discussions of problems, 109

predictor variable, 204, 205, 209
Preferred Reporting Items for
　　Systematic Reviews and
　　Meta Analyses (PRISMA)
　　publication standards, 83
preliminary literature search,
　　undertaking, 5
　　keeping track of the papers
　　　found, 6
　　literature, searching, 5–6
　　search results, 6
pre-drawing conversation, 139
primary realist research, 91
principlism, 57
PRISMA publication standards *see*
　　Preferred Reporting Items
　　for Systematic Reviews and
　　Meta Analyses (PRISMA)
　　publication standards
probability, 48
probability of pass, 209
probability sampling *see* random
　　sampling
'problem-gap-hook' method, 256
procedural ethics, 58
　　data management, 61
　　de-identifying data, 60–61
　　documentation required, 59–60
　　guidance on compliance with
　　　ethical principles, 61
　　online data collection, 61
professional society, membership
　　of, 274, 275
profile, maintaining, 278
profile papers, 221
　　defined, 214
programme theory, 74, 90, 95–97
　　'final', 93
　　initial, 93
　　'more refined', 93
　　and realist analysis, 93
project feedback, 240
project initiation phase, 236–238
project management, 235, 236
　　closing, 242–243
　　executing, 241
　　　accountability, 241
　　　productivity, 241
　　initiation, 236
　　　defining the project, 237–238

integrating the project
　　plan, 239
　　project stakeholders, 238
　　risk register, 238–239
monitoring and controlling,
　　241–242
planning, 239
　　project phases, 239
　　project tasks, 239–241
project team, assembling, 79–80, 95
proofreading, 251
proportional stratified random
　　sampling, 49
proportion of variance, 209
prospective cohort study, 214
pseudonymisation, 61, 218
pseudonymised data, 218
pseudo-r^2 type measures, 209
psychological theories of
　　learning, 32
Public and Patient Engagement
　　Evaluation Tool (PPEET), 41
p-value, 201, 205, 208

Q

QI projects *see* quality
　　improvement (QI) projects
qualitative and quantitative study
　　components, integration of,
　　103–104
qualitative data, 24
qualitative data analysis software,
　　119, 176
qualitative paradigm, 165
qualitative research, sampling
　　in, 50
　　common qualitative sampling
　　　strategies, 52
　　data collection, 51–52
　　data saturation, 51
　　manageable amount of data, 51
　　mapping the sample to the
　　　study, 51
qualitative systematic reviews, 73
quality improvement (QI)
　　projects, 254
quantitative data, 80, 96, 183,
　　201–203, 213
quantitative research, sampling
　　in, 47

number of participants, 50
random sampling, 48–49
sampling decisions and their
　　effects on generalisability,
　　49–50
quantitative systematic reviews,
　　70, 72
questionnaire, 16, 183
quick ethnography, 148

R

RAMESES quality standards, 92
randomised controlled trials
　　(RCTs), 72, 81, 83,
　　156, 214
randomness, 193–194, 201
random sampling, 48
ranking items, 186
rapid ethnography, 148
reading, 274
read write web, 115
realism, 89
realist analysis, 92–95
　　programme theory and, 93
realist approach, 89, 91–93, 110
realist evaluation, 91, 96, 109
realist research, 89–90
　　primary, 91
　　programme theory and realist
　　　analysis, 93
　　researching complex intervention/
　　　phenomenon, 92
　　research question/aim, 92
　　secondary, 91
　　stakeholders' involvement in
　　　realist projects, 95–96
realist research project, designing,
　　96–97
realist reviews, 69, 74, 80, 91
　　context in, 74
　　goal of, 74
　　mechanism in, 74
　　outcome in, 74
　　as 'theory-driven', 74
realist synthesis, 91
recruitment, 42, 52, 62, 116
　　participant information, 53–54
　　potential participants, 52–53
RECs *see* Research Ethics
　　Committees (RECs)

reference management software, 232
Reflect–Plan–Act–Observe–Reflect stages, 108, 113
reflexive thematic analysis, 167–171
reflexivity, 27, 28, 63, 132–133, 170, 246
  as an ethnographer, 150
regression analysis, 206, 208
  linear, 209
  logistic regression, 209
  multiple, 208
regression model, 209
relational ethics, 57, 62
  external stakeholders, 62–63
relationship-building efforts, 42
relationships
  between positionality and reflexivity, 36
  cause-and-effect, 25
  identifying, 206
  positive, 44
  pre-existing, 25
relevance to research in clinical education, 58
Reporting Guidelines for Social Media Research (RESOME), 119
representativeness, 119
reproducibility and generalisability, 25, 26
research, 3
  aims, 7
  defined, 3
  objectives, 7
  questions, 7
research design, 21, 22
  constructivist
    data collection and analysis, 27–28
    dimensions of problem, 25–26
    'good' research, conducting, 28
    knowledge, 26–27
    methodology, 27
  post-positivist
    data collection and analysis, 24–25
    dimensions of problem, 23–24
    'good' research, conducting, 25

knowledge, 24
methodology, 24
researcher bias, 169, 170
researcher subjectivity, 169–172
researcher- generated photo-elicitation, 141
Research Ethics Committees (RECs), 58–59, 227, 229–230
research fellowships, 277
research governance, 59, 61
research independence, establishing, 278
  funding, 278
  independent, becoming, 278–279
  profile, maintaining, 278
research participants, 139
research project
  conducting
    keeping on top of references, 232
    papers, accessing, 232–233
    supervisor, making good use of, 233
    using exemplars and reporting standards, 233
    writing, 231–232
  designing
    getting the research question right, 230
    keeping it small, focused, and achievable, 231
    letting the methods follow, 230
    planning for all eventualities, 231
    seeking feedback on proposal, 230–231
  preparing for, 227
    choosing supervisor wisely, 228
    methods versus subject expertise, 228
    preliminary sources of information, 227–228
    project approval, 228–229
    proposal, developing, 228
    research ethics committees, 229–230
research protocol, 217
research questions, 13, 92
  beyond the question, 16–17

case studies, 34–36
defining the problem, 14–15
evaluating, 18
FINER, 15, 16
getting help, 16
good research question, 15–16
limitations in, 17
  comparing something with nothing, 18
  learner reactions, focusing on, 17
  self-reported outcome data, using, 17–18
  shared understandings, assuming, 18
  turning problem to be solved into, 108–109
RESOME *see* Reporting Guidelines for Social Media Research (RESOME)
resources, available, 7–8
resources and support, 42–43
result dissemination, 240
results, of research article, 256
review articles, 6, 41, 254
rich pictures, 137–139
  how to use 139
  key considerations when using, 138–139
roles of clinical education, 272

S
safe haven, 217–218
  defined, 214
salami-slicing, 64
Sample, Phenomenon of Interest, study Design, Evaluation, Research type (SPIDER), 82
sample size calculations, 50
sampling
  cluster, 49
  common purposive sampling strategies, 52
  common sampling reporting weaknesses, 53
  convenience, 49
  opportunistic, 52
  proportional stratified random sampling, 49
  in qualitative research, 50

sampling (*cont'd*)
    data collection, 51
    data saturation, 51
    manageable amount of
      data, 51
    mapping the sample to the
      study, 50–51
  in quantitative research, 47
    generalisability, 49–50
    number of participants, 50
    random sampling, 48–49
    sampling bias, 47
    stratified, 48–49
    systematic random, 48
sampling bias, 47
scattergrams, 220
scatter plot, 206, 207
scholarly literature search engines,
    5–6
scope creep, 241–242
scope of clinical education
    research, 4
scoping review, 73–74
screening and selecting documents,
    83–84
SD *see* standard deviation (SD)
search results, 6, 79, 255
secondary realist research, 91
self-critical reflection, 107, 109
self-reported outcome data, using,
    17–18
semi-structured data, 213
semi-structured interviews, 129,
    130, 133, 139, 147
sentiment analysis, 120
shared-meaning-based
    interpretative story themes,
    167–168
shared understandings, 18,
    42, 241
short-term ethnography, 148
simple linear regression, 208
situational ethics, 61–62
  insider research, 62
skewness, 202, 210
small pots of funding, accessing,
    274–275
small q qualitative research, 165
'snail-mail' surveys, 189
snowball sampling, 52, 62

social media (SoMe), 115, 117–119,
    259, 265–266
socio-cultural theories, 32, 33,
    35–36
sociological dimensions, 160
software and coding, 215, 218
specific, measurable, appropriate,
    realistic, and time specific
    (SMART), 7
SPIDER *see* Sample, Phenomenon
    of Interest, study Design,
    Evaluation, Research type
    (SPIDER)
SPSS *see* Statistical Package for the
    Social Sciences (SPSS)
squared correlation, 208
stakeholder groups, 41, 43, 74, 80,
    82, 84, 85, 95, 110, 238
stakeholders, 39
  as collaborators, 41
  considerations when
    involving, 42
    involved stakeholders,
      similarity of, 43
    logistics, 42
    power differentials and
      tokenism, 43
    resources and support, 42–43
  as consultants, 41
  controlled research, 41
  identifying, 41–42
  involvement, 39–41
    contributing to a culture of, 44
    facilitating capacity
      building, 40
    leading to use of the
      findings, 40
    supporting effective research,
      39–40
  involvement in realist projects,
    95–96
  potential stakeholders, examples
    of, 40
  recruiting, 109
  roles in clinical education
    research, 41
  strategies for involving
    stakeholders, 43
    communication of roles, goals,
      and expectations, 43–44

    compensation, providing, 44
    necessary training, providing,
      43
    relational practices, engaging
      in, 44
standard deviation (SD), 203
standard errors, 208, 209
statistical analysis, 201, 220
  with corresponding research
    questions and variable
    types, 210
  descriptive statistics, 201
    central tendency, 202
    dispersion, 202–203
    frequency distribution, 202
    graphic presentations, 203–204
    types of data, 201–202
  inferential statistics, 204
    choosing inferential statistical
      tests, 205
    correlation, 206
    determining statistical
      significance, 204–205
    independent and dependent
      variables, 204
    logistic regression, 209
    multiple comparisons, 205–206
    regression analysis, 206–209
    relationships, identifying, 206
    uncertainty and bias, 209–210
Statistical Package for the Social
    Sciences (SPSS), 218
statistical test,168, 195, 204–206, 210
storyboarding, 247
strategy, writing, 257
stratified sampling, 48–49
structured data, 213
  defined, 214
structured interviews, 130
student reactions, 17
Student's *t*-test, 204, 205, 210
study design, 17
style, language, and structure,
    256–257
subjectivity and interpretation,
    dealing with, 177–178
substantive theory, 91, 93
supervision meeting, 178
supervisor, 16, 179, 276
  choosing supervisor wisely, 228

co-supervisors, 228, 230
  making good use of, 233
  potential, 228
survey design, 183
  common errors in, 188
  reporting results, 187
  six principles of, 184
    cognitive work, 184
    conversation between you,
      survey designer, and your
      respondents, 185
    good decisions and bad
      surveys, 185
    pretesting survey to know
      how it functions, 185
    questions shaping the
      answers, 184
    respondents, 184–185
  six-step process for designing a
    high-quality survey, 185
  cognitive interviewing, 188
  interviews and focus
    groups, 186
  pilot testing, 186–187
  pretesting the survey and
    survey items, 187–188
  searching the literature,
    185–186
  survey items, writing,
    186–187
  survey administration, 187
survey uses (and misuses),
    183–184, 189
systematic, education research
    as, 4
systematic random sampling, 48
systematic reviews, 69–70, 72, 75
  mixed methods, 73
  qualitative, 73
  quantitative, 72

T
tangible incentives, 53, 62
teaching approaches, 255
team reflexive exercises, 238, 242
technical action research, 107
template analysis, 169
text mining, 83
thematic analysis, 168
  codebook, 169

coding reliability, 168
  reflexive, 168–169
thematic analysis approaches,
    28, 165
  diversity of, 170–172
  quality research, 170–172
  researcher's role in, 169–170
  spectrum of, 165–166
theme, 166–169, 176–177
theme conceptualisations, 166–168
theoretical basis, education
    research having, 4
theory, 31–32
  choice of, 32
  grand theories, 32
  illustrative case studies, 33–36
    context, 33–34
    methodological choices,
      34–36
    positionality, 33–36
    research question, 34–36
    unit of analysis, 35, 36
  middle-range theories, 32
  programme theory, 93
  putting theory to work, 31
  socio-cultural theory, 35
  working with learning theory,
    32–33
think-aloud process, 188
3D technology, 48
Timeboxing, 249
time-management techniques, 249
  choosing the setting, 249
  digital tools, making the most of,
    249–250
  voice
    genre, 248
    tone and, 248–249
  writer's block, 250
titles, 255
tokenism, 43
tone and voice, 248–249
topic guide, 130–131
topic of interest
  defined, 7
  identifying, 5
traditional seated one-on-one
    interview, 130
transferability, 28, 178
transparency, 4–5, 26

triangulation, 104, 109, 116, 149
trustworthiness, 133
t-test *see* Student's *t*-test
Twitter, 8, 118, 119, 265

U
UK Medical Education Database
    (UKMED), 215, 217, 219
umbrella reviews, 75
uncertainty and bias, 209–210
unit of analysis
  case studies, 35, 36
  identifying, 34
univariate analysis, 204
unstandardised coefficients, 208
unstructured data, 213
unstructured interviews,
    129, 130

V
verisimilitude, 157
video interview, 129
video meeting, 132
video recording, of interview, 131
vignettes, 130
Violin plot, 203
virtual meetings, 265
virtual reality simulation, 193
visual abstracts, 259
  advantages of, 138
  photo-elicitation, 139, 140
    how to use, 141
    key considerations when
      using, 141
  point of view video elicitation,
    141
    how to use, 142
    key considerations when
      using, 142
  rich pictures, 138, 139
    how to use 139
    key considerations when
      using, 138–139
visual elicitation, 137
visual ethnography, 149
visual metaphors, 138
voice
  genre, 248
  tone and, 248–249
vulnerable group, 121

W

walking interview, 130
web-based research
    communities, 259
we-enquiry, 111
work–life balance, 49
workshops, 263, 264
workshops and conferences,
    attendance at, 274
world wide web, 115
writer's block, 250
writing, 84–85, 231–232
    academic, 248–249, 253

for different formats to achieve
    impact, 251
writing for publication,
    253
    abstract, 255–256
    article type, 254–255
    discussion, 256
    ethical issues, 255
    getting started, 253–255
    graphics, 257
    introduction, 256
    methods, 256
    results, 256

    style, language, and structure,
        256–257
    submitting the paper, 257
        decoding the decision, 258
        peer review, 257–258
        publication journey, 258–259
    title, 255
    where to publish, 253–254
    writing strategy, 257
writing well, 149

Y

YouTube, 116, 261, 267